THE

OMEGA Rx ZONE

By Dr. Barry Sears

The Zone

Mastering the Zone

Zone-Perfect Meals in Minutes

Zone Food Blocks

The Anti-Aging Zone

The Soy Zone

A Week in the Zone

The Top 100 Zone Foods

The Omega Rx Zone

Zone Meals in Seconds

What to Eat in the Zone

THE OMEGA Rx ZONE

THE MIRACLE OF THE NEW HIGH-DOSE FISH OIL

DR. BARRY SEARS

ReganBooks

HarperTorch
An Imprint of HarperCollinsPublishers

This book is not intended to replace medical advice or to be a substitute for a physician. If you are sick or suspect you are sick, you should see a physician. If you are taking prescription medication, you should never change your diet (for better or worse) without consulting your physician, because any dietary change will affect the metabolism of that prescription drug.

Prevention will always be the best medicine. However, prevention can be undertaken only by the individual, and that includes eating correctly. This is the foundation of a healthy lifestyle. You have to eat, so you may as well eat wisely.

Although this book is about food, the author and publisher expressly disclaim responsibility for any adverse effects arising from following the advice given in this book without appropriate medical supervision.

HARPERTORCH
An Imprint of HarperCollins*Publishers*
10 East 53rd Street
New York, New York 10022-5299

Copyright © 2002 by Dr. Barry Sears
ISBN: 0-06-074186-4

First HarperTorch/ReganBooks paperback printing: January 2005
First ReganBooks trade paperback printing: June 2003
First ReganBooks international trade paperback printing: September 2002
First ReganBooks hardcover printing: May 2002

The ReganBooks hardcover edition contains the following Library of Congress Cataloging in Publication Data:
Sears, Barry, 1947–
   The Omega Rx zone: the miracle of high-dose fish oil / Barry Sears.
      p. cm.
1. Fish oils in human nutrition.   2. Fish oils—Therapeutic use.   I. Title.
QP752.F57 S43 2002
613.2'84—dc21   2002017891

HarperCollins ®, HarperTorch™, and ❦™ are trademarks of HarperCollins Publishers Inc.
Printed in the United States of America
Visit HarperTorch on the World Wide Web at www.harpercollins.com

10 9 8 7 6 5 4 4 3 2 1

To my wife, Lynn, and my daughters, Kelly and Kristin,
who gave me the love, support, and tolerance during
my twenty-year odyssey to understand the Zone

Acknowledgments

No book is ever written alone, and the books I have written about the Zone are no different. As in all of my books, my wife, Lynn, who does much of the editing for my books, and my brother, Doug, who helps me translate my scientific ideas into easily understood terms for the general public, have been my primary pillars during the past two decades in which I have been developing my Zone technology. I also want to especially thank Deborah Kotz for her continuing excellent editorial input and Mel Berger for his thoughtful advice. Also important was the trust of my colleagues, such as Dan Ward and Rene Espy, who were willing to apply my dietary concepts to their patients.

Finally, I wish to thank the great team that I have at ReganBooks, and in particular Cassie Jones for her excellent final editing of this book. As always, my greatest thanks go to Judith Regan for the courage and foresight to support and publish my Zone concepts.

Contents

THE OMEGA$_x$ ZONE

Introduction

Although the Zone has been around for seven years, I still find that its basic concepts are misunderstood or misinterpreted by both the medical profession and the general public. First of all, the Zone is not a fad diet or a marketing gimmick. It is a term I came up with to describe the physiological state your body is in when it has the proper balance of hormones— a balance that results in optimal health. The Zone can be readily measured and quantified by a number of blood tests that your doctor often routinely orders during an annual physical.

How to get to this Zone is an entirely different matter. Entering the Zone and staying there require you to treat your diet as if it were a drug. In fact, food may be the most powerful drug you will ever encounter because it causes dramatic changes in your hormones that are hundreds of times more powerful than any pharmaceutical.

People often ask me if I would change anything if I could write my first book, *The Zone,* again. The only thing I would do differently is to emphasize the critical need for supplementation with high-dose pharmaceutical-grade fish oil. This product wasn't around when I first wrote *The Zone*. After using it for the past three years, I've come to the conclusion that it may be the miracle drug for the twenty-first century. In my opinion, high-dose pharmaceutical-grade fish oil will radically change how medicine is practiced in the future.

The Omega Rx Zone describes how high-dose fish oil will allow you to reach the full potential of the Zone. I believe that the concepts outlined in this book will have a far greater impact than any concept currently discussed in biotechnology, including gene therapy. Fish oil was the crucial dietary factor that enabled our ancestors to evolve into modern humans some 150,000 years ago. And I think it is the crucial missing link that will enable us to age with our mental capabilities completely intact—free from dementia and depression.

However, high-dose fish oil will be able to alter our future only if we know how to harness its potential correctly by also keeping the hormone insulin within the Zone. Only by constantly controlling insulin levels can you ultimately control those magical hormones known as eicosanoids that are the key to preventing disease and, more important, maintaining wellness. Although very few physicians understand the power of eicosanoids, these hormones will take center stage in twenty-first-century medicine because they affect everything in your body, including your heart, your mind, and even your emotions.

This book represents my continuing exploration of how food affects hormonal responses, and how those responses can be manipulated to allow you to reach your full potential in terms of health, intellect, and emotional well-being. This book will explain how you can use my dietary program to enter the Zone and reach virtually any goal you have for your body and your brain. Those goals might include better health (including the prevention or reversal of heart disease, diabetes, neurological disorders, and cancer), better physical performance, or even better relationships. I'm sure you never imagined that the path to a more fulfilling life would be paved with fish oil!

To reach the Zone, you need three distinctive dietary components. The first is *insulin control.* You need some insulin to survive, but excess insulin leads to a wide range of disease conditions. I was not the first to recognize this fact, but I do believe I was the first to discover why: elevated levels of insulin lead to pushing eicosanoids out of the Zone. My first book, *The Zone,* was based on this premise. Unfortunately, at the time it was written the thought of using your diet to control insulin was exceptionally controversial, and virtually no one knew how to pronounce *eicosanoids* (eye-KAH-sah-noids), let alone understood how they worked. So the world came to believe that the Zone was only about insulin control and weight loss. Nothing could be further from the truth, because insulin is only part of the overall hormonal control technology that gets you to the Zone.

The second part of my dietary program is *calorie restriction* without hunger or deprivation. This is the only proven way to reverse the aging process, as I explain in chapter 7 and have explored in greater detail in my book *The Anti-Aging Zone.*

The final and most important part of my program is *supplementation with fish oil,* and lots of it. The emphasis on high-dose fish oil will be even more controversial than my earlier emphasis on controlling the protein-to-carbohydrate ratio of every meal in order to maintain appropriate insulin levels. Today, mainstream medicine and the general public are just beginning to accept the concept of insulin control.

Now it's time to bring the public's attention to the critical role of eicosanoids, and how high-dose fish oil can manipulate them. In time, I believe, the medical community will also accept this initially controversial aspect of my dietary program. Once it is accepted, we will enter a new era of medical care based primarily on the food we eat, not the drugs we take. This is the foundation of the Omega Rx Zone.

If high-dose fish oil is so important, why doesn't it get more respect? After all, it was recognized more than two hundred years ago as a revolutionary treatment for arthritis. Furthermore your grandmothers told your parents that fish oil was brain food, and in line with this belief, every kid had to take cod liver oil. How could something so common (and simultaneously so unpalatable) be considered cutting-edge biotechnology?

Actually, genetic research is forcing scientists to rethink their concepts about the central role of fish oil in the evolution of modern humans. Genetic analysis has led to the theory that consumption of high-dose fish oil may be the underlying reason now modern humans mysteriously appeared 150,000 years ago, and that consumption of higher levels of fish oil was the defining development that gave this new species the brain power to conquer the earth. Furthermore, new medical research is beginning to indicate that virtually every chronic disease is affected by an imbalance of eicosanoids, which can be altered by high doses of fish oil. In essence, our future as the dominant species on the planet is intimately tied to understanding why this strange elixir works.

How I got involved with fish oil and its effect on hormonal control is a strange journey in itself. I'm a lipid chemist, and proud of it. Lipids is a fancy word for fats. Lipids aren't sexy, and they're hard to work with. Lipids smell, oxidize easily, and are hard to clean up. That's why there are actually very few people in lipid science. We simply get no respect. My own start in lipid research began when I was a graduate student at Indiana University. My professor, Gene Cordes, decided that since lipids were so hard to work with, he would just pretend that soapsuds were like lipids—and it was a lot easier doing this type of research because it was simple to clean the test tubes.

I wasn't too keen on the idea of spending my time working with soapsuds, so Gene told me I could work with one of his new postdoctoral fellows, Mahrenda Jain, who was trying to purify real lipids and make biological membranes with them. That was a very lucky break for my scientific career, since Mahrenda turned out to be one of the smartest individuals I have ever met in science. After working a few weeks with Mahrenda, I quickly found out why Gene was working with soapsuds. These natural lipids were nasty. Once you isolated them, they would immediately start breaking down, and you have to pay meticulous attention to detail and clean up after each experiment. But I stuck with it and soon developed a love affair with lipids.

After earning my Ph.D. degree, I received a National Institutes of Health postdoctoral fellowship to the University of Virginia Medical School, which at that time was the center of lipid research in the United States. This was another extraordinarily lucky break, since all the fundamental research in understanding the physics of lipids was being done there. These labs were a hothouse of creativity; virtually nothing was known at the time about how lipids interact. Working with incredibly intelligent professors such as Tom Thompson and Chsien-chsien Huang, along with other creative postdoctoral fellows such as Lenny Davidowicz, I was like a kid in a candy store.

My first task at Virginia was to start making synthetic

lipids, since natural lipids tend to oxidize easily and would continually mess up precise biophysical experiments. Because stability was the name of the game, I created my lipids with saturated fats, which had no potential to become rancid by oxidation. (The food industry has known this for years, and that's why lard was the fat of choice for deep-frying foods.)

While my own research was an attempt to create highly stable lipids for biophysical experiments, I was also becoming aware of some remarkable epidemiological data showing that Greenland Eskimos were virtually free of heart disease even though they ate a lot of fat. Since heart disease runs rampant on the male side of my family, I was keenly interested. The only explanation for the fact that Eskimos weren't dying of heart disease (and the fact that they had virtually no depression, cancer, or multiple sclerosis) seemed to be that they consumed a lot of fish oil.

This was one of those defining times in science when different technologies cross over and affect each other. The early research on eicosanoids was finally unfolding, and that provided the answer to the Eskimo paradox. The Eskimos' high intake of fish oil was changing their levels of eicosanoids, thus virtually eradicating heart disease, along with a wide variety of other chronic diseases. As a lipid scientist, I became hooked on fish oil. And I wasn't the only one.

In the mid-1980s fish oil was the hot item in the health food industry, but the craze soon died. Why? There were two reasons. First, the amounts of fish oil used in the experiments were far too low to have consistent effects. Second, elevated levels of insulin would obliterate many of the benefits offered by any level of fish oil supplementation. At the same time as fish oil entered the scene, we began an era of high-carbohydrate, low-fat diets. These diets caused an epidemic of elevated insulin that would offset any hormonal benefits of fish oil.

My first book, *The Zone,* explained that to control eicosanoids, you have to control insulin and provide some level of fish oil. However, I didn't recognize, then, the levels of fish oils that were ultimately needed to bring about a revolution in health care. That last bit of knowledge had to wait until I had access to pharmaceutical-grade fish oils. The fish oils that are commonly available are basically the sewer of the sea, and there is only so much you can take before you get severe intestinal problems like bloating and diarrhea. I had no idea how far you could push the envelope of eicosanoid control until I had access to these newest pharmaceutical-grade materials. My recent research in the past three years with high-dose pharmaceutical-grade fish oils has demonstrated to me beyond a shadow of a doubt that the combination of consistent insulin control coupled with high-dose fish oil may be a true miracle cure for the twenty-first century. I hope that after reading this book you will agree.

The Omega Rx Zone

This book is arranged in four parts. Part I sets the foundation for understanding the importance of high-dose fish oil in terms of the continuing evolution of the Zone concept. This part will describe not only how the long-chain omega-3 fatty acids found in fish oil enabled our ancestors to become human, but also why they became the key to understanding wellness for both the brain and the body in the twenty-first century. By the end of Part I, you will know that the Omega Rx Zone is far beyond simply a diet; it is a new vision to help understand why chronic diseases develop.

Part II provides you with the basic plan to get into the Omega Rx Zone and the understanding of what types of fish oil are available to reach a higher state of wellness. More important, you will learn the blood tests that define the Omega Rx Zone so that you can retake control of your physical and mental health.

In Part III, I make specific recommendations for use of high-dose, pharmaceutical-grade fish oil for a variety of chronic disease conditions. Part IV shows you how to reach your full genetic potential in the Omega Rx Zone.

chapter 1

The Continuing Evolution
of the Zone

The distinguishing feature that makes us human is our constant search to understand the world around us. In that search, there are two types of questions you can ask. One is how things work the way they do, and the other is why things occur in the first place. The "how" questions are the backbone of science, whereas the "why" questions are usually the foundation of philosophy. In medicine, the "why" questions are rarely asked because there are no obvious answers, and the chances for success are very low. Furthermore, even if you do successfully answer a "why" question, your answer is likely to generate a violent reaction in the medical community if it in any way suggests a significant deviation from the status quo.

In my own case, I have pondered a very basic "why" question for the past twenty years: Why do we develop chronic disease? Although the medical establishment has developed a massive infrastructure to treat the symptoms of chronic disease, we have made very little progress in understanding its underlying cause.

I reasoned many years ago that the best chance I had for success at answering this fundamental "why" question was to understand the world of hormones. Until recently, most people used the word *hormones* only to describe puberty or an overactive sex drive. Now hormones are the subject of many a cocktail party conversation because they appear to be the magical elixir that will keep you young and vital: hormone replacement therapy for females and testosterone and replacement for males. Hormones are so important because they orchestrate an incredibly complex flow of biological information in the body. I truly believed that hormones were the overriding factor that determined whether we would be chronically sick or well. Controlling these hormones, I theorized, would be the key to preventing chronic disease. I also speculated that hormonal control could be achieved primarily through our diet.

All my Zone books are based on the premise that you have the power to control your hormones through your diet. Hormones are the key to your future, and in particular to longevity, optimal health, and ultimately remaining human. In fact, improved hormonal control is like a philosophers' stone that allows you to enjoy better health, better performance, better relationships, and a longer life.

Once you learn to control your hormones, you have a magical "drug" that can:

- Prevent heart disease
- Reverse cancer
- Reduce pain and inflammation
- Treat neurological disease

But if you can treat those diseases with this "drug," then the same "drug" can also:

- Reverse the aging process
- Make you smarter
- Make you thinner
- Improve your physical performance
- Improve your relationships with others

If controlling your hormones is the way to a longer and better life, is there any drug out there that allows you to do this consistently and with no side effects? Fortunately a "drug" exists that takes you off the path to disease and puts you on the path to wellness. It's not a pill or injection or even a gene transplant; it's the food you eat. But for this "drug" to work you have to take it at the right time and at the right dosage for the rest of your life.

HOW IS THE OMEGA RX ZONE DIFFERENT FROM THE ZONE?

I first introduced the Zone seven years ago. The Zone is not some mystical place; it is a physiological state of your body in which the hormones that can be controlled by the diet are balanced for optimal health. Furthermore, the Zone is defined by very precise clinical parameters in the blood. These blood tests are based on the dynamic balance of two key hormonal systems (insulin and eicosanoids) that can be controlled by my dietary program. My earlier recommendations still remain the best way to control insulin, but only the new emphasis on high-dose fish oil can truly allow you to achieve the full potential of the Omega Rx Zone. This is because the Omega Rx Zone is ultimately about improved eicosanoid control. In essence, you should think of the Omega Rx Zone as a top of a mountain, and my dietary recommendations as the best pathway to it.

As I mentioned in the introduction, there are three components to my dietary plan:

1. Balancing protein and carbohydrate at *every* meal
   This controls insulin levels.
2. Calorie restriction without hunger or deprivation
   This is the only proven way to increase longevity.
3. Supplementation with high-dose fish oil
   This alters eicosanoids.

The first two components follow my original dietary recommendations to move a person toward the Zone. The third component is completely new and boosts the health benefits obtainable in the Omega Rx Zone to new heights.

People in the medical community may raise their eyebrows when they hear how much fish oil I'm suggesting to reach the full potential of the Omega Rx Zone. My recommendations, however, are backed up by sound science. Equally important, I have had the opportunity to use high-dose fish oil in a number of seemingly hopeless situations, and each time I have been amazed at the results. There are patients with dementia who returned from the living dead. There are cancer patients who can now look forward to a much longer life than they ever expected. There are young children with severe attention deficient disorder who had a complete reversal of behavior within three weeks. There is a patient who was scheduled to have both feet amputated because of nonhealing diabetic ulcers—yet after four months of using high-dose fish oil, the wounds healed completely and the amputations were never done. There was a housebound woman with chronic pain who was on oxygen twenty-four hours a day because of obstructive pulmonary disease; within four weeks of starting to take high-dose fish oil, she was off oxygen, walking, and pain-free. There was a woman who had such severe fibromyalgia that she rarely got out of bed, but within twenty-four hours of using high-dose fish oil, she was able to resume a normal life. These stories sound very much like those told by snake oil salesmen in the nineteenth century, but they are true and, as you will read later, backed by cutting-edge science.

When I first advocated balancing protein and carbohydrates to control insulin in *The Zone*, it was an extremely controversial concept. Now it is widely accepted. I think that, in time, the need for supplementation with high-dose fish oil will likewise be recognized.

THE MIRACLE OF HIGH-DOSE FISH OIL

Why haven't you heard about the miracle of high-dose fish oil until now? There are five primary reasons that fish oil hasn't really taken off in the medical world:

1. Traditional fish oils taste terrible.
2. We've never used enough fish oils to see dramatic benefits.
3. High-carbohydrate diets obliterate many of the benefits of fish oil.
4. The amount of impurities and toxins in standard fish oils was so great that no one would ever risk consuming the levels needed to see benefits.
5. Only recently has pharmaceutical-grade fish oil become available.

As I will show you in the coming chapters, high-dose fish oil can remarkably change our view of medicine, and especially the treatment and prevention of chronic disease, particularly neurological disorders. High-dose fish oil has the power to take our minds to a much higher state while simultaneously addressing our health concerns as we grow older. With high-dose fish oil, we have the opportunity to reverse heart disease, cancer, diabetes, pain, dementia, and even aging itself.

More important, you will be able to control your emotions, give your mind the opportunity to express the full potential of human creativity, and give your body the opportunity to perform at peak physical levels.

You're probably thinking that it can't be this easy—or, if it is, why haven't we heard about it before? Well, the studies have been published for decades, but no one had a systematic approach to putting it all together. The Omega Rx Zone is that approach. It is based on treating food *as if* it were a prescription drug. If you want to reach your full genetic potential and lead a longer life, this is a proven technology to help you attain that goal.

If you want to jump ahead and get started on the program, go immediately to Part II, which begins on page 57. You'll begin to see results in fourteen days or less.

Of course, I don't want you to simply take my word for it. I want you to understand why my dietary recommendations work, because once you do, your life will be changed forever. That's why it is useful to read the next few chapters. Knowing how my dietary program works to improve both the mind and the body begins with understanding the dietary events that led us to become human in the first place, more than 150,000 years ago.

chapter 2

The Beginnings of Modern Man

Humankind's evolutionary split from our great ape ancestors occurred about five million years ago. As it turns out, the primate order (which includes monkeys, apes, and humans) hasn't been a particularly successful evolutionary branch—more than 97 percent of all primate species have died out since our early ancestors first stood and walked upright on two feet. Even though the genetic difference between modern humans and apes is less than 2 percent, apes are a dying species, while we are thriving. With the exception of humans, all primates are on the verge of extinction. Today there are only four species of great apes still left on the earth—gorillas, orangutans, chimpanzees, and pygmy chimpanzees—and it is unlikely that they will still exist in their natural habitats fifty years from now. With such a losing pedigree, how did we become successful?

To understand why we succeeded, you have to go back in time to the beginning of modern man, *Homo sapiens,* approximately 150,000 years ago. For the previous three million years, our primate ancestors had been living without any great increase in intelligence or impact on the planet. Even when early relatives of humans learned to make and use fire some million years ago, that didn't improve their lot very much. Then something happened virtually overnight to turn this rather insignificant species into the dominant player on the planet.

About 150,000 years ago the earth's climate was much cooler, and our immediate ancestors were isolated into two groups. One species, known as the Neanderthals, inhabited Europe, and the other species remained in Africa. The Neanderthals adapted to the cold weather by becoming more muscular, shorter, and stockier to conserve heat, whereas our African ancestors simply began to die out. Our immediate ancestors in East Africa eventually numbered fewer than 10,000, and they were ready to take the road to Extinction City. It was at this precipice overlooking extinction that modern humans made their sudden appearance.

Within a few thousand years, these modern humans made more progress than their ancestors had made in the previous three million years. Fifty thousand years later, this completely new species started making its way from Africa to conquer the rest of the world. Then, some forty thousand years ago, there was one final cognitive leap that resulted in an explosion of art, culture, religion, social organization, and tool making never seen before on this planet. Soon afterward, other species that had survived for hundreds of thousands of years under the most brutal conditions suddenly became no match for this previously undistinguished bit player in the soap opera of evolution. When the otherwise evolutionarily successful Neanderthals encountered this new species, it was no contest. The last of the Neanderthals died out some thirty thousand years ago, disappearing with the other 97 percent of unsuccessful primate species before them.

Throughout evolution, the size of the prehuman brain was steadily increasing. What uniquely characterizes modern humans, however, is their ability to think and to restructure their environment. To do so requires manipulation of sensory inputs into an action plan for improved survival. Before 150,000 years ago, our ancestors weren't very good at this. Modern humans, though, had an evolutionary advantage: a rapid increase in the size of the frontal cortex, where thinking and reasoning take place. The better your rational thinking, the more rapidly you can adapt to new environments and conditions. But if evolution usually takes so long, how were modern humans able to develop in the equivalent of a blink of an eye in evolutionary time?

Many scientists believe that the starting point separating modern humans from the ragtag band of earlier species was the diet that our ancestors adopted in the East African Rift Valley. In essence, they stumbled on brain food. This brain food caused their thinking skills to expand with incredible speed, giving them a tremendous advantage over every other species on the planet. Within an incredibly short time, they became able to dominate the earth.

Fat is the most likely candidate for the brain food that initiated this mental development. This was not just any type of fat, however, but a rare type of fat that would have been in short supply on the plains of Africa but was found in great abundance in the lakes of the East African Rift Valley.

Ironically, this rare dietary fat had been available since the beginning of life on the planet some three billion years ago, when the first life-forms were a very simple single-celled organism known as algae. Simple as these organisms were, they developed the unique ability to synthesize that rare type of fat.

The trouble was that there wasn't a lot of water on the savanna; this made it very difficult for our primate ancestors to find a lot of algae, even by scavenging. The amounts of algae-derived fats that our prehistoric ancestors were consuming were still insufficient to enable their brains to evolve to a higher level. Without adequate amounts of these fats, brain evolution, in terms of cognitive skills, advanced at a snail's pace. It wasn't until our ancestors stumbled onto brain food in the East African Rift Valley that the evolution of the mind went into warp speed.

THE MOTHER OF US ALL

In trying to determine exactly how modern humans evolved, fossil hunters use sophisticated tools like carbon dating. Yet even with these tools, they can only piece information together from fragments of bones. From these fragments come often conflicting theories of evolution. About twenty years ago, however, a new tool of genetic analysis became available. Mutations in the genetic code occur with a somewhat consistent frequency, although not all these mutations lead to successful evolutionary changes—in fact, many of them can lead to extinction. We can take a living species, such as humans, and use genetic analysis to trace its origins.

Although the DNA in your body comes from both your mother and your father, there is a special type known as mitochondrial DNA that comes only from your mother. By studying the number of mutations in mitochondrial DNA, you can determine two things: (1) the approximate time the species first developed, and (2) whether the species developed in a single location or simultaneously in different locations.

The data are starting to show clearly that every man, woman, and child on the planet can trace his or her ancestry to a single woman who lived nearly 150,000 years ago. That woman has been called Eve. Here begins the history of modern humans—and it reads like a B-movie science fiction script.

As I pointed out earlier, it appears that our immediate ancestors were perhaps only one or two generations from complete extinction, just like the other 97 percent of previous primate species. But something happened that gave them a second chance: they learned to scavenge a new food source that wouldn't have been found in the African savanna. This food was the shellfish found along the shores of the lakes in the East African Rift Valley. Shellfish consume algae and therefore can accumulate algae-derived fats in higher concentrations, in turn giving our immediate ancestors more of these algae-derived fats than have been consumed at any time in history.

Catching fish is a pretty difficult task, and it would not be mastered for about another 100,000 years later but collecting shellfish from the lakeshore was definitely within the abilities of the premodern humans. They also had the tools to open the shellfish and extract the protein, which would be rich in accumulated algae-derived fats. Of course, after a million years of scavenging for protein from land animals, eating shellfish would have been completely alien to them. But in desperate situations, like the threat of extinction, you tend to do whatever it takes to survive. The first courageous soul was the one who ate these strange creatures and began the process that spawned a new species: modern humans. With an increasing intake of algae-derived fats, the development of the frontal cortex (the site of thinking in the brain) began to accelerate, which allowed cognitive skills to explode. And soon this small ragtag group of primate survivors that had been close to extinction embarked on the conquest of the world.

It took them nearly 50,000 years to consolidate their forces and mount their comeback from near extinction, but it is clear that approximately 100,000 years ago our true ancestors left Africa to begin to populate the globe. Surprisingly, although their brain development was dramatically enhanced, their tool-making ability didn't increase as rapidly. They continued to use the same tools—but they had learned to use them much better.

The most recent chapter in our evolutionary drama began about 40,000 years ago with the appearance of the Cro-Magnon. Except for being taller, more muscular, and possibly more intelligent than humans today, they would be virtually indistinguishable in any modern city. The Cro-Magnon ushered in a dramatic explosion not only in tool making but also in art, religion, and social behavior—all the things we use to define civilization. This leap in cognitive development appeared to coincide with one hunting skill modern humans had at last developed: fishing. Since fish are at the end of the food chain that starts with algae, they can accumulate even larger amounts of these algae-derived fats than shellfish. By eating more fish, modern humans had even greater access to this new brain food, and the world has not been the same since.

THE PALEOLITHIC DIET

If simply consuming large amounts of fish is the key to mental greatness, then whales, not humans, should be ruling the world. Obviously, there must be something else. First, we needed to have free use of our arms to have the ability to make tools. Walking on two feet was one of the defining events that led to our development. Once we stood upright, our arms were free to make tools. Other mammals never reached that point, or, as with whales, their forelimbs became flippers.

The other piece of the puzzle is the structure of the brain.

In particular, we needed to have a frontal cortex. Even the most primitive primates, like monkeys, have the beginnings of a frontal cortex, whereas other mammals do not. Without that piece of anatomy, rational thinking and reasoning are impossible.

But even if that piece of anatomy is present, our development still depends on a continual supply of glucose. The brain requires glucose in order to function, and glucose must be constantly extracted from the blood sugar. In fact, about 70 percent of blood sugar goes to supply the brain. Without this fuel source, maximum cognitive function can never be developed. Therefore, an evolutionary push also came when we began consuming a diet that maintained a constant supply of blood sugar to the brain. Only then would we have been able to set in motion the appropriate orchestration that allowed the frontal cortex to develop when exposed to adequate levels of algae-derived fats.

What exactly was this diet that our ancestors consumed some 10,000 to 40,000 years ago, when the human mind flowered fully? Scientists' best estimate is that this diet was very different from what we're consuming today. The Paleolithic diet was rich in low-fat protein and moderate in carbohydrates, and it provided adequate levels of algae-derived fats. The latest research has also indicated that it probably took about 65 percent of its calories from animal sources and 35 percent from plant sources. Since agriculture had not yet been developed, the only carbohydrate sources were fruits and vegetables, which are exceptionally rich in vitamins, minerals, and antioxidants.

When this diet is broken down into percentages of protein, carbohydrate and fat, it comes to approximately 40 percent carbohydrates, 30 percent protein, and 30 percent total fat. That is, in essence, the same dietary balance I put forth in *The Zone,* the balance I developed to maintain blood sugar levels to control insulin levels in both cardiovascular and diabetic patients and improve athletic performance in world-class athletes. This helps to explain the apparent paradox in anthropology that Paleolithic humans were taller, stronger, and leaner than humans today.

Our dominance of the world is based more on good fortune than anything else. Our lucky break occurred when we started eating a lot of shellfish nearly 150,000 years ago, probably out of desperation, since traditional food supplies were rapidly being eliminated by the increasingly colder climate. This increase in the consumption of algae-derived fats, coupled with a consistent supply of blood glucose for a constantly glucose-hungry brain, laid the foundation for the emergence of a new species: modern humans.

The diet that made us human is the one that will keep us human. That diet was rich in fruits and vegetables and contained virtually no grains. It was also rich in high-quality protein, especially fish and lean protein. But most important, it was rich in algae-derived fats. Our diet has the power to radically improve or impair our intelligence. To understand why, you have to learn more about the fats that made us smart.

chapter 3

The Fats That Made Us Human

Fat has become a foul three-letter word in our society. We've become a nation of fat phobics, and some of us try to avoid this nutrient at all costs in an effort to lose weight and improve our health. Yet this war on fat has been completely misguided.

Fat is the essential ingredient that made us human and is the dominant feature of our brain. In fact, more than 60 percent of the dry weight of the brain is fat. Much of this fat is required for the electrical insulation of the nerves (to preserve the fidelity of their messages) and for the connections (synapses) between nerves that allow information to be exchanged with ease throughout the brain.

More important, life itself would be impossible without fat. Fats hate water and spontaneously group together to form remarkable structures called membranes. The water environment inside these membranes is now separated from the water outside them, and this separation gives rise to cells, the primary structure of biological life. Consider the 60 trillion cells in your body. If there were no membranes to keep the enzymes, proteins, carbohydrates, and DNA separate from the rest of the body, you would collapse into a puddle of paste.

Three billion years ago, the only living things on the planet were algae, which consisted of a single membrane composed primarily of fat. But the membranes formed by algae-derived fats are far from static; they dance a rhythm controlled by the fluidity within the fat molecule itself. That fluidity is governed by the number of double bonds in the fat molecule. Double bonds in fats result when hydrogen atoms have been extracted from the carbon-to-carbon bonds that are the backbone of all fats. This extraction is done in a very specific way by enzymes so that each double bond (called a *cis* double bond) forms a kink in the molecular structure of the fat as shown below.

The more unsaturated a fat molecule is, the more double bonds it has, and the more fluidity it imparts to the membrane. This fluidity is the key to understanding why algae-derived fats made us smart.

But before we get to this lesson in biochemistry, let's take a leap back in time to about 550 million years ago, when there was an explosion in biological diversity as mul-

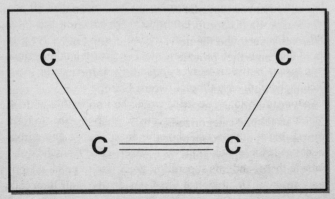

ticell organisms were starting to evolve from single-cell algae. These new organisms had to develop a communication system so their specialized cells could transmit messages to one another. One way was to build nerve connections between specialized cells. Another involved the use of hormones.

The first hormones developed by living organisms were known as eicosanoids, and they used fats in cell membranes as their building blocks. These eicosanoids don't use just any type of fat for their synthesis; they require the long-chain highly unsaturated (polyunsaturated) fat found only in algae-derived fats. These were the same fats that made us smart 150,000 years ago, and the eicosanoids that are derived from those fats control our health today.

THE STRUCTURE OF FATS

If you managed to avoid taking a college-level biochemistry course, you're headed for a taste of what you missed. The reason I refer to *fats* rather than *fat* in this chapter is that there are many different types of fat, and these fats are very complex. Depending on the function of a particular cell, your body needs specific types of fats to keep the cell membranes in their appropriate fluidity zone. For example, the cells that surround the nerves in your brain need to be very rigid because they provide insulation to maintain the fidelity of the electronic signals. On the other hand, the cells in the retina of the eye have to be extremely fluid to allow visible information to pass into the brain.

Fats can be categorized by their fluidity; they are either saturated (solid at room temperature), monounsaturated (liquid at room temperature, but cloudy in a refrigerator), or polyunsaturated (liquid in a refrigerator). The number of double bonds contained within the fatty acid determines these designations. The more double bonds a fat has, the more fluid (unsaturated) it is. However, the more unsaturated a fat is, the more prone it is to be attacked by free radicals, which causes rancidity. Since fish oils contain high levels of polyunsaturated fats, they are quite likely to become rancid. Do you ever wonder why fish gets a fishy smell after a day or two in your refrigerator? That's due to its high content of polyunsaturated fats, which are becoming oxidized.

Within the classification of polyunsaturated fats, there is one further subdivision: omega-3 and omega-6 fats. This distinction has to do with the position of the double bonds in the fat, which determine its three-dimensional structure. This ultimately determines the type of eicosanoids that can be made from fats. Furthermore, the length of the polyunsaturated fatty acid is critically important, because only the longer-chain polyunsaturated fatty acids (20 carbon atoms) have the number of double bonds that can provide the fluidity necessary for cells in the retina to transmit visual images to the brain, for nerve synapses to transfer information throughout the brain, and for the brain's mitochondria to produce optimal amounts of energy. In addition, only the long-chain polyunsaturated fats (both omega-6 and omega-3) can be used in the manufacture of eicosanoids, which are the keys that ultimately control human health.

I call these long-chain polyunsaturated fats Jekyll and Hyde fats, because, as you will see in chapter 4, they can be synthesized into either "good" or "bad" eicosanoids. Long-chain omega-3 fatty acids (found in fish oil) are the building blocks necessary to help manufacture "good" eicosanoids. On the flip side, long-chain omega-6 fatty acids (found in high concentrations in vegetable oils) are the building blocks used to manufacture "bad" eicosanoids. The balance of "good" and "bad" eicosanoids will be the primary factor

Molecular Structure of Long-Chain

Omega-3 and Omega-6 Fats

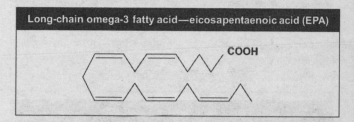

Long-chain omega-3 fatty acid—eicosapentaenoic acid (EPA)

COOH

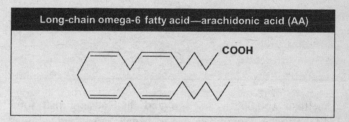

Long-chain omega-6 fatty acid—arachidonic acid (AA)

COOH

determining your physical and mental health. My dietary recommendations were developed to control that balance.

As you may have already guessed, fish oils are rich in long-chain omega-3 fats. The central features of my dietary plan are the long-chain omega-3 fats called eicosapentaenoic acid (EPA) and docosahexaenoic acid (DHA). DHA is the key fat for the brain, whereas EPA is the key fat for health. Fish oil is rich in both.

With this short background about fats, we can look at the algae-derived fats and begin to understand why they were so important for the emergence of modern humans.

First, these algae fats were rich in long-chain omega-3 fatty acids. Since algae is at the bottom of the food chain, our prehistoric ancestors would have gotten these fats from marine sources that ate algae—probably beginning with

Molecular Structure of EPA and DHA

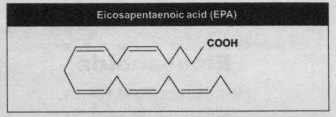

Eicosapentaenoic acid (EPA)

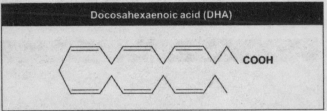

Docosahexaenoic acid (DHA)

shellfish 150,000 years ago and then adding fish some 40,000 years ago. Once we began consuming higher amounts of these long-chain omega-3 fats, our frontal cortex (which controls thinking and reasoning) began to expand rapidly. This is because DHA is the critical long-chain omega-3 fatty acid required for the building of neural tissue. Furthermore, it appears that only DHA can stimulate the growth of nerve cells. This probably explains why DHA is preferentially transported across the placenta into the fetal circulation for maximum impact on brain development.

The second reason high-dose fish oil is so important is that it also contains EPA, the other long-chain omega-3 fat that controls our health by modulating the balance of "good" and "bad" eicosanoids. How that happens is explained in chapter 4.

chapter 4

Eicosanoids

Hormones That Harm,
Hormones That Heal

If you've read *The Zone,* you probably have a better under-standing of eicosanoids than most physicians. If you're read-ing my work for the first time, you're probably unfamiliar with this remarkable group of hormones.

When you think of the word *hormone,* testosterone and estrogen probably come to mind. Insulin is another hormone that people are becoming familiar with. But then there are the mysterious hormones—eicosanoids—which I call the phantoms of the hormone world. Eicosanoids arise, do their job, and then self-destruct, all in a flash. Eicosanoids are extremely difficult to measure with a blood test, because they were never designed to circulate in the blood.

Yet eicosanoids play an integral role in your health. Just ask the Nobel Prize committee, which awarded the 1982 prize in medicine for the discovery of how eicosanoids con-trol virtually every function in the human body, and how aspirin, the wonder drug of the twentieth century, works by altering their levels. A search of the literature for eicosanoids will yield more than 87,000 articles published in peer-reviewed journals. Given all this, it is unclear why these hormones aren't better understood by physicians and the general public.

I first started writing about these hormones more than seven years ago—and I continue to write about them—because they are key to our future. I want you to understand the power of these hormones and how to harness this power to benefit your health.

Eicosanoids were the earliest hormones; they were first produced by living organisms some 500 million years ago. They are also the most powerful hormones, since they affect the synthesis of virtually every other hormone in your body. In a sense, you can think of eicosanoids as "superhormones" capable of bringing great health benefits ("good" eicosanoids) or great harm ("bad" eicosanoids), depending on which one a cell produces. Other hormones are produced by particular glands, but every cell in your body is capable of producing eicosanoids. In essence, you have about 60 trillion eicosanoid glands, and your job is to maintain an appropriate balance of "good" and "bad" eicosanoids in each of them.

When I talk about "good" and "bad" eicosanoids, keep in mind that these terms describe very powerful, opposite physiological actions generated by different eicosanoids. In appendix D I go into far greater detail about the molecular definitions of these eicosanoids and how they work. Just keep in mind that you need a *balance* of "good" and "bad" eicosanoids for optimal health. This is no different from talking about "good" and "bad" cholesterol. If you had no "bad" cholesterol, you would die. What you need is an appropriate balance between "good" and "bad" cholesterol to reduce the risk of heart disease. You can think of eicosanoids the same way, but you should realize that they're even more important than cholesterol in terms of their impact on your overall health. The reason is clear from the table below.

What Do "Good" and "Bad" Eicosanoids Do?

"Good" Eicosanoids	"Bad" Eicosanoids
Prevent blood clots caused by platelet aggregation	Promote blood clots caused by platelet aggregation
Cause dilation (opening) of blood vessels	Cause constriction (closing) of blood vessels
Reduce pain	Promote pain
Decrease cell division	Promote cell division
Enhance the immune system	Depress the immune system
Improve brain function	Depress brain function

You can see from this table that the "bad" eicosanoids appear to have very few redeeming characteristics, and many chronic diseases can be viewed as an excessive production of "bad" eicosanoids. Here are some examples of chronic diseases that result from such an excess:

- Heart attack
- Stroke
- Hypertension
- Arthritis
- Cancer
- Chronic infection
- Depression
- Alzheimer's disease

Why not just eliminate all the "bad" eicosanoids, so that you never get a heart attack or cancer? It's not quite that easy. Let's take a heart attack as an example. If you don't have enough "bad" eicosanoids, you would probably bleed to death, because you need some "bad" eicosanoids to form a clot that stops bleeding. Of course, if you are producing too many "bad" eicosanoids, your platelets will clot in the wrong place, such as the middle of an artery which causes a heart attack. The same is true for understanding high blood pressure, cancer, pain, immune disorders, and neurological disease—what you need is a balance of "good" and "bad" eicosanoids.

Most chronic diseases stem from an imbalance of eicosanoids, not a deficiency. Although there are drugs that can inhibit the production of "bad" eicosanoids, these medications have significant side effects, because they can't discriminate very well between "good" and "bad" eicosanoids. It's like destroying an entire village in order to save one house. Aspirin was considered the wonder drug of the twentieth century because it could change the levels of eicosanoids. Other early wonder drugs were corticosteroids like cortisone and prednisone. However, if these powerful drugs are used for more than thirty days, your immune system begins to shut down, since they knock out "good" and "bad" eicosanoids indiscriminately.

The only "drug" that can give you the appropriate balance of "good" and "bad" eicosanoids—with no side effects—is following my dietary recommendations. Once you maintain that balance, you are squarely in the middle of the Omega Rx Zone.

MAKING THE DIETARY CONNECTION

As powerful as eicosanoids are, they are ultimately controlled by the diet. All "bad" eicosanoids are derived from the long-chain omega-6 fatty acid, called arachidonic acid (AA). Enhanced production of "good" eicosanoids requires the presence of eicosapentaenoic acid (EPA), found in fish oil, because it inhibits the production of AA (see appendix D for a more detailed explanation). Unlike traditional drugs that treat the symptoms of chronic diseases after the diseases have taken hold in the body, my program works directly to alleviate the ultimate cause of these chronic diseases, which is an eicosanoid imbalance. In the process, you will also move toward a state of wellness that can be monitored with a powerful new blood test that has recently become available. This blood test measures your ratio of AA to EPA and is the best way to estimate the ratio of "bad" to "good" eicosanoids throughout your body. This test and the others that clinically define the Omega Rx Zone are described in chapter 9.

HORMONAL CROSS TALK

Hormonal systems don't operate independently of one another: what affects one system is bound to have an influence on another. The term used to describe this hormonal interaction is *cross talk,* and that's exactly what is occurring. Hormones from one system communicate with hormones in another system. Nowhere is this clearer than with insulin and eicosanoids—this is why controlling both is so critical for the success of my dietary program.

How Insulin Affects Eicosanoids

Insulin is a key regulator of many of the most important enzymes in the body. For example, it activates the critical enzyme responsible for making cholesterol in the liver. The pharmaceutical industry takes in more than $10 billion a year by selling drugs called statins that inhibit this same enzyme. Yet by simply reducing insulin levels, you will reduce cholesterol production by the liver. By reducing cholesterol production, you will eventually decrease the production of "bad" cholesterol (LDL cholesterol). Of course, if you don't reduce insulin, then you are going to have to take a lot of the statins to lower cholesterol levels.

One of the best indicators that you are making too much insulin is that you're overweight and shaped like an apple. The increasing rate of obesity in the United States is really an epidemic of excess insulin production (hyperinsulinemia). Recently a panel of experts on cholesterol warned us that our obesity crisis is causing increasing cholesterol levels, and that this is setting us up for an epidemic of heart disease. Their solution? Widespread use of cholesterol-lowering statins. I personally think that lowering excess insulin by following my dietary program would have no side effects and be far more effective and far cheaper than taking statins for the rest of your life.

Just as elevated insulin levels can profoundly affect the synthesis of cholesterol, the production of eicosanoids can also be adversely affected. In particular, the key enzyme that produces arachidonic acid (the building block of "bad" eicosanoids) is stimulated by elevated insulin, as shown on the next page.

The delta 5-desaturase enzyme (stimulated by insulin) transforms the omega-6 fatty acids in your diet into the building block (arachidonic acid) for the "bad" eicosanoids. By now, you know why this is not good for your health.

Simply by lowering insulin levels, you can significantly decrease the generation of the building blocks for "bad" eicosanoids. Of course, the door swings both ways. Increasing insulin levels will increase the production of the building blocks for "bad" eicosanoids, and in the process accelerate the development of a wide array of chronic diseases.

Until I came to that realization many years ago, I was always puzzled about why elevated insulin levels seemed to be associated with so many diverse disease conditions. The

Effect of Insulin on Essential Fatty Acid Production

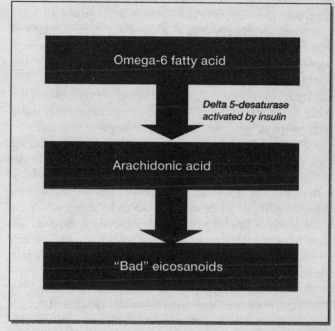

"smoking gun" was eicosanoids. Then it all made sense, because only eicosanoids could have such a widespread impact on human physiology. But although this was obvious to me, it still has not become obvious to the medical establishment.

How Eicosanoids Affect Insulin

"Good" eicosanoids decrease the production of insulin in the pancreas, whereas "bad" eicosanoids increase the production of insulin. You can get yourself into real hormonal trouble by eating a high-carbohydrate diet that consistently generates high levels of insulin. The excess insulin increases the levels of "bad" eicosanoids, causing the pancreas to generate even more insulin. This, in turn, will cause your body to produce greater amounts of arachidonic acid, putting you into a downward spiral toward hormonal hell. You have to control both insulin and eicosanoids simultaneously to have precise control over your body.

Trying to control only one hormonal system without the other is like driving a car in which one front wheel is going forty miles an hour and the other one is going four miles an hour. You can do it, but it sure takes a lot of effort. Imagine how much easier it is to have both wheels moving at the same speed. That's why my plan is based on controlling both eicosanoids (through high doses of fish oil) and insulin (by eating lots of fruits and vegetables balanced with adequate levels of low-fat protein). Maintaining a constant balance in your intake of protein, carbohydrate, and fat can enable you to control the most powerful agents known in medical science: hormones.

To this day, very few medical experts understand the ongoing cross talk of these two hormonal systems. But even though the medical experts might not be aware of this science, you can bet your bottom dollar that both hormonal systems are communicating back and forth to push you either toward wellness or toward chronic disease. And all this communication is controlled by your diet. If you want to take control of the cross talk between insulin and eicosanoids, then my dietary program is your best "drug."

By now you should have a good understanding of why fish oil is so critical for our future. First, it contains the long-chain omega-3 fats (like DHA) that are critical for our brain function. Second, it supplies the long-chain omega-3 fats (like EPA) that allow us to make more "good" and fewer "bad" eicosanoids, and this is critical for our health. As our ancestors found out some 150,000 years ago, eating certain marine animals that are rich in fish oil makes us smarter and healthier at the same time.

The unique fats found in fish oil provided the molecular foundation that dramatically increased our brain function. Once our ancestors began to consume higher levels of these fats, they altered the course of evolution forever. The same fats that gave rise to modern humans thousands of years ago will be the key to twenty-first-century medicine because it can induce the body to make more "good" and fewer "bad" eicosanoids. Conversely, without enough of these long-chain omega-3 fatty acids we are going to have a difficult time in the future both cognitively and medically.

chapter 5

What Is Wellness?

When you think of "wellness," you probably think of the absence of disease. If you're not sick, you must be well. Right? Wrong. Even if you have no outward signs of disease, you may still be heading into a downward spiral that will cause chronic disease later in life.

Doctors have no trouble defining chronic disease, but defining wellness is far more complex. The following table illustrates that difficulty.

Definitions

Chronic Disease	Wellness
Depression	Happiness
Heart disease	Healthy heart
Chronic pain	Pain-free
Cancer	Cancer-free

As you can see, virtually none of the usual definitions of wellness can be quantified easily. How do you prove that you don't have a single cancer cell in your body, or that your arteries are clear of atherosclerotic plaque? The medical establishment has succeeded very well at describing and testing for various chronic diseases—and it has developed a corresponding number of drugs to treat them. Defining wellness, though, has never been a priority, because its definitions are too amorphous. I believe that promoting wellness can be a cornerstone of twenty-first-century medicine. In order for this to happen, we must get a better handle on describing and quantifying it.

There are really three distinct stages of chronic disease. The first stage is wellness. The second stage is subchronic disease. With subchronic disease, you know you aren't well, but you aren't sick enough to be considered truly ill. This is the gray area that most of us live in. The third stage is the manifestation of some type of chronic disease. Only then is the full armament of today's medical establishment thrown at you in an effort to drive you back into subchronic illness, where the overt symptoms of chronic disease become temporarily submerged. The real goal of twenty-first-century medicine should be to move us all the way back to wellness—if only we could define it.

Part of the reason current medicine seems so complex is that we sometimes make it more difficult than it really is. Instead of micromanaging disease, we should focus on macromanaging wellness and let the body take care of itself. I came to this line of reasoning twenty years ago and found that the best way to keep the body moving toward wellness is to accomplish one primary goal:

- Decrease inflammation

If you accomplish this goal, then virtually every chronic disease will improve. Here are some examples:

Chronic disease	Goal
Heart	Decrease inflammation
Stroke	Decrease inflammation
Arthritis	Decrease inflammation
Alzheimer's disease	Decrease inflammation
Multiple sclerosis	Decrease inflammation
Chronic pain	Decrease inflammation

Decreasing inflammation can be achieved in only one way: by increasing the production of "good" eicosanoids and decreasing the production of "bad" eicosanoids. By using my dietary program to control eicosanoids, you will begin to macromanage wellness instead of micromanaging disease, because you can now alter the levels of eicosanoids that control inflammation. To do so effectively, though, you need to have blood tests that define wellness so that you know where you're starting from and can measure your progress. It's not enough to assume that if you're not sick, you must be well. You need a scientific way to prove that your body is in a state of wellness. The blood tests that define the Omega Rx Zone (which are described in chapter 9) are the same blood tests that define wellness.

In the past, the Zone has mistakenly been described as a weight-loss diet. While it's true that being in the Zone will help you lose excess body fat, the Zone really is about the simultaneous control of both eicosanoids and insulin, and how balancing these two hormonal systems will improve your health. However, these two hormones don't necessarily play equal roles in the prevention and treatment of chronic diseases. Below I list the relative impact these two hormones have on specific diseases.

Optimal Health Matrix

Condition	Impact of Insulin	Impact of Eicosanoids
Fat loss	90%	10%
Diabetes	75%	25%
Heart disease	40%	60%
Cancer	30%	70%
Brain function	25%	75%
Skin	15%	85%
Inflammatory pain	10%	90%

You can see from this table that apart from fat loss and control of diabetes, most of the health benefits of being in the Omega Rx Zone are derived from improved eicosanoid control. What's not quite as obvious from the table is that the greater the impact of eicosanoids on a condition, the more you have to supplement your diet with high-dose fish oil to obtain benefits. That's because high-dose fish oil primarily influences eicosanoid levels.

Of course, by controlling insulin and eicosanoids simultaneously, you'll achieve the full range of health benefits of the Omega Rx Zone. Following my dietary recommendations allows you to cover all your bases. So if you, say, want to reduce arthritis pain or prevent depression, you'll get all the other benefits (like fat loss) at the same time. More important, you'll be moving toward a state of wellness, a state that can be defined with laserlike precision through certain blood tests.

TAKE THIS SIMPLE WELLNESS TEST NOW

Get a first indication that you're on the path to wellness by taking a basic cholesterol blood test that measures your levels of triglycerides and HDL ("good") cholesterol. This test is given during your annual physical, which you should be getting anyway. The ratio of triglycerides to HDL is an indirect marker of both your insulin status and your eicosanoid status. Your aim is to have a high level of HDL cholesterol compared with triglycerides. If the ratio of triglycerides to HDL is less than 2, you've got a rough indicator that you're relatively healthy. If your ratio is greater than 2, you've got a flashing warning light telling you that you're already in the area of subchronic illness and you're headed toward one (or more) chronic disease conditions in the future. Chapter 9 describes even more precise (though less widely used) blood tests that will tell you your likelihood of developing heart disease, cancer, or dementia, years ahead of their actual development. If you are at risk, don't despair, because following my dietary program you can change that future within thirty days.

If promoting wellness is the key to twenty-first-century health care, then ultimately that means keeping insulin and eicosanoids within the Omega Rx Zone. One of the hardest concepts for physicians and the rest of us to understand is the power of food to alter our hormonal responses (especially insulin and eicosanoids), for better or worse. Since hormones are hundreds of times more powerful than drugs, learning to harness hormones will be the key to having a longer and better life by maintaining yourself in the Omega Rx Zone. The clinical definitions that describe the Zone are universal. It's like the top of a mountain; it doesn't change. Many lifestyle paths can lead to the Zone. Some paths, however, will provide much easier ways to reach the peak than others. I believe my dietary plan is simply the easiest and fastest way to reach the Zone. Getting yourself on that pathway will be a snap if you follow the program described in Part II.

chapter 6

Brain Wellness

With growing frequency, news items appear about the benefits of fish oil—especially about studies showing that fish oil helps the brain in some way. Fish oil has been said to thwart depression, lessen the effects of Alzheimer's disease, and keep a host of other brain disorders at bay. The central theme of this book is that consumption of high doses of fish oil dramatically alters our brain function (how we think, focus, and reason) and quite probably boosts our intelligence.

In chapter 5, I put forward the critical need to define wellness if we are to make it the goal for twenty-first-century medicine. The brain operates under the same conditions as the body. Just as you want to achieve a state of wellness for your body, you also want to achieve a state of wellness for your brain. Your brain isn't in a state of wellness just because you don't have some obvious neurological problem, like depression or attention deficit disorder. Your brain is in a state of wellness only if you're thinking at peak efficiency. This means you're unhampered by mental fuzziness, jittery nerves, inability to complete tasks, or a sense of doom and gloom. Ask yourself these questions to see if your brain is in a state of wellness:

1. Do you have a hard time concentrating on your daily tasks?
2. Do you find yourself moving from project to project without ever completing the one at hand?
3. Do you have a hard time getting organized or remembering things?
4. Do you find it difficult to look forward to the future?
5. Are you feeling down more often than you're feeling good?
6. Are you finding yourself acting less civil to others?

If your answer to any of these questions is "yes," your brain is in a state of subchronic illness. I could list dozens of additional questions about your mental health, but you get the idea. You *know* when you're operating in slow motion or just not feeling the mental zip that you had when you were younger. You might even blame your mental decline on advancing age. I can't tell you how many forty- and fifty-year-olds tell me that their mental capacity is diminishing as they reach middle age. I tell them that their brainpower may be diminishing, but this has nothing to do with their age. They're simply not maintaining the brain in a zone of wellness.

Because of its amazing complexity, the human brain remains shrouded in mystery. We're not exactly sure how it works. As a result, when the brain goes wrong we feel powerless to fix it. There are two points in your life when your brain is most vulnerable: when you're an infant, and it is still developing; and when you reach old age, and it begins to fail. In one case, your brain can be robbed of reaching its full potential; in the other, you lose your ability to take a lifetime of experiences and integrate them into a cohesive and meaningful mosaic. This is why our greatest fear, as we age, is that the brain will give out before the body.

My dietary program can dramatically alter brain function at both ends of the age spectrum and in all the years between. By following this plan, you give your brain what it loves and avoid giving it what it hates. As a result, you keep it humming at peak efficiency at every stage of your life. As hokey as it sounds, if you're good to your brain, your brain will be good to you.

Just like body wellness, brain wellness depends on increased blood flow and decreased inflammation. In order to achieve both, you have to give the brain what it loves and avoid the things it hates. Fortunately, the list is pretty short.

Brain Loves	Brain Hates
Adequate blood flow	Inflammation
Stable blood sugar	Loss of key neurotransmitters
Docosahexaenoic acid (DHA)	Excess cortisol

Let's look at each one of these items in more detail. You'll begin to see just how much dietary control you have over your brain's state of wellness.

WHAT THE BRAIN LOVES

Adequate Blood Flow

The most important thing the brain needs is an excellent supply of oxygen, and this comes only from adequate blood flow, since your blood cells carry oxygen to your brain and the rest of your organs. Your brain's energy, as well as the energy in the rest of your body, is made by energy power-houses called mitochondria that are found in each cell. Oxygen enables mitochondria in your brain cells to pump out an energy chemical, adenosine triphosphate (ATP). Without adequate levels of ATP, your brain has an energy drain, and its function decreases.

As you age, the mitochondria become less efficient at pumping out ATP, and a primary reason for this is decreased blood flow to the brain. Although the brain represents only about 2 percent of your total body mass, it accounts for more than 25 percent of the blood flow. Without adequate blood flow, your brain is deprived of oxygen and thus is unable to manufacture enough ATP to operate at peak efficiency. Below a critical level of ATP production, brain cells can begin to die. A stroke is an extreme example of this: blood flow and oxygen to a portion of the brain are restricted, and brain cells in that region die off.

The best way to increase blood flow to the brain (and every other organ, for that matter) is to generate more "good" eicosanoids (which are powerful vasodilators that widen the opening of arteries, veins, and capillaries) and fewer "bad" eicosanoids (which are powerful vasoconstrictors that have the opposite effect). The long-chain omega-3 fatty acid contained in fish oil, EPA, will increase the production of "good" eicosanoids by decreasing the levels of arachidonic acid (the building block of "bad" eicosanoids). The higher the level of EPA in the diet, the more your cells will be induced to make more "good" eicosanoids (see appendix D).

Stable Blood Sugar

Even if you have adequate oxygen flow to the brain, you still need a stable supply of glucose, since the brain also needs this fuel to make ATP. The only way to maintain a steady supply of glucose to the brain is to control insulin levels.

Having a spike in your insulin levels (which comes from eating too many carbohydrates) can drive glucose levels down so low that your brain function is compromised. That's why you feel so sleepy two hours after eating a huge pasta meal. Your thinking becomes fuzzy, you have difficulty concentrating, and all you want to do is take a nap.

At this point, your brain, deprived of adequate levels of blood sugar to make ATP, is desperately seeking any way possible to get more blood sugar. As a result, you are driven by an almost manic urge to eat carbohydrates. That's your brain's way of telling you that you have to get some glucose into the bloodstream quickly—or else. The more carbohydrate-rich that food is, the faster it can reach your bloodstream and then your brain. Candy bars, soft drinks, and other types of junk food are just a quick way to self-medicate the low blood sugar induced by elevated insulin levels from your last meal. These carbohydrate fixes temporarily solve the problem of low blood sugar but create a new cycle of increased insulin levels, and you soon find yourself with one bout after another of craving carbohydrates. To keep yourself out of this vicious circle, you need to prevent your brain from sending out the distress call in the first place. The way to do that is to keep it supplied with steady amounts of glucose by maintaining insulin levels within a defined zone that is neither too high nor too low.

As I will explain in chapter 7, the only way to stabilize blood sugar levels is by maintaining a relatively constant protein-to-carbohydrate balance every time you eat. You need some insulin to drive glucose into your cells for storage, but too much insulin reduces blood sugar to such low levels that brain function is impaired. By stabilizing insulin in the blood, you won't have a dizzying drop in blood sugar. And there's an added benefit: steady insulin will enable your body to maintain a steady level of the hormone glucagon, which releases stored blood sugar from the liver, allowing a constant supply of blood sugar for the brain. Carbohydrates stimulate the release of insulin, and protein stimulates the release of glucagon; that is why I always recommend balancing these two nutrients at every meal and snack.

Docosahexaenoic Acid

The final thing the brain loves is an adequate level of docosahexaenoic acid (DHA). This is one of the two long-chain omega-3 fatty acids found in fish oil (EPA is the other). More than 60 percent of the weight of the brain is fat, and most of the long-chain omega-3 fatty acids in the body are concentrated in the brain. Virtually all of this long-chain omega-3 fat, however, is in the form of DHA, since the brain contains very little EPA. One reason the brain demands such high levels of DHA is that it's critical for certain cell membranes such as the synapse (to transfer information), the retina (to receive visual inputs), and the mitochondria (to make ATP). Thus, the key brain cells can't perform at peak levels without adequate DHA in their membranes.

Trying to maintain your brain function without adequate DHA is like trying to build the sturdiest brick house in town without enough bricks. You might have the best architect, the best location, and the best contractor, but if you don't have enough bricks, the dream house will never be built properly. Without adequate DHA, your brain can't function adequately and can't form new neural connections, let alone maintain old ones.

WHAT THE BRAIN HATES

Inflammation

While you're providing your brain with the important things it needs, you also have to avoid giving it what it hates. And your brain absolutely despises inflammation. Inflammation appears to be the underlying condition associated with the development of Alzheimer's disease. All inflammation is ultimately caused by the increased production of "bad" eicosanoids. What's more, many of the proinflammatory cytokines (proteins produced by immune cells) lead to the production of more "bad" eicosanoids, and vice versa. So bad begets worse, and the inflammation cycle continues unabated.

The best way to stop this cycle is to consume high doses of fish oil to provide adequate levels of EPA. Not only will you choke off the production of "bad" eicosanoids (by decreasing the production of arachidonic acid), but you'll also decrease the production of inflammation-promoting cytokines. This is a real win-win situation for your brain.

Loss of Key Neurotransmitters

The second thing the brain hates is any loss of key neurotransmitters. Those are the chemicals that control the flow of information transfer from one nerve cell to the other as they cross the gap (synapse) between different nerve cells. Without adequate levels of neurotransmitters, information slows dramatically. Two of the most important neurotransmitters are serotonin and dopamine. Consider serotonin to be your stress-adaptation hormone and dopamine to be your action hormone. When serotonin levels are low, depression and violent or impulsive behavior become more likely. When dopamine levels are low, there's an increased likelihood of Parkinson's disease (decreased motor skills) or attention deficit disorder (decreased ability to focus on immediate tasks).

A multibillion-dollar drug market has been developed to provide a wide variety of pharmaceuticals that are intended to increase either serotonin or dopamine. Unfortunately, if a drug increases one of these neurotransmitters, it often depresses the other. There is, however, one natural "drug" that can increase both dopamine and serotonin simultaneously. That "drug" is high-dose fish oil. By taking high doses of fish oil, you can maintain adequate levels of both neurotransmitters.

Excess Cortisol

Your brain also detests excess cortisol—the hormone your body releases in response to long-term stress. The more stress (which includes chronic pain or inflammation) you have in your life, the more cortisol is released to control it. Unfortunately, nothing kills brain cells (especially those in the hippocampus, where memories are stored) faster than excess cortisol. Excess cortisol also inhibits short-term memory, like remembering where you put your keys.

My dietary recommendations reduce excessive cortisol production in two ways. First, EPA in fish oil decreases the production of arachidonic acid, which in turn decreases the production of "bad" eicosanoids. As the levels of "bad" eicosanoids decrease, the need for the body to produce cortisol also decreases. Second, my dietary program stabilizes insulin levels, thus shutting down the need for production of excess cortisol. Cortisol is sometimes released to stimulate the release of stored sugar into the blood when blood sugar levels dip too low. This occurs if you are not producing adequate levels of glucagon (the primary hormone to stimulate the release of stored carbohydrate), which can be suppressed by high levels of insulin. Although cortisol gives your brain what it needs for the moment (more blood sugar), you then have the problem of excess cortisol levels flowing through the bloodstream, causing damage to the memory center in the hippocampus in the brain.

The table below summarizes your brain's desires and aversions—and what impact insulin and fish oil have on them.

Brain Loves and Hates

	Impact of Insulin Control	Impact of High-Dose Fish Oil
Brain Loves		
Blood flow		✓
Stable blood sugar	✓	
DHA		✓
Brain Hates		
Inflammation		✓
Loss of neurotransmitters		✓
Excess cortisol	✓	✓

As you can see, insulin control accounts for about 25 percent of your brain function, whereas eicosanoid control accounts for about 75 percent. Thus, you need a combination of dietary measures (balancing carbohydrates and protein) and high-dose fish oil to give your brain what it loves and avoid what it hates. This is the foundation of my dietary program, which I outline in Part II.

Getting to the Omega Rx Zone

Part II gives you all the dietary elements you need to get into the Omega Rx Zone. My basic plan consists of three elements: my dietary plan to stabilize your insulin levels, a calorie restriction program without hunger or deprivation, and my recommendations for fish oil supplementation. You need all three to fully realize the benefits of being in the Omega Rx Zone. You'll also learn everything you need to know about fish oil supplements, including the reasons that pharmaceutical-grade fish oil should be your primary choice if you supplement your diet with fish oil. And you'll get a detailed plan for monitoring your progress in the Omega Rx Zone, including blood tests you can take that will measure any health improvements and self-evaluations that you can do at home.

If you're otherwise healthy and would like to lose some excess body fat and see a significant gain in physical and mental energy, this part of the book will give you the comprehensive program you need. If you're at increased risk of developing heart disease, cancer, Alzheimer's disease, or some other chronic disease, or if you already have a chronic disease, you'll need to use Part II as your basic plan and then use my recommendations in Part III to supplement that basic plan. Part IV shows you how to reach your full potential in the Omega Rx Zone in terms of boosting your brainpower, athletic performance, and sense of well-being.

Ready to enter the Omega Rx Zone? Let's begin.

chapter 7

The Basic Plan

The word *diet* usually implies some type of short-term weight loss program. In fact, a diet should be considered a systematic lifelong approach using food to reach your desired goal. That's why we talk about the American Heart Association diet, the American Cancer Association diet, the American Diabetes Association diet, and so on. All these diets are meant to be followed for a lifetime to reduce the likelihood of developing some type of chronic disease. My dietary program is no different, because you use it to control your hormones for a lifetime in order to reduce the likelihood of developing all types of chronic disease.

In reality, there are only four types of diets you can follow.

Types of Diets	Examples
Very low carbohydrate, high fat, high protein	Atkins
Moderate carbohydrate, moderate fat, moderate protein	Omega Rx Zone

Types of Diets	Examples
High carbohydrate, moderate fat, moderate protein	USDA, American Heart Association
Very high carbohydrate, very low fat, very low protein	Ornish

The only diet that recommends a moderate amount of each of the three macronutrients—carbohydrate, fat, and protein—is the one based on my dietary recommendations. It's a dietary approach that works to help you shed excess body fat permanently because it lowers elevated levels of insulin. Despite this fact, my program has been mislabeled a "high-protein" diet for years. When you follow my dietary recommendations, you *never* eat more than 3 or 4 ounces of low-fat protein at any one meal. That's exactly what every nutritionist in America recommends.

Let's look at the two types of diets at the extremes. High-protein diets, such as the Atkins diet, allow you to eat virtually unlimited amounts of protein and fat with virtually no carbohydrates. In the absence of a minimal amount of incoming carbohydrates, the body is quickly set into an abnormal metabolic condition known as ketosis. This condition occurs when there is not enough carbohydrate to metabolize fat completely, and waste products known as ketone bodies begin to accumulate in the blood. People often feel cranky and irritable on these high-protein diets because the brain can't function properly without an adequate amount of carbohydrates. The diets at the other extreme—the high-carbohydrate, low-fat diets such as those advocated by Dean Ornish—allow you to eat virtually no fat and very little protein. These high-carbohydrate diets can cause an increase in insulin levels, the very thing you're trying to avoid. Common sense dictates that diets at the extremes (Atkins and Ornish) are difficult to follow for a few weeks, let alone for a lifetime.

We're left with only two candidates for lifelong diets, differing only in the amount of daily carbohydrate that should be consumed: the moderate-carbohydrate diet and the high-carbohydrate diet. When it comes to getting your hormone levels balanced, it makes sense to aim for moderation in all types of food rather than tip the scales to favor one nutrient over another.

As I have emphasized in my previous books, carbohydrates don't just consist of breads, pasta, and other grains. Carbohydrates also include fruits and vegetables. This is a revelation to most Americans. The carbohydrates you consume on my dietary program consist mainly of fruits and vegetables, because it's easier to stick to a moderate-carbohydrate diet by eating fruits and vegetables rather than eating carbohydrate-dense foods like bagels, pasta, and potatoes. As I will show, making a switch from one form of carbohydrates to another can have profound hormonal consequences that will dramatically affect every aspect of your health and longevity.

My dietary plan, however, is more complex than simply reducing excess carbohydrate intake. Its centerpiece is the consumption of high-dose fish oil. On my dietary program, you eat lots of fruits and vegetables, balanced with lean protein and supplemented with high-dose fish oil. I want to state up front that the medical community at large may not initially embrace my recommendations for taking high-dose fish oil. But the science involved makes it clear to me that the use of high-dose fish oil will radically change how medicine will be practiced in the twenty-first century. That's because it allows you to alter those hormones (eicosanoids) that will keep your mind and body in peak condition for the future.

Controlling your hormones may seem confusing and difficult at first. If endocrinologists can barely understand their complexity, how are you going to be able to orchestrate your own hormonal symphony? The truth is that you don't really need to understand all the inner workings of your hormone systems to get the balanced level of hormones that your body needs. All you have to do is follow some very basic dietary rules to reach the Omega Rx Zone and keep yourself there. As I stated in chapter 1, my dietary program consists of three distinct components: insulin control, calorie restriction, and eicosanoid modulation. Doing all three simultaneously is a lot easier than you think.

INSULIN CONTROL

Let's start with controlling insulin, since it is the primary factor in losing excess body fat and preventing type 2 diabetes, as shown in the Optimal Health Matrix on page 44. Insulin control is achieved through balancing protein and carbohydrate at each meal to maintain stable blood sugar levels for the next four to six hours. Think of it as like balancing the ratio of air and gas in the carburetor of your car to get the best possible mileage. Likewise, you are trying to get the best possible hormonal mileage for each meal. Hormonally you are only as good as your last meal, and you will be only as good as your next meal. This means that you have a dietary decision to make every four to six hours.

Following is a quick review of my dietary technology for lifelong insulin control. First, begin thinking of food in terms of its three major categories: protein, carbohydrate, and fat. Only then can you easily master the basic rules of controlling insulin. How can you use these components of food to get yourself into the Omega Rx Zone? Just follow the commonsense approach your grandmother taught you: *balance* and *moderation*. Balance your plate at every meal and never eat too many calories in one sitting. The only tools you need to achieve both these goals are the palm of your hand and your eye—that is why I call this the hand-eye method.

Step 1: Start with Protein

Every meal or snack in my dietary plan starts with an adequate serving of low-fat protein. Your body needs a constant supply of dietary protein to replace the protein that is lost on a daily basis. What's more, eating protein stimulates the release of the hormone glucagon, which has a hormonal action opposite to that of insulin. Glucagon tells your body to release stored carbohydrates from the liver to replenish blood sugar levels for the brain. Without adequate levels of glucagon, you'll always feel hungry and mentally fatigued because your brain is short of its primary fuel—blood sugar. This is why adequate protein at mealtime is critical for optimal brain function.

Finally, you need to choose your protein selectively to avoid choices that are high in arachidonic acid—the building block of "bad" eicosanoids. In general, low-fat protein sources like fish, chicken, turkey, egg whites, and soy imitation meat products are low in arachidonic acid. Protein sources that are rich in saturated fat and cholesterol like organ meats (liver, pâté, foie gras), fatty cuts of beef and pork, and egg yolks are also rich in arachidonic acid.

How much protein should you consume at any one meal? Here's an easy rule of thumb: consume only as much protein as the size and thickness of the palm of your hand. For the average American female, this amount is 3 ounces (20 grams) of low-fat protein at a meal; for the average American male, it is about 4 ounces (30 grams) of low-fat protein. Unless you are very physically active, your body can't utilize any more protein than that at a single sitting, and any excess protein you eat will be converted to fat. Here are some low-fat protein choices:

Low-Fat Protein Choices

Protein Source	Amount for 20 Grams of Protein (typical for a woman)	Amount for 30 Grams of Protein (typical for a man)
Fish	4.5 ounces	6 ounces
Chicken	3	4
Turkey	3	4
Egg whites	6	8
Very low-fat beef	3	4

Now divide your plate into three portions. Your low-fat protein portion should cover about one-third of your plate.

1/3 of the Plate

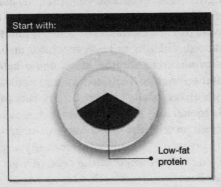

Start with:

Low-fat protein

Step 2: Balance with Carbohydrates

Once you have the protein portion of your meal, you need to balance it out with carbohydrates, primarily fruits and vegetables. Yes, fruits and vegetables are carbohydrates. In fact, they are the primary sources of carbohydrates in my dietary plan. Fruits and vegetables have several advantages over bread, pasta, rice, and potatoes. First, they are the richest source of vitamins, minerals, and have a host of antioxidant phytochemicals. What's more, they have a much lower density of carbohydrates than starches; this means that, ounce for ounce, you get more food (and nutrients) for fewer carbohydrates and calories. For example, you can fill your plate completely with steamed vegetables and still not equal the amount of carbohydrates you'd find in one small serving of rice.

Fruits and vegetables also contain much more soluble fiber per gram of carbohydrate than bread and pasta; soluble fiber helps keep your insulin levels on an even keel by slowing the early rate of carbohydrates so that you won't get the quick spikes in your blood sugar and subsequent spikes in your insulin levels that can come from eating highly processed carbohydrates. This lowered insulin response will keep blood sugar levels stable over time, so your brain will have an adequate and more consistent supply of energy. The combination of the two factors—lower carbohydrate density and greater soluble fiber content—is why fruits and vegetables are the primary major carbohydrate choices if you want to reach the Omega Rx Zone.

Your best carbohydrate choices are shown below.

Carbohydrate Choices

Best Choices

> Most vegetables
> Most fruits (berries are the best)
> Selected grains rich in soluble fiber (slow-cooked oatmeal and barley)

Poor Choices

> Starches and most grains (bread, pasta, rice, pota-
> toes, and so on)
> Some fruits (bananas)
> Some vegetables (corn and carrots)

For a more complete listing of carbohydrates and their effects on insulin levels, see appendix E.

Add enough fruits and vegetables to cover the other two-thirds of your plate.

Balanced Plate

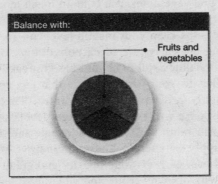

Balance with:

Fruits and vegetables

Step 3: Add Monounsaturated Fat

Now your plate is completely covered. Protein takes up one-third of the space and low-density carbohydrates take up the other two-thirds. Where does fat come in? Fat is what makes food taste great. But not all fat is the same. On my dietary program you use primarily monounsaturated fat—whether it's the teaspoon of olive oil that you cook your vegetables in or the avocado slices or handful of slivered almonds that you put on top of your salads. Without some monounsaturated fat, you can't have a complete Omega Rx Zone meal. But the amount of monounsaturated fat I am talking about would be considered a dash.

Monounsaturated fat has no direct effect on insulin, nor does it have any effect on glucagon. It does, though, act like a control rod in a nuclear reactor, slowing the rate at which carbohydrates enter your bloodstream. In addition, it causes the release of another hormone—cholecystokinin, or CCK—that tells your brain to stop eating. Thus, fat gives you a feeling of satiety and helps blend the flavors that give great meals their exquisite taste, with the added bonus of lowering your insulin response to carbohydrates in that meal.

Fats to Avoid

The fats you should minimize or avoid are the saturated fats, trans fats, and omega-6 fats.

- You find saturated fats in fatty cuts of red meat and high-fat dairy products such as cheddar cheese, butter, and ice cream. These will make your cell membranes more rigid, causing the liver to produce more cholesterol to break up this rigidity.

- Trans fats are found in margarine and other partially hydrogenated oils that are used in many processed snack foods. These artificial fats can act as inhibitors to the enzymes needed to synthesize the longer-chain essential fatty acids, thereby disrupting eicosanoid formation. This is probably the main reason that high intakes of trans fats are associated with increased heart disease.

- Polyunsaturated fats like soy, corn, and safflower oils are rich in omega-6 fats, which in excess are far worse for you hormonally than either saturated fats or trans fats. I consider omega-6 fats the really "bad" fats because they can lead to the increased formation of arachidonic acid, the building block of all the "bad" eicosanoids.

Fats to Choose

The best monounsaturated fats to add to an Omega Rx Zone meal are those found primarily in olive oil, selected nuts, and avocados, as shown below.

Fat Choices

Good Choices
Olive oil
Nuts rich in monounsaturated fats (almonds, cashews, macadamia nuts)
Avocados

Poor Choices
Saturated fats (whole milk, full-fat cheeses, cream, ice cream)
Trans fats (margarine, partially hydrogenated vegetable oil)
Omega-6 fats (soybean oil, safflower oil, sunflower oil, corn oil)

Finally, add a dash (that's a small amount) of "good" fat to complete your meal.

A Quick Review of Your Plate

Now that you have an idea what types of protein, carbohydrate, and fat you will be using to make meals and snacks on my program, let me review how easy it really is. Just divide your plate into three sections. On one-third of your plate, choose one of the low-fat protein foods—no bigger than the size and thickness of your palm. Then fill the other two-thirds of the plate to overflowing with fruits and vegetables. Finally, add a dash of good fat. There you have it: a meal designed to get you to the Omega Rx Zone.

Note: How can you tell if your last meal was hormonally correct? You aren't hungry, and you have peak mental acuity four hours after your last meal.

You'll find yourself eating a large quantity of food on my program: three meals and two snacks a day. When you are composing your meals, use a dinner-size plate. When you are composing your snacks, use a dessert plate. It couldn't be any easier.

This part of the plan seems like common sense, and it is. More important, it guarantees you insulin control and stable blood sugar levels for the next four to six hours. When you visualize the composition of your plate as a food pyramid, it looks like this:

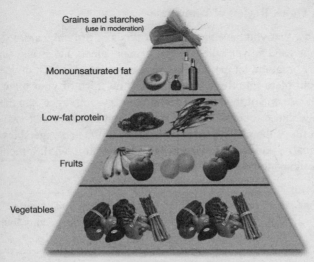

Grains and starches
(use in moderation)

Monounsaturated fat

Low-fat protein

Fruits

Vegetables

Zone Food Pyramid

Notice that you are eating a lot of fruits and vegetables and adequate amounts of low-fat protein, always adding some monounsaturated fat, and keeping starches and grains to a minimum. I don't ban pasta, rice, bread, and other grains outright, but I do advise you to use these starches as condiments rather than as the full carbohydrate portion of your meal or snack. The two grains that I recommend in small amounts are slow-cooked oatmeal and barley, since both are rich in soluble fiber, which slows the rate of entry of any carbohydrate into the bloodstream.

If you compare the insulin-control component of my dietary program with that recommended by the USDA, you get a very different picture, as shown here.

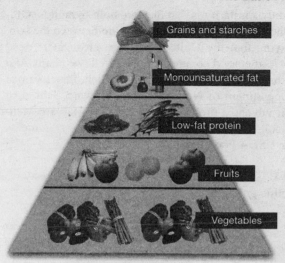

Zone Food Pyramid

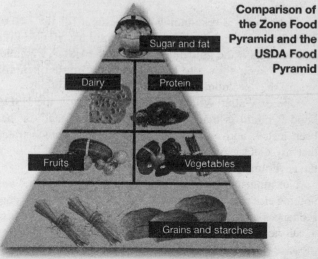

Comparison of the Zone Food Pyramid and the USDA Food Pyramid

USDA Food Pyramid

The only similarity is that they are both pyramids. Otherwise, there appears to be no relationship between the two. Am I saying that the United States government is dead wrong in its dietary recommendations? Well, yes, I am. And I'm not the only one saying it. Walter Willett, the chairman of the Department of Nutrition at the Harvard School of Public Health and a professor of medicine at Harvard Medical School, has recently made the following statements about the USDA Food Pyramid:

> "The USDA Pyramid is wrong. It was built on shaky scientific ground."

> "The USDA Pyramid offers wishy-washy, scientifically unfounded advice."

> ". . . nor has it ever been tested to see if it really works."

Not exactly a resounding endorsement for the USDA Food Pyramid. In fact, research at Harvard has yielded little data to support the guidelines found in the USDA Pyramid. It hasn't been shown to have more than limited benefits against the development of chronic disease conditions.

One of Walter Willett's major objections to the USDA Food Pyramid is that it was never tested. Actually, it has been tested, and every published study has demonstrated that my dietary recommendations are superior to those of the government. Let's look at the facts.

Nutritionists often say that "a calorie is a calorie," and nothing else counts. In contrast, I say that the hormonal consequences of a calorie of protein are different from those of a calorie of carbohydrate, which are different still from those of a calorie of fat. My dietary recommendations are based on hormonal thinking, whereas the USDA Food Pyramid, the American Heart Association diet, and many other medically endorsed diets are based on caloric thinking.

The only way to determine who is correct is to have individuals follow diets with exactly the same number of calories, but with different protein-to-carbohydrate ratios. If the USDA, the American Heart Association, and nutritionists are right, then your weight and health shouldn't change no matter which diet you're following. If I am right, you'll see dramatic differences in your body fat and your health if you choose one diet over another.

The USDA Food Pyramid recommends eating 55 percent of your calories as carbohydrate and 15 percent as protein. Since carbohydrates and protein have the same number of calories per gram, you can see that the USDA recommends consuming almost four times the amount of carbohydrates for every gram of protein. On the other hand, using the hand-eye method of my dietary program will give you only slightly more than a gram of carbohydrates for every gram of protein consumed. This is why the USDA diet is a high-carbohydrate diet and my program is a moderate-carbohydrate diet. Therefore, it should be easy to take diets with different carbohydrate-to-protein ratios but the same number of calories and compare them clinically to see which one wins.

The results are already published. Studies from the Harvard Medical School have found that a moderate-carbohydrate diet like my dietary recommendations generated superior hormonal responses after a single meal compared to a high-carbohydrate meal like those advocated by the USDA and the American Heart Association. Other studies from the Harvard Medical School have shown that a moderate-carbohydrate diet provides better metabolic responses and greater appetite suppression than high-carbohydrate diets. Other investigators have found improved lipoprotein levels and greater fat loss (nearly twice as much) on moderate-carbohydrate diets, compared with high-carbohydrate diets. At some point, the bureaucrats at the USDA should simply give up and tell the American people they were dead wrong in recommending a high-carbohydrate diet.

CALORIE RESTRICTION WITHOUT HUNGER OR DEPRIVATION

The research data indicate quite clearly that in controlling insulin the moderate-carbohydrate content in my dietary program is superior to the high-carbohydrate content recommended by the USDA. Furthermore, the Harvard Medical School and I have the same opinion on the scientific credibility of the USDA Food Pyramid. But what about the second component of my program: calorie restriction? This part of the plan doesn't sound like much fun, since people don't want to deprive themselves of food and feel hungry even if it makes them live longer. I can assure you that you won't be hungry on this plan. In fact, you may actually need to remind yourself to eat every five hours, because you won't be hungry. Once you see the amount of food you're allowed at every meal, you'll know that you won't ever be deprived.

First let me summarize the science behind calorie restriction. Calorie restriction is the only proven way to reverse the aging process. There is no scientific argument on this point, and I have devoted an entire book (*The Anti-Aging Zone*) to this subject. Here's a brief explanation of why calorie restriction works.

First, by reducing calorie intake (especially high-density carbohydrate foods such as starches, grains, bread, and pasta), you will automatically reduce insulin levels. Second, the reduction in calories you consume decreases the formation of free radicals that can attack both DNA and polyunsaturated fats. Third, calorie restriction decreases production of the stress hormone cortisol as an indirect consequence of lowering insulin levels. And finally, the reduction of carbohydrate intake will decrease the formation of carbohydrate-protein complexes known as advanced glycosylated end (AGE) products. These carbohydrate-modified proteins stick in all the wrong places, like the capillaries that feed the eye and the kidney, and are associated with accelerated heart disease and potentially Alzheimer's disease. I call these the four pillars of aging, since any dietary intervention that reduces (1) insulin levels, (2) free radical levels, (3) cortisol levels, and (4) the formation of AGE proteins will slow down the rate of aging. The actual physiological improvements in calorie restriction are listed below.

Physiological Changes with Calorie Restriction

Increased	Decreased
Maximum life span	Insulin levels
Learning ability	Heart disease
Immune function	Cancer
Kidney function	Diabetes
Female fertility	Autoimmune disease
	Body fat
	Bone loss

This is a pretty impressive list of benefits. However, no one wants to be hungry and deprived, no matter what the health benefits. Neither do I. When you follow my moderate-carbohydrate, moderate-protein, moderate-fat program, you'll never feel hungry between meals. Feeling less hungry on fewer calories is a phenomenon that I call Zone paradox. You'll find yourself living this paradox once you start eating more fruits and vegetables and eating fewer starches and grains. Suddenly, you'll be automatically restricting calories without even thinking about it.

If you have balanced your plate according to my hand-eye method, you are automatically practicing calorie restriction, but without hunger or deprivation. Let's do the numbers by comparing my plan with the newly published dietary recommendations of the American Heart Association (AHA). According to the AHA, a person should eat 50 to 100 grams of protein per day. I recommend that a person should eat 75 to 100 grams of protein per day. So both diets recommend roughly the same amount of protein at the upper end. The American Heart Association states that proteins should be approximately 15 percent of your total calories and carbohydrates should be about 55 percent of the total calories, with the rest of the calories (30 percent) as fat. On my dietary plan, you always consume more carbohydrate than protein, but not nearly as much as on the American Heart Association plan. You also get most of your carbohydrates from fruits (berries being the best) and vegetables. And you add a dash (that's a small amount) of heart-healthy monounsaturated fat to every meal. On my plan, you are not a slave to percentages, but you are looking to approximate the right amount of protein, carbohydrate, and fat at every meal and snack.

Let's see how an average male who would need 100 grams of protein per day would stack up on both diets.

Omega Rx Zone		American Heart Association
Protein	100 grams	100 grams (15 percent of calories)
Carbohydrates	140 grams	367 grams (55 percent of calories)
Fat	60 grams	90 grams (30 percent of calories)
Calories	1,500	2,667

If you want to play the percentage game as recommended by the American Heart Association (and the USDA, for that matter), you eat a lot of calories. In fact, this typical male would be eating 44 percent fewer calories on my dietary program than are recommended by the American Heart Association, even though both plans advocate *exactly* the same amount of low-fat protein. With this reduction in calories come all the longevity benefits of calorie restriction. But what about hunger? Who could live on so few calories? Actually, a better question would be, how can you eat all the food you are supposed to on my dietary plan? Let me give an example of meals and snacks that a typical male requiring 100 grams of protein would consume on my program.

Breakfast
Egg white omelet consisting of
- 8 egg whites or 1 cup of egg substitute
- 2 teaspoons of olive oil
- 3 sun-dried tomatoes

1 cup slow-cooked oatmeal

1 cup strawberries

Lunch
Chicken Caesar salad with 4 ounces skinless chicken breast and 12 olives

2 cups steamed vegetables

1 apple

Afternoon snack
2 hard-boiled eggs with the yolks removed and filled with hummus (mashed chickpeas and olive oil)

Dinner
>   6 ounces grilled salmon
>   ½ teaspoon slivered almonds
>   4 cups steamed vegetables
>   1 cup mixed berries

Late-night snack
>   1 ounce low-fat cheese
>   4 ounces red wine

Although that's a lot of food, it is still only about 1,500 calories. The calorie-restriction component of my dietary plan is based on changing the composition of the carbohydrates you eat. You consume more low-density carbohydrates such as fruits and vegetables and fewer starchy, high-density carbohydrates such as pasta, potatoes, rice, and grains. Medically, this is known as reducing the glycemic load, and it's explained in greater detail in appendix E. To illustrate the impact of changing the types of carbohydrate you eat on the glycemic load, let's use the serving sizes recommended by the USDA to see how much food you would need to consume to reach the 140 grams of carbohydrates on my dietary program for the average male consuming 100 grams of protein per day.

The USDA recommends 3 to 5 servings of fruits and vegetables per day. My dietary plan recommends 10 to 15 servings per day. The USDA also recommends 6 to 11 servings of starchy carbohydrates per day, whereas my plan recommends only 2. Let's see how this plays out mathematically.

Omega Rx Zone

Carbohydrate Type	Servings	Grams of Carbohydrate
Grains, pasta, rice	2	40
Fruits	5	50
Vegetables	10	50
Total	17	140

USDA

Carbohydrate Type	Servings	Grams of Carbohydrate
Grains, pasta, rice	11	220
Fruits	2	20
Vegetables	3	15
Total	16	255

As you can see, on my dietary plan you consume more servings of carbohydrates (and thus more actual food) but much lower amounts of total carbohydrates. If you followed the guidelines of the American Heart Association for the male who needed 100 grams of protein per day, you would still have to come up with an additional 130 grams of carbohydrates to meet the carbohydrate recommendations. That's a lot of carbohydrates. Bottom line: the more carbohydrates you eat, the more insulin you produce.

One of the first signs of excess insulin production is the accumulation of excess body fat (remember, insulin is a storage hormone). No wonder obesity has become epidemic in our country—it's probably because our population is desperately trying to follow the government's advice for a "healthy" diet that is high in carbohydrates.

When you follow my dietary recommendations, you practice calorie restriction without hunger or deprivation. How does this work? By controlling insulin, you are also stabilizing blood sugar, so you aren't hungry, because the brain is getting a constant supply of fuel. As a result, you don't eat as many calories at your next meal. This phenomenon has been confirmed by the Harvard Medical School studies that I outlined earlier. Somehow, I trust hard science from Harvard Medical School more than the USDA, whose primary responsibility is to promote the agricultural industry, namely grain farmers. But most important, by lowering insulin you are also decreasing the body's production of arachidonic acid (AA), the building block of the "bad" eicosanoids.

CONTROLLING EICOSANOIDS

The most important part of my dietary program is the modulation of eicosanoids, and this can be done only with high-dose fish oil. This is what distinguishes the advice in this book from that in my previous Zone books. Take a look again at the Optimal Health Matrix on page 44. It should be obvious that the key to optimal health is improved eicosanoid control. This is best done by consuming an adequate amount of long-chain omega-3 fatty acids, while simultaneously reducing your intake of omega-6 fatty acids. This one step will have a greater impact on your health than any other dietary intervention you could make—and move you toward a state of wellness, as I discussed in chapter 5. However, controlling your insulin levels should go hand in hand with increasing your intake of long-chain omega-3 fatty acids. This is because excess insulin can induce the body to make more of the long-chain omega-6 fatty acids (arachidonic acid) that will drive you away from wellness and toward the development of chronic disease. Thus, controlling insulin will amplify the extraordinary benefits of taking high-dose fish oil.

Just how much fish oil do you need? It's a lot more than you may have read about in magazine articles or even in many published research articles. This is what makes my dietary recommendations controversial yet also makes them so powerful. But before I get into the details, let's see what the government has to say about fish oil.

In April 1999, a National Institutes of Health conference tried to determine the amount of fish oil we should have in our diet. The consensus of the conference was that people should try to consume 3 grams per day of long-chain omega-3 fatty acids. This is slightly more than what your grandmother gave your parents when they had to consume a tablespoon of cod liver oil every day. Even if you ate one serving of fatty fish per day, that would provide you with only a little more than 1 gram of long-chain omega-3 fats. Therefore, to match the amount of long-chain omega-3 fatty acids found in 1 tablespoon of cod liver oil, you would have to eat a lot more fish, as shown below.

Long-Chain Omega-3 Fatty Acid Content in Fish

Fish (3.5-ounce servings)	Total Omega-3 (grams)	Servings Required to Equal 1 Tablespoon of Cod Liver Oil
Mackerel	1.8	1.4
Lake trout	1.6	1.6
Herring	1.5	1.7
Sardines	1.4	1.8
Tuna (fresh)	1.3	1.9
Salmon	1.1	2.3
Trout (others)	0.5	5.0
Catfish	0.4	6.2
Cod	0.3	8.3
Snapper	0.2	12.5
Tuna (canned)	0.2	12.5
Sole	0.1	25.0

As you can see, the fish that most people tend to eat are relatively low in long-chain omega-3 fatty acids. Except for salmon, the ones that have the highest content of long-chain omega-3 fats tend not to be Americans' favorites. To get the same amount of long-chain omega-3 fatty acids per day as your grandmother did by taking 1 tablespoon of cod liver oil, you would have to eat more than ½ pound of salmon per day. I love salmon, but there are limits to that love. And if you ate sole, you would have to consume more than 5 pounds per day to meet the government's recommendations!

Fish don't make long-chain omega-3 fatty acids very well, but algae do a very good job of it. Fish are simply at the end of the food chain that starts with algae, and thus they tend to collect algae-derived long-chain omega-3 fatty acids in their fatty tissue. By the same token, they also collect and concentrate other lipid-soluble toxic substances such as organic mercury, PCBs, and DDT in their fatty tissue. The fattier the fish, the more omega-3 fatty acids it contains— and, unfortunately, the more organic mercury, PCBs, and DDT it will also contain. Everything we dump into our oceans eventually gets concentrated in fish.

More than twenty years ago, researchers found that fish caught off the Greenland coast had relatively high levels of PCBs. You can run from polluted waters, but you can't hide from them if you are eating fish. And the more polluted the waters, the higher the levels of contamination in the fish. This is why a few decades ago, pregnant women were warned not to eat any fish caught in Lake Erie. Now the government is again warning pregnant women not to eat such ocean fish as king mackerel, swordfish, and tuna because of high levels of organic mercury. Furthermore, many of the potential cardiovascular benefits of eating fish are attenuated with the increasing intake of organic mercury, which accelerates the development of heart disease.

How do you get adequate levels of long-chain omega-3 fatty acids without ingesting toxins such as organic mercury, PCBs, and DDT? One possible solution to this problem was the development of farmed factory-raised fish. Theoretically, by farming fish, you could control the levels of contamination. But frankly, these farmed fish were far inferior in taste and color to their wild cousins. The color could be addressed by adding coloring agents (natural or artificial). This is often done with chickens to give them a more "golden" color. More ominous, though, is that the fatty-acid composition in these farmed fish changed, reducing the level of long-chain omega-3 fatty acids and increasing the amounts of the harmful arachidonic acid (AA). The trouble is that cheaper soybean oil, not fish oil or algae, is frequently used as a fat source for these farmed fish. Soybean oil is rich in omega-6 fats, which can be further metabolized into arachidonic acid. Thus, the AA content of farm-raised fish can be many times higher than the content found in their cousins raised in the wild. This is shown below in the ratios comparing AA content with a type of long-chain omega-3 fatty acid called eicosapentaenoic acid (EPA) in isolated fish oil from salmon, wild salmon, and farm-raised salmon. The smaller the ratio, the greater the content of EPA. The larger the ratio, the greater the content of AA.

AA/EPA Ratio of Various Types of Salmon Oil

Source of Fish Oil	AA/EPA
Isolated salmon oil	0.05
3.5-ounce fillet of wild salmon	0.83
3.5-ounce fillet of farmed salmon	1.86

Source: United States Department of Agriculture (USDA)

When you eat fish, you're actually eating fish muscle, which tends to be richer in arachidonic acid (AA) than fish oil. This is why the AA/EPA ratio is so low in isolated salmon oil compared with a salmon fillet. Furthermore, the AA/EPA ratio is more than twice as high in farmed fish as in wild salmon, and it is 35 times higher in farmed fish than in isolated salmon oil. One of the primary reasons for following my dietary program is to decrease your AA intake. The more fish flesh (especially farmed fish) you consume, the more AA you take in. So by eating farmed fish instead of taking isolated fish oil you unfortunately move toward a less favorable eicosanoid balance. Eating wild salmon will move you toward a more favorable eicosanoid balance, although not as much as consuming the isolated salmon oil.

Another major problem with increasing our fish consumption is price. As our demand for fish increases, the supply of fish dwindles because of overfishing, and the price of fish goes up. What's more, many Americans find fish difficult to cook compared with beef and chicken, because it can be overcooked to a mushlike consistency or become unappetizingly dry. Compared with recipes for fish, recipes for chicken and beef can seem downright simple.

Nonetheless, by eating more fish, you will still be improving the balance of eicosanoids, owing to their better balance of AA/EPA compared with other animal sources. This is why populations who consume a lot of fish (like the Japanese) are among the healthiest in the world. Taking isolated fish oil will accelerate the movement toward wellness, since fish oil contains the lowest amount of arachidonic acid.

Even if you can find a way to eat one or two fish meals a day, you still wouldn't be doing enough to optimally control your eicosanoids for maximum health. That's because you still need to radically reduce the amount of AA and other shorter-chain omega-6 fatty acids in your diet. This has been shown to have a dramatic effect on the reduction of fatal and nonfatal heart attacks in the Lyon Diet Heart Study that I describe in chapter 11. Thus, you still need to decrease your consumption of animal protein (especially fatty red meats, organ meats, and egg yolks, which are all rich in AA) and increase your consumption of low-fat animal protein (chicken, turkey, and egg whites) and isolated soy protein, such as that found in soy imitation meat products.

Although soy is a great source of protein, the fat that soybeans naturally contain is rich in omega-6 fatty acids. Using defatted soy products solves that problem, since the omega-6 fatty acids have been extracted in order to make isolated soy protein. Soy imitation hamburgers and sausages made from defatted soy protein are now found in many supermarkets, making it easier to reduce your arachidonic acid intake. And they finally taste pretty good!

Once you have lowered your arachidonic acid intake, you still have to make sure that most of the fats you add to your diet are monounsaturated fats, such as olive oil, nuts, and avocados, which are also very low in omega-6 fatty acids. This simple dietary change further reduces the potential overproduction of arachidonic acid. Not surprisingly, people in Italy, Greece, and Crete who consume large amounts of monounsaturated fats are generally considered healthier than Americans.

How Much Fish Oil Do You Really Need?

How much fish oil you need depends on how well you are—and only your blood values can really tell you that, as I'll describe in chapter 9. If you are well, then the maintenance dose I recommend is 2.5 grams of pharmaceutical-grade fish oil (approximately 1 teaspoon or 4 capsules), which contains the same amount of long-chain omega-3 fatty acids that was found in the tablespoon of cod liver oil your grandmother dispensed fifty years ago. On the other hand, if your blood values, as described in chapter 9, indicate that you have sub-chronic illness or if you already suffer from certain neuro-logical disorders, like Alzheimer's disease, attention deficit disorder, or severe inflammatory pain, you will need much more fish oil. In Part III I give specific recommendations for dealing with chronic disease. And you can find names and sources for brands of pharmaceutical-grade fish oil in appendix G.

Now that you've seen all three components of my dietary plan, I can describe it in terms of a more comprehensive Omega Rx Zone Food Pyramid:

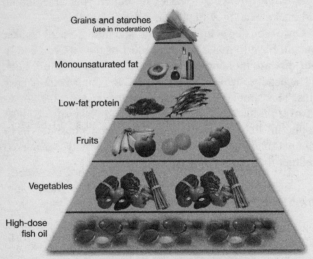

Grains and starches
(use in moderation)

Monounsaturated fat

Low-fat protein

Fruits

Vegetables

High-dose
fish oil

Omega Rx Zone Food Pyramid

You can see that the most important dietary intervention you can make to move toward wellness is taking high-dose fish oil on a daily basis. However, if you also follow my dietary guidelines to control insulin and restrict calories, you position yourself squarely in the Omega Rx Zone, where life is always better.

THE BASIC OMEGA RX ZONE RULES

Now that you know what goes into my dietary plan, you need to know a few other simple rules in order to maintain yourself in the Omega Rx Zone for a lifetime.

1. Always eat an Omega Rx Zone meal within one hour after waking.
2. Every time you eat, go for a balance of protein, carbohydrates, and fat, using my hand-eye method.
3. Try to eat five times per day: three meals and two snacks. Afternoon and late-evening snacks (which are really minimeals) are important to keep you in the Omega Rx Zone throughout the day.
4. Never let more than five hours go by without eating a meal or snack—whether you are hungry or not. In fact, the best time to eat is when you aren't hungry, because not being hungry means you have stabilized your insulin levels.
5. Eat more fruits and vegetables (yes, they are carbohydrates) and ease off the bread, pasta, grains, and other starches. Treat these "high-density" carbohydrates like condiments.
6. Always supplement your diet with high-dose fish oil, as described in chapter 8.

My dietary plan is not exactly rocket science. All you have to do is be consistent in taking your "drug" at the right time and dosage throughout the day. The most important part is the type of fish oil you use, and chapter 8 will give you the information you need to know if you want to get all the benefits of being in the Omega Rx Zone.

chapter 8

Fish Oil Supplements
Knowledge Is Power

As you know, I am a big proponent of supplementing your diet with high-dose fish oil. I always use myself, my family, and my staff to test out any new dietary concept before I ever recommend it. Furthermore, I have been testing high-dose fish oil in a large number of patients over the past three years, and in every case the results have been dramatic, as you will see in Part III.

Since the doses of fish oil I recommend are pretty high by conventional standards (though not by historical standards), I only advise taking what I refer to as *pharmaceutical-grade* fish oil. This type of fish oil exceeds my rigorous standards for purity, meaning that toxins like PCBs or DDT have been reduced to exceedingly low levels, and it has been refined so that gastrointestinal problems associated with lower grades of fish oil are no longer present. You aren't going to find pharmaceutical-grade fish oil in a health food store or super-market, because the extra refining simply makes it too expensive. But your brain and body deserve nothing less. At the levels of fish oil supplementation that I recommend, less pure fish oil will cause a buildup of toxic impurities like PCBs, which have been shown to disrupt your hormonal system, possibly giving rise to cancerous tumors, not to mention significant gastrointestinal problems like gas, abdominal pain, and diarrhea.

THE HISTORY OF FISH OIL

Since you'll be taking a lot of fish oil on my dietary program, a little education about its manufacturing is in order. To extract fish oil, the fish are boiled until the oil rises to the top of the vat, a process known as rendering. Unfortunately, this crude fish oil represents the sewer of the sea, since anything eaten previously by the fish that is water-insoluble will become part of that rendered oil. This includes toxins like PCBs, DDT, and organic mercury compounds. The big problem is how to make fish oil suitable for human consumption.

The first recorded production of fish oil occurred in 1775 in England. When cod was brought back from America, the livers were slapped onto the filthy streets of London, and the oil would ooze out. This was collected—along with anything else on the streets—and sold as cod liver oil. Disgusting as it was, this crude cod liver oil was considered a miracle cure for arthritis.

Obviously, we've come a long way from letting cod livers ooze their content into the gutters, but I still consider the cod liver oil sold in today's drugstores pretty vile. Although modern cod liver oil isn't contaminated by street sewage, it's still full of industrial contaminants like mercury and PCBs that pollute the waters where cod live. And it has the same foul taste that turned the stomach of every child in America who took it two generations ago. So while it's true that 1 tablespoon of cod liver oil supplies 2.5 grams of long-chain omega-3 fatty acids—what I consider a maintenance dose—it also supplies contaminants and a high dose of vitamin A, which is stored in the body's fat tissues and can cause toxic effects like hair loss if taken in high enough doses.

In the 1980s, fish oil manufacturing took a technological leap. Manufacturers began extracting the oil from the body of the fish instead of the liver, and this solved the problem of vitamin A toxicity, since the liver contains all the vitamin A. These fish body oils, however, tasted just as bad as cod liver oil, so consumers were loath to try them. Manufacturers solved this problem by encapsulating the oil in soft gelatin capsules, which could be swallowed whole.

But that posed another problem. To get the same amount of long-chain omega-3 fatty acids provided by 1 tablespoon of cod liver oil, you needed to consume eight 1-gram capsules of fish body oil per day. To get the amount of long-chain omega-3 fatty acids used in the Harvard Medical School study to treat bipolar depression (see chapter 10), you would have to take more than thirty 1-gram capsules per day. None of us wants to spend the day popping capsules, but the one or two capsules a day that most of us are willing to take were essentially like a placebo, since the amount of long-chain omega-3 fatty acids found in that dose is extremely small. And even that small amount of health-food-grade fish oil can cause significant gastric problems.

Now you can understand why the fish oil mania that swept our nation in the mid-1980s burned out so quickly. People were not seeing any perceptible health benefits, because the amounts they were taking were too low to have any positive effect. Furthermore, any small benefits that might have occurred would have been canceled out by our changing dietary habits. Remember, we were in the midst of a passionate love affair with carbohydrates in that decade (fat-free cookies, anyone?), and this would have caused a surge in our insulin levels, which in turn would lead to an increase in arachidonic acid formation. This was exactly the opposite of what the fish oil was expected to do. Adding insult to injury, after the capsule dissolved in the stomach, many people were bothered by a fishy taste on their breath for hours. If that wasn't enough, other contaminants (usually weird fatty acids made by algae) present in the fish oil would usually cause bloating and diarrhea.

Although the vitamin A was removed from the fish body oil capsules, there was still the lingering problem of PCBs. To deal with this problem, some manufacturers applied a technology called molecular distillation, which removed some (but not all) of the PCBs. Since molecular distillation also removed cholesterol, it was possible to market these fish oil products as cholesterol-free. (Actually they weren't, but the amount of cholesterol dropped below a certain limit required by the government to make that statement.) Although molecular distilled fish oils are better than less refined health-food-grade fish oils, I'm still not a great fan of them, because they do have enough contaminants to cause problems when taken in high doses.

The next innovation in fish oil was the removal of some of the saturated fats by distillation. These "fractionated" fish oils contained slightly increased levels of long-chain omega-3 fatty acids. However, their purity was still not up to what I define as pharmaceutical standards. Furthermore, the cost of producing these newer fish oils was simply too high for the health food industry. No consumer was willing to pay considerably more for a product that provided only a minimal improvement in health benefits. Thus, this slightly improved version of fish oil didn't go anywhere in the marketplace.

The final breakthrough in fish oils was the development of what I consider a pharmaceutical-grade product. This requires advanced chemical engineering that begins with the removal of most of the saturated fat by fractional distillation and the removal of virtually all the PCBs (measured in parts per billion) by more sophisticated molecular distillation. With these innovations, a new type of fish oil was created, one that could deliver a concentrated amount of long-chain omega-3 fatty acids without unwanted by-products like chemical contaminants or harmful fatty acids. Pharmaceutical-grade quality required that more than 99 percent of the health-food-grade starting material be discarded (actually, it was just resold as health-food-grade fish oil). Only with the use of pharmaceutical-grade fish oil can you deliver high enough levels of long-chain omega-3 fats to your brain and body. Once you do, remarkable things begin to happen within thirty days, if not sooner.

It was this type of pharmaceutical-grade fish oil that I started using in my studies on patients with Alzheimer's disease and other neurological conditions. In chapter 10, I describe the almost miraculous effects that high-dose pharmaceutical-grade fish oils had on these patients. With the pharmaceutical-grade oils—unlike typical health-food-grade oils, even those that had been molecularly distilled—I have not seen any reported side effects. No one complains about gastrointestinal problems like bloating or diarrhea or has any problems with a bad taste in the mouth, even after taking the liquid fish oil using a tablespoon.

Pharmaceutical-grade fish oil is really high-tech cod liver oil—producing results without the contaminants, taste, or gastric side effects. Equally important, you'll experience the benefits of taking pharmaceutical-grade fish oils within thirty days. (This is important, since that is the maximum time most of us will give to notice a difference.) If your grandmother

had only had access to pharmaceutical-grade fish oil instead
of the old elixir, cod liver oil, the health care crisis we are currently facing might never have occurred in the first place.
Now a mere teaspoon of pharmaceutical-grade fish oil packs
a larger punch—omega-3 fatty acids—than a tablespoon of
cod liver oil, without the harmful contaminants and trouble-
some side effects.

STANDARDS FOR PHARMACEUTICAL-GRADE FISH OIL

What are the standards for pharmaceutical-grade fish oil?
There are three criteria that have to be met. Unfortunately,
these criteria aren't required to be listed on the label of the
fish oil product. This means you have to rely on the integrity
of the brand, and such reliance is always risky in the health
food business. At the time this book went to press, there
were only two products in the United States that met the criteria, but I am sure that in time more products will meet
these standards. These current pharmaceutical-grade products are listed in appendix G on page 343. Shown below are
the criteria.

Criteria for Pharmaceutical-Grade Fish Oil

Total long-chain omega-3 fatty acids	more than 60 percent of the total fatty acids
Mercury	less than 10 parts per billion (ppb)
PCBs	less than 30 parts per billion (ppb)
Dioxins	less than 1 part per trillion (ppt)

These are very stringent criteria. In fact, the upper levels
for contaminants for a pharmaceutical-grade fish oil are
hundreds, if not thousands, of times lower than new proposed standards for health-food-grade fish oils.

1. In natural fish oil, only 5 to 20 percent of the fatty acids are a combination of EPA and DHA, the beneficial long-chain omega-3 fatty acids. The vast majority of the fatty acids in fish oil are saturated fats, and they include some fatty acids that are disruptive to your gastrointestinal tract. These weird fatty acids made by algae are rarely found in plant or animal sources, and your body simply wasn't meant to digest them. Removing them from fish oil can help prevent gastrointestinal distress without sacrificing any health benefits.

2. Crude fish oil should be considered the sewer of the sea. Anything that is water-insoluble, such as PCBs, dioxins, and organic mercury compounds, will be found in crude fish oil. Mercury has a powerful negative impact on cardiovascular and neurological function. PCBs are known carcinogens, and dioxin is the active ingredient in Agent Orange—used to defoliate entire forests during the Vietnam War—and is a primary contaminant in toxic waste sites such as Love Canal. These are chemicals you simply don't want to be ingesting.

TEST THE QUALITY OF YOUR FISH OIL PRODUCT

A manufacturer may state that fish oil is "pharmaceutical grade," but there really is no standard definition for this. The laws that govern the supplement industry in the United States are extremely lax and allow manufacturers to put whatever they want on a product label, as long as it doesn't promise to cure or prevent a particular disease.

If you decide to buy a fish oil supplement that isn't

listed in appendix G, I say buyer beware. I also urge you to conduct what I call a first pass pharmaceutical-grade "test." Pour a few teaspoonfuls of liquid into a cup and place it in your freezer for five hours. (If you have capsules, cut a few capsules in half and squeeze the liquid out.) If the oil remains liquid after that time, it may be pharmaceutical grade. If the oil is frozen solid, it's definitely not pharmaceutical grade. (Remember: saturated fats freeze at cold temperatures, whereas polyunsaturated fats do not.)

Unfortunately, this test will tell you only if the product is fractionated, not whether it has an unacceptable level of PCBs or an appropriate AA/EPA ratio. If the label does not state the level of PCBs to be less than 1 part per trillion (ppt), then the fish oil probably contains significant amounts of PCBs, which should be cause for concern. In appendix G, I list the current manufacturers whose products meet my pharmaceutical-grade standards.

You don't necessarily have to swear off health-food-grade fish oil altogether. After all, it's cheaper and easier to obtain. I think it's probably OK if you consume no more than three or four 1-gram capsules of fish oil per day—which will give you a dose of 1 gram of long-chain omega-3 fatty acids.

A special note on cod liver oil: It tends to be even less pure than health-food-grade fish oil, and it also contains high levels of vitamin A, which can be toxic in high dosages. Although cod liver oil is the most inexpensive form of fish oil, it is definitely not recommended for the high doses on my dietary program. And it tastes wretched.

HOW MUCH MONEY CAN YOU EXPECT TO SPEND?

Producing fish oil with pharmaceutical-grade purity definitely costs more. Take a look below to see the relative cost difference between cod liver oil and the various qualities of fish oil.

This cost figure is somewhat deceptive because it includes all the fatty acids found in these supplements—not just pure long-chain omega-3 fatty acids. So while health-food-grade fish oil may be much cheaper than pharmaceutical-grade oil, you're also getting much less long-chain omega-3 fatty acids. Thus, you would have to take more of these supplements to get the same amount of omega-3 fatty acids you'd find in a pharmaceutical-grade product. (What's more, you get a heaping dose of contaminants and strange fats from algae that can lead to significant gastric side effects.)

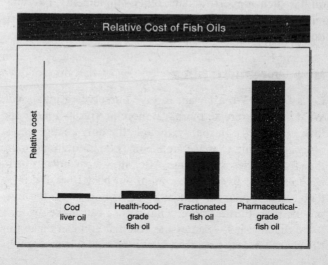

Relative Cost of Fish Oils

Taking 1 teaspoonful of pharmaceutical-grade fish oil will cost you a little more than $1 a day. That dose will give you 2.5 grams of long-chain omega-3 fatty acids. This is what I call a maintenance dose to maintain good health and to reduce the risk of future chronic disease. You may balk at paying a little more than $1 a day for a dietary supplement. If so, consider how many times you've shelled out $3 for coffee from Starbucks!

Furthermore, the recent GISSI clinical trial (see chapter 11) has demonstrated conclusively that pharmaceutical-grade fish oil significantly reduces mortality from existing heart disease. In the same trial, vitamin E was shown to be ineffective. There are other trials, which have shown that vitamin E has no benefits in the treatment of heart disease, even though people who go into a health food store know in their hearts that it must. If you are buying a supplement, at some point you have to ask yourself, "Where are the research data that support it?" Pharmaceutical-grade fish oil has such supporting data; other supplements, like vitamin E, don't. If you are going to spend money for a nutritional supplement, make sure it works.

MY FIVE-MINUTE RULE

Let's face it: We all want to give ourselves a makeover. We'd like to exercise more, eat more nutritious foods, and lower our stress. In reality, though, the only changes most of us are willing to make are the ones that require no more than five minutes of our time. After all, we can always manage to squeeze five minutes out of our busy lives. Taking a daily dose of pharmaceutical-grade fish oil meets the five-minute rule. Furthermore, a daily dose can make up for a lot of dietary sins. I can assure you that you can make this life change in less time than it takes to read this paragraph.

RECOMMENDATIONS FOR FISH OIL FOR THE OMEGA RX ZONE

My basic rule is always to take the *least* supplemental fish oil that you need to maintain a state of wellness. Start with the maintenance dose of 2.5 grams of pharmaceutical-grade fish oil (equivalent to the amount of long-chain omega-3 fatty acids in a tablespoon of cod liver oil) every day. See how you feel after about three weeks, and then adjust your dose upward in small increments. If you continue to see a significant benefit in your mental and physical performance as you increase the amount of fish oil, your body needs a higher dose. Once the increase in benefits levels off, you know you've found the optimal dose and you can stop increasing.

If you don't see any changes after you increase your initial dose, try going in the other direction by reducing the dosage until you observe a drop-off in your mental or physical performance, or deterioration in your blood chemistry. My recommendations for the balance of protein to carbohydrate can be applied almost universally, but the amount of high-dose fish oil an individual needs varies from person to person. This means you'll have to do some experimentation to find the dose that works best for you. Of course, you can always use the blood tests discussed in chapter 9 to give you a precise definition of your need for fish oil.

Frankly, any amount of fish oil you can consume will benefit your health. Compared with estimates of the intake of long-chain omega-3 fats by Eskimos (7 to 10 grams per day) and even with a tablespoon of cod liver oil (2.5 grams per day), the current intake by Americans is dismal. The newest guidelines put forward by the American Heart Association call for two servings of fatty fish per week. That would be equivalent to taking about 250 mg of long-chain omega-3 fatty acids per day, and it would effectively double the average American's intake, which is currently about 125 mg of long-chain omega-3 fatty acids per day. However, the recommendations of the American Heart Association are still ten times less than what your grandmother supplied to your parents with a tablespoon of cod liver oil. These ranges of daily intake of long-chain omega-3 fatty acid intakes over the years are summarized below.

Relative Intakes of Long-Chain Omega-3 Fatty Acids

	Amount per Day (grams)
Harvard Medical School study for bipolar depression	10
Eskimos	7 to 10
Neo-Paleolithic humans	3
One tablespoon cod liver oil	2.5
New AHA recommendation	0.25
Current American intake	0.12

On the basis of my own research and what has already been published, I've come up with different recommendations for the amount of pharmaceutical-grade fish oil you should take, depending on your unique health concerns. (Specific health problems are discussed further in Part III.)

However, follow these recommendations only if you are taking pharmaceutical-grade oil. Health-food-grade fish oils contain far too many impurities to be used at these levels.

Recommendations for Taking Pharmaceutical-Grade Fish Oils

Goal	Amount of Long-Chain Omega-3 Fats
Maintenance	2.5 grams per day (1 teaspoon or 4 capsules)
Improved cardiovascular health	2.5 to 5 grams per day (1 to 2 teaspoons or 4 to 8 capsules)
Enhancement of brain function, reduction of chronic inflammation, and achievement of optimal health	5 to 10 grams per day (2 to 3 teaspoons or 8 to 16 capsules)
Treating neurological disease	10 to 25 grams per day (1 to 3 tablespoons)

MORE FISH OIL, MORE CALORIES?

If you begin taking high doses of fish oil, do you need to adjust your calorie consumption to make up for the calories in fish oil? Probably not. First of all, pharmaceutical-grade fish oil doesn't contain that many calories in addition to the amounts that you'll be taking on my dietary plan. My maintenance dose of 2.5 grams of long-chain omega-3 fatty acids (1 teaspoon or 4 capsules at pharmaceutical-grade fish oil) per day is about 40 calories. Increasing to 10 grams a day will provide an additional 160 calories, and 20 grams will add an additional 320 calories.

But you have to remember that fat (especially long-chain omega-3 fat) doesn't make you fat. Increased insulin levels do that (see chapter 13). However, on my dietary plan you're eating only about 1,200 to 1,500 calories a day, so even if you take the highest dose of fish oil that I recommend, you'll still be eating far fewer calories than you were when you weren't following my program. If you're going to indulge in extra calories, let them come from pharmaceutical-grade fish oil! Your brain will be eternally grateful.

THE PAYOFFS OF HIGH-DOSE FISH OIL

What can you expect when you begin taking high-dose fish oil if you're relatively healthy and have no chronic illnesses like heart disease or Alzheimer's disease? You will notice that your mental abilities are enhanced and that your emotions are on a more even keel. Taking significant doses of long-chain omega-3 fatty acids increases your body's production of the two neurotransmitters dopamine and serotonin. Dopamine spurs you to action, enhancing your brain's ability to concentrate on the task at hand and allowing you to organize yourself more efficiently. Serotonin is your morality or "feel good" hormone. It gives you a sense of well-being and allows you to handle stress more easily. As I explain in chapter 10, when you have depleted these neurotransmitters, you're at greater risk of developing attention deficit disorder (low dopamine levels) or depression (low serotonin levels).

Here's my promise to you. Within thirty days of taking 1 to 2 teaspoons (or 4 to 8 capsules) of pharmaceutical-grade fish oil and following the rest of my dietary recommendations for the Omega Rx Zone, you can expect to find yourself thinking more clearly with a greater sense of concentration, owing to increased dopamine production. In addition, your ability to handle stress will be greatly increased, owing to increased serotonin production. Finally, you will see an improvement in your physical capacity for exercise, especially in terms of greater endurance, owing to better blood flow. Most important, however, you are keeping yourself in the Omega Rx Zone, ensuring a longer and better life.

But what if you have a chronic disease or neurological disorder? Would you benefit from even greater levels of long-chain omega-3 fatty acids? In Part III, I provide a separate plan for each disease condition with specific recommended doses. For now, let me just say this: Patients with neurological disorders like Alzheimer's, attention deficit disorder, depression, multiple sclerosis, and Parkinson's disease (to name a few) appear to require higher levels of these fatty acids—on the order of 10 to 25 grams per day. I've seen an incredible improvement in symptoms in patients who take these higher doses; I've also found that when they drop their dose to below 10 grams of long-chain omega-3 fatty acids per day, their neurological symptoms invariably reappear.

TAKING ENOUGH FISH OIL

Patients who take such high doses would find it inconvenient to swallow 10 or more fish oil capsules a day. They need to take fish oil straight from the bottle, delivered by the tablespoon (just as your grandmother did). The purity of pharmaceutical-grade fish oil makes that a realistic possibility, especially if the fish oil is kept in the freezer (remember, it won't freeze). Women have a much more highly developed sense of smell than men. Therefore, here are some tricks I have learned to make taking liquid high-dose fish oil easier. (Of course, if you are taking a maintenance dose, then the capsules work just fine.)

The Citrus Trick

Suck on a slice of citrus fruit (lime, lemon, or orange) for five seconds before taking the liquid fish oil. The acidity of the citrus fruit (especially lime) will dampen the receptors in your taste buds, so you won't taste the fish oil.

Big Brain Shake

My favorite way to consume fish oil is in my Big Brain Shake. It is an incredibly tasty way to get your daily dose of fish oil, and it's also a complete Omega Rx Zone meal. Each teaspoon of pharmaceutical-grade fish oil you add will give you a little more than 2.5 grams of omega-3 fatty acids, so a 3-teaspoon serving of fish oil will give you about 8 grams. I developed separate recipes for men and women to conform to my dietary recommendations.

Big Brain Shake for Men

2 cups mixed berries (fresh or thawed frozen)
30 grams of protein powder
*1 to 3 teaspoons flavored pharmaceutical-grade fish
    oil*

Blend and drink.

Big Brain Shake for Women

1⅓ cups mixed berries (fresh or thawed frozen)
20 grams of protein powder
*1 to 3 teaspoons flavored pharmaceutical-grade fish
    oil*

Blend and drink.

You can see that my Big Brain Shake is not very difficult to make. In fact, you can probably make it, consume it, and clean up the blender in five minutes, and that time allotment meets my five-minute rule—a lifestyle change you should be able to fit in without too much hassle. In fact, I guarantee that making my Big Brain Shake will take less time than brewing a cup of coffee in the morning. That's why it's the ideal breakfast on my dietary program. You can even make it the night before so it's waiting for you in the refrigerator. Now your morning time commitment has dwindled to about two minutes. Not a bad price to pay for a better brain, a better body, and a longer life.

SHORT-CHAIN VERSUS LONG-CHAIN OMEGA-3 FATTY ACIDS

Not all omega-3 fatty acids are created equal. Only the long-chain omega-3 fatty acids have the maximum impact on balancing your eicosanoid levels while also providing DHA, a long-chain omega-3 fatty acid that's food for your brain. You can get these long-chain fatty acids only from fish oil. Short-chain omega-3 fatty acids, such as alpha linolenic acid (ALA), which is found in flaxseed oil and other seed oils, have the potential to be made into their longer-chain relatives, such as EPA and DHA. The trouble is that the biosynthetic process is incredibly long and difficult (see appendix D for a more detailed description), so you can't really get much long-chain fatty acid from short-chain fatty acid. In fact, you would need to consume nearly 30 grams of ALA to make 1 gram of EPA and 0.1 gram of DHA. This is not a very good return on your dietary investment.

HIGH-DOSE FISH OIL: TOO GOOD TO BE TRUE?

After reviewing more than 2,600 articles on fish oils, the Food and Drug Administration has come to the conclusion that consuming up to 3 grams per day of long-chain omega-3 fatty acids is "generally recognized as safe." This is actually slightly more than my recommendation of a maintenance dose of 2.5 grams per day. Safety, though, depends on the type of fish oil you are using. If you use health-food-grade fish oils, I would not recommend more than 1 gram per day of long-chain omega-3 fatty acids. (This equals three to four 1-gram capsules.) In reality, you'd have a tough time exceeding that amount because at higher doses you'd probably experience gastrointestinal side effects like bloating and diarrhea.

Is it possible to take too much fish oil—even if it's pharmaceutical grade? Of course. Fish oil does contain calories, and these calories can add up if you sit around eating fish oil capsules all day. But consuming a maintenance dose of fish oil (2.5 grams of omega-3 fatty acids per day) will provide you with about an extra 40 calories per day if you are using pharmaceutical-grade fish oil. Even consuming 10 grams of long-chain omega-3 fatty acids per day would add less than 200 calories per day.

Potential Side Effects

Pharmaceutical-grade oil has been studied for years in well-designed research trials and is considered extremely safe. As with any food or supplement, however, there are always potential side effects, especially at high doses. I have identified seven possible side effects that you should be aware of. Although I have not seen them over the past three years in patients taking very high doses of pharmaceutical-grade fish oil, that doesn't mean they shouldn't be addressed.

Potential Side Effects of High-Dose Fish Oil

1. Excessive bleeding
2. Increased LDL cholesterol levels
3. Depression of the immune system
4. Excess production of "good" eicosanoids
5. Increased blood sugar levels in type 2 diabetics
6. Increased incidence of stroke
7. Reduction of antioxidant levels

Excessive Bleeding

While it's true that fish oil thins the blood, I haven't seen any evidence that it poses a danger in terms of excessive bleeding from cuts or injuries. This concern may have cropped up from the observation by European explorers that Eskimos who were shot tended to bleed more readily than Europeans. More controlled trials have yet to confirm this interesting observation. On the more scientific side, we do know that there is no difference in the time it takes for blood to clot after a wound (bleeding time) between those who take 2 to 3 grams per day of long-chain omega-3 fatty acids and those who take no fish oil. Studies using 7 grams of long-chain omega-3 fatty acids to prevent restenosis (the closing of an artery after an angioplasty) reported no increase in bleeding times. Even when fish oil was combined with aspirin or Coumadin (a blood-thinning drug used to prevent clot formation), there were no adverse effects on the bleeding time.

In one study by Garrett FitzGerald at Vanderbilt University, normal individuals who took 10 grams of EPA per day had the same bleeding times as those who took a single aspirin. Another study by Gary Nelson of the USDA demonstrated that consumption of 6 grams of pure DHA per day had no effect on the bleeding time. It's true that Eskimos have, on average, a longer bleeding time than Danes (the Eskimos also have much lower levels of heart disease); but when Eskimos and Danes both took an aspirin, the Danes' bleeding times exceeded those of the Eskimos. In fact, the Eskimos' bleeding times decreased!

The only study that found even a slight increase in bleeding times was one in which the participants took more than 20 grams of long-chain omega-3 fatty acids per day. That study, done twenty years ago, used health-food-grade fish oils, since pharmaceutical-grade oils weren't available then. A more recent study using 18 grams of long-chain omega-3 fatty acids in cancer patients found no increase in bleeding times. In our studies of patients with Alzheimer's disease, which I will describe in chapter 10, we found no increase in bleeding times with pharmaceutical-grade fish oil, even though some patients were taking 25 grams of long-chain omega-3 fatty acids per day.

Frankly, there just isn't any good evidence that taking high-dose pharmaceutical-grade fish oil will have any more of an effect than taking an aspirin per day.

Increased LDL Cholesterol Levels

Another possible adverse effect is an increase in low-density lipoprotein (LDL) cholesterol. This "bad" cholesterol is associated with a higher risk of heart disease. With increased consumption of fish oil, the average increase in LDL cholesterol is on the order of 5 to 10 percent. On the other hand, high-dose fish oil causes a massive drop in triglyceride levels, thereby lowering the TG/HDL ratio. This is important, because the TG/HDL ratio indicates which type of LDL particle you have. There are two types of LDL particles—the small, dense "baseball"-shaped particles, *bad* "bad" cholesterol, that are highly associated with heart disease and the big fluffy "beach ball" particles, the *good* "bad" cholesterol, that have no impact on heart disease.

Two Types of LDL Particles

Good "bad" cholesterol	Bad "bad" cholesterol
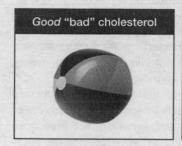	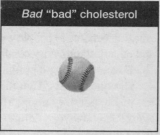

As your triglyceride levels drop, more of your LDL particles get converted from the small, dense baseball type that is more likely to form atherosclerotic plaques on your arteries into the fluffy "beach ball" form that is far less likely to clog your arteries. How can you tell which type of LDL particles you have? Look at the ratio of triglycerides to HDL cholesterol in your latest blood test. If it is less than 2, you have primarily the fluffy beach balls. If it is more than 4, you have mostly the small, dense baseballs. The importance of this triglyceride-to-HDL (TG/HDL) ratio has been confirmed by recent studies showing that if the TG/HDL ratio is less than 2, then even if you smoke, have hypertension, or are sedentary, your risk of developing heart disease is still as low as those who have much better lifestyles or normal cholesterol levels. So even if the LDL levels go up slightly, you have a far better proportion of *good* "bad" cholesterol. Of course, if you are controlling insulin at the same time, then your LDL cholesterol will decrease. On my dietary pro-

gram, you get the best of both worlds: lowered LDL cholesterol and more fluffy beach balls.

Depression of the Immune System

Another potential side effect of high-dose fish oils is suppression of the immune system. As I point out in chapter 14, which
is about chronic pain, long-chain omega-3 fatty acids can offer
amazing benefits to people with arthritis, autoimmune diseases,
and other inflammatory conditions. They do this by depressing
"bad" eicosanoids and pro-inflammatory cytokines.

The question is: Can the immune system be depressed
too much, possibly giving rise to cancer or dangerous infections? The answer is almost certainly no, since high-dose
fish oil has been shown to have great benefits in the treatment of a wide variety of cancers. There is one report in the
literature, which discusses the possibility that fish oil lowers
the level of immune cells called natural killer cells. However, that single report used health-food-grade fish oil, which
would have far greater levels of contaminants than
pharmaceutical-grade fish oil.

One reason that high-dose fish oil might adversely affect
the immune system is a possible decrease in the production of
"good" eicosanoids. But there is an easy way to circumvent
that possibility. The building block of many of the "good"
eicosanoids is gamma linolenic acid (GLA). Taking high
doses of fish oil can sometimes decrease the activity of the
enzyme that is needed to produce GLA. You can, however,
get GLA into your diet. All you have to do is eat two bowls of
slow-cooked oatmeal (not the instant kind) every week. You
could also take a dietary supplement containing evening primrose oil or borage oil, both of which are available in health
food stores. You need to take only about one capsule *per
week*. A typical bottle might last one or two years.

If something like GLA is good, then wouldn't more be better? Not necessarily. With any more than the very low levels (1 to 5 mg per day) I recommend, there is a good chance that this extra GLA will be metabolized into excess arachidonic acid (see appendix D) and destroy all the hormonal benefits that you are trying to produce. Although there are a few diseases (alcoholism and premenstrual syndrome) and goals (enhanced performance for elite athletes) for which more GLA might be required, most individuals need very small amounts.

Excess Production of "Good" Eicosanoids

Making too few "good" eicosanoids with high-dose fish oil is possible, but it is also possible to make too many "good" eicosanoids. The consumption of long-chain omega-3 fatty acids will increase "good" eicosanoids, but consuming too much fish oil could tip the balance toward too many "good" eicosanoids. Then your body will no longer have the balance between "good" and "bad" eicosanoids that keeps you in the Omega Rx Zone. How will you know if this balance is upset? The most likely indication would be an increase in flatulence and perhaps diarrhea. The easiest way to address the potential problem of overproduction of "good" eicosanoids is simply to cut back on the amount of high-dose fish oil you are taking.

Increased Blood Sugar Levels in Type 2 Diabetics

The jury is still out on whether too much fish oil can increase blood sugar in type 2 diabetics. One early study reported that adverse effects were observed at high doses of fish oil (20 grams per day), but later studies have shown no adverse effects at levels up to 3 grams per day. (They also found no improvement in blood sugar levels.) However, my own studies with type 2 diabetics (see chapter 13) indicate that those who follow my dietary recommendations will significantly decrease their blood sugar levels.

Increased Incidence of Stroke

The possibility of an increased likelihood of stroke has been raised by numerous researchers studying high-dose fish oils. This is because the epidemiological data regarding Greenland Eskimos indicated that they seemed to have higher stroke rates than Danes. This potential side effect of high-dose fish oil was addressed by studies that compared Japanese fishing villages and farming communities twenty miles away. The researchers found a much lower incidence of stroke in the fishing villages (where people consumed more fish) than among the farmers (who consumed much less fish and therefore less fish oil). The residents of the fishing villages had an AA/EPA ratio of 1.5 in their blood, the lower limit that I recommend. See chapter 9. In a more recent study, Greenland Eskimos who suffered hemorrhagic strokes had an AA/EPA ratio of 0.5, three times below the lower limits that I recommend, while those who had not suffered strokes had an AA/EPA of 0.8—which is still twice as low as the lower limits that I recommend. If the AA/EPA ratio is three times lower than my recommendations, then there might be an increased risk of stroke. However, even Alzheimer's disease patients taking 25 grams of long-chain omega-3 fatty acids rarely had their AA/EPA ratios drop below 1.5.

Reduction of Antioxidant Levels

Finally, there is the potential problem that high-dose fish oil will deplete the levels of antioxidants in your body; fish oil is prone to oxidation, owing to its high degree of polyunsaturation. But this is not a problem if you follow my dietary program, since you consume 10 to 15 servings of fruits and vegetables per day. Research from Tufts Medical School has shown that the amount of antioxidants in this number of servings is more than adequate to maintain excellent levels of free-radical-scavenging antioxidants in the bloodstream.

Another way to circumvent this potential problem is to use extra-virgin olive oil whenever possible. Extra-virgin olive oil is exceptionally rich in antioxidants compared with other monounsaturated oils, since it is derived from a fruit (olives) instead of a seed. Olive oil contains a very potent antioxidant called squalene that has been shown to virtually eliminate any increase in oxidation products in the bloodstream that may occur with high-dose fish oil. That's why monounsaturated fats, especially olive oil, are a major constituent of my dietary plan.

Of course, taking 100 to 400 I.U. of vitamin E per day as a supplement is another way to circumvent this potential problem. Even though vitamin E has not been shown to reduce the likelihood of heart disease, it provides a very cheap insurance policy because it helps maintain adequate levels of antioxidants in the body in the presence of high-dose fish oil.

Avoiding Side Effects: A Summary

Even though there might be some potential side effects with the consumption of high-dose fish oil, I have shown they can be easily circumvented if you do three things:

1. Make sure you are using pharmaceutical-grade fish oil.

2. Add small amounts of gamma linolenic acid (GLA) to your diet by eating two bowls of slow-cooked oatmeal each week.

3. Ensure adequate intake of antioxidants by consuming lots of fruits and vegetables and by using extra-virgin olive oil or taking supplemental vitamin E.

Knowing which type of fish oil to use and how much of it to use can be very complex—unless you have all the facts. The main thing is to seek out a pharmaceutical-grade fish oil that meets the criteria I discussed earlier in this chapter. While it's OK to use small amounts of health-food-grade fish oil, I would never recommend more than three to four capsules per day (which contain the equivalent of 1 gram of long-chain omega-3 fatty acids). Although this isn't enough to give you the full benefits of the Omega Rx Zone, something is always better than nothing.

I keep talking about all the benefits you'll see on my dietary plan, such as improved mental and physical performance, enhanced relationships, and a greater sense of well-being—to say nothing about the alleviation of certain neurological and inflammatory diseases. But these benefits can be subjective, if there are no blood tests to measure them directly.

A skeptic might wonder whether high-dose fish oil is just a placebo. All I can say is that your blood doesn't lie. Blood tests can measure the exact effects that the high-dose fish oil is having on your body and, more important, can predict your future. Chapter 9 describes those tests in detail.

chapter 9

Your Blood Will Tell Your Future

What if you could quantify your wellness by a single blood test that would predict your future health and longevity? In particular, what if that one blood test would tell you your likelihood of suffering from dementia, having a heart attack, or getting cancer? Would you take it? Perhaps, but only if you could use the results to change your destiny.

Such a test does exist, and with it and a few other blood tests, you can determine whether you're in the Omega Rx Zone. As I stated earlier, the Omega Rx Zone is not some mystical place—it is a state of hormonal balance that can be quantified with laserlike precision by testing your blood. The Omega Rx Zone is the way I define wellness. It's the goal that you're heading toward. Being out of the Omega Rx Zone means that you're already moving toward some sort of chronic disease in the future. Although you may not develop the disease itself until decades later, you're still putting yourself at increased risk. Getting yourself back into the Omega Rx Zone is the only sure way to reduce this risk and increase the likelihood that you'll be healthy in later years.

Even if you're already stricken with a chronic condition like arthritis, heart disease, cancer, or Parkinson's disease, you don't need to give up hope of achieving a state of wellness. Getting into the Omega Rx Zone can speed your recovery and put you back on the path to health.

THE BLOOD VALUES YOU NEED TO HAVE

All my promises mean very little without clinical validation. I first became convinced of the benefits of high-dose fish oil when I saw how dramatically they altered virtually hopeless chronic disease conditions. Furthermore, those benefits could be tracked by certain blood tests. I am now even more convinced by a new blood test that's become available only in the past few years. For the first time, we now have an excellent way to estimate the balance of "good" and "bad" eicosanoids in the bloodstream. If you take only one blood test in your life, this should be it.

This unique blood test measures the ratio of arachidonic acid to eicosapentaenoic acid in the phospholipids in the blood. Remember, AA is the building block of "bad" eicosanoids, whereas EPA is a beneficial long-chain omega-3 fatty acid necessary for the production of "good" eicosanoids. Thus, the AA/EPA ratio will be a very good indicator of the balance of "good" and "bad" eicosanoids throughout the body. The balance of these eicosanoids controls virtually everything else in your body.

As you'll see, this one test is exceptionally powerful in predicting disease, and it also accurately charts progress in the treatment of chronic disease. More important, it will give you proof positive that following my dietary progam really works to alter your health profile from a state of illness to a state of wellness—within thirty days. Unfortunately, this test is not yet routinely offered by doctors, but in appendix G you can find a list of laboratories that do it; I also provide information about a test kit that you can take to your doctor's office for drawing the small amount of blood necessary for the test.

Before you begin my dietary program, you should also consider having two routine blood tests to get a baseline measure of your state of wellness (or lack of it). You might already have these tests in your medical records, and if the results are less than six months old, they can serve as your baseline.

Fasting Lipid Profile

The first blood test is a fasting lipid profile. Among other things, this test contains the information to calculate your ratio of triglycerides to HDL cholesterol (TG/HDL). Just take the triglyceride level and divide by the HDL cholesterol level. You will have to do this yourself, since it won't be on the test results. This ratio is an indirect marker of both eicosanoid and insulin levels. An increased level of triglycerides and a decreased level of HDL indicate that you probably have too many "bad" eicosanoids and not enough "good" ones and that your insulin levels are probably elevated.

The TG/HDL ratio also gives you a measure of your risk of developing heart disease, according to several recent studies in which this test was administered to healthy individuals who were then followed for years to see who eventually developed heart disease. On the basis of these studies, the TG/HDL ratio is a significantly better predictor of future heart disease than total cholesterol or even LDL cholesterol was. The fastest way to lower the TG/HDL ratio is to follow my dietary program; you will reduce triglycerides by balancing your carbohydrate and protein intake and even more by supplementing your diet with at least 2.5 grams a day of long-chain omega-3 fatty acids.

Fasting Insulin Blood Test

The other test I'd like you to take is a fasting insulin blood test to determine your baseline insulin level before you begin my dietary program. Although not as routine (or as cheap) as a fasting lipid profile, the fasting insulin blood test is a standard screening test for diabetes. Many physicians neglect to order it because it's expensive and managed care companies are loath to pay for it. So you may need to twist your doctor's arm a little to get this test administered. Since an elevated level of insulin causes an elevated TG/HDL ratio, you can treat the TG/HDL ratio as a surrogate marker for elevated insulin if you are unable to get a fasting insulin test.

AA/EPA Test: The Gold Standard

After you begin my dietary program, you should consider getting a measurement of your AA/EPA, the gold standard test for monitoring your eicosanoid levels. This test will tell you whether you have too many "bad" eicosanoids or too many "good" ones. A ratio between 1.5 and 3 indicates that your "good" and "bad" eicosanoids are in balance and that you are in the Omega Rx Zone of wellness. (Keep in mind that the average American has an AA/EPA ratio of about 11, whereas the average Japanese has a ratio of 1.5.) This test is also useful in helping you adjust your daily dose of fish oil, especially if you are taking very high doses. Since the optimal dose of fish oil varies from person to person, you need to monitor your blood or your physical symptoms periodically (see my Eicosanoid Status Report on page 123) to see if you're taking the right level of long-chain omega-3 fatty acids.

A SUMMARY OF MY RECOMMENDATIONS FOR TESTING

1. Before you begin my dietary program, get a baseline measurement of your ratio of triglycerides to HDL and your fasting insulin levels. If you had these tests done in the past six months, use the results in your medical records. If not, have the blood tests administered by your doctor.

2. A month after beginning my program, have these blood tests taken again to verify that your blood values are changing as you comply with the program. If you are feeling better, why not validate it? These tests will also show you if you need to increase your dose of fish oil. Have these tests once or twice a year to continue to monitor your progress.

3. If you want to have a laserlike pinpointing of your eicosanoid levels, have the AA/EPA test a month after beginning my dietary program. As I recommend in Part III, *you should have this test done if you're taking more than 5 grams of pharmaceutical-grade omega-3 fatty acids per day*. This test will show if you're producing too many "good" eicosanoids—if you are, you should cut back on your daily dose of fish oil.

These tests will tell you whether you're well, subchronically ill, or chronically ill. Here's a guideline for interpreting your results.

Interpreting the Tests

Test	Diseased: Already have a chronic disease	Poor: On a path to chronic disease	Good: On the path to wellness	Ideal: State of wellness
Triglyceride/HDL	4 or greater	3	2	1
Fasting Insulin (uU/ml)	15 or greater	13	10	5
AA/EPA	15 or greater	10	3	1.5

These numbers are based on clinical research studying normal individuals for a number of years and then determining what values predict the development of chronic disease. For example, if your fasting insulin levels are greater than 10, your risk for developing heart disease increases dramatically. Likewise, if your TG/HDL is less than 1.7, your likelihood of developing heart disease is dramatically reduced, even if you smoke, are sedentary, have elevated LDL levels, or have hypertension. The Japanese are the longest-lived people in the world, and their average AA/EPA ratio is 1.5.

FINE-TUNING YOUR FISH OIL INTAKE

Now that you have the blood values that define wellness (and also define the Omega Rx Zone), you have a very precise way of determining the amount of pharmaceutical-grade fish oil that's optimal for you.

Begin with a daily maintenance dose of 2.5 grams of long-chain omega-3 fatty acids (equivalent to 1 teaspoon or 4 capsules of pharmaceutical-grade fish oil). Through my experience, I've found that this is the best starting dose of fish oil for most people who are in good health and have no chronic diseases. Once you've taken this dose for a month, you should repeat the triglyceride/HDL blood test or have

an AA/EPA test to determine if you need to adjust your
intake of fish oil upward or downward.

The best direct test to monitor your progress is the one
that measures the ratio of AA/EPA, and ideally you want to
keep that ratio between 1.5 and 3. If your AA/EPA ratio is
within the ideal range, you know you're taking the optimal
dose of fish oil. If the AA/EPA ratio is greater than 3, you
need to increase your dose of fish oil. You have a little lee-
way in how much you increase it at a time, but I usually recommend taking an extra two to four capsules a day (an
increase of 1.25 to 2.5 grams of long-chain omega-3 fatty
acids) or an extra teaspoon (2.5 grams of long-chain omega-
3 fatty acids). Add this to your baseline daily dose of 2.5
grams of long-chain omega-3 fatty acids.

The other reason the AA/EPA test is the gold standard is
that it's the only test that will tell you if your level of "good"
eicosanoids is too high, which would indicate that you have
to lower your dose of fish oil. *I strongly recommend that
people taking more than 5 grams of long-chain omega-3
fatty acids per day on a continual basis should have the
AA/EPA test just to ensure that they're not tipping their
eicosanoid balance too much the other way.* If your ratio is
less than 1.5, you need to decrease the amount of fish oil
you're taking. Use your own judgment as to how much to
decrease it. You might need to decrease it by only a capsule
or two a day, or you might need to decrease it by four capsules a day—depending on how much fish oil you were taking before.

If you have trouble getting the AA/EPA test, you can use
your TG/HDL ratio to determine if you need to take more
fish oil. This ratio won't tell you if you're taking too much
fish oil, but it'll do in a pinch. You want to keep the
TG/HDL around 1. That means you're taking the optimal
dose of pharmaceutical-grade fish oil. If the TG/HDL ratio

is greater than 2, take more fish oil. Try taking an extra one to four capsules a day if your ratio is below 4 or an extra four to eight capsules a day if your ratio is above 4.

The reason I strongly advocate having these three blood tests is that they take the guesswork out of following an eating or nutritional supplement plan. Unlike other diets, my program is the product of clear-cut science— science you can verify for yourself through your own blood values. If food is to be treated as if it were a "drug," then there is a need to have blood tests available to confirm your success in using that "drug." Your blood doesn't know how to lie.

ARE YOU IN THE OMEGA RX ZONE? TRY THESE FREE TESTS

If for some reason you don't want to have a blood test, there are other ways to determine if you're in the Omega Rx Zone. These methods are far from precise, but they can give you a rough estimation of your state of wellness.

A quick way to tell if you are producing too much insulin is to stand naked in front of a mirror. If you are overweight and carry your fat mostly on your waist (that is, you're shaped like an apple), then your insulin levels are almost certainly too high. You can, however, be thin and still have elevated levels of insulin. That's why this is far from a perfect test. You might be able to tell if you're in trouble, but you can't determine that you're completely fine.

If you already have a chronic illness (such as heart disease, type 2 diabetes, cancer, or arthritis), then you can assume that neither your AA/EPA ratio nor your insulin level or both are not in the ideal range.

Measuring your percentage of body fat can give you a slightly more precise indication of your insulin levels. In appendix H, I outline a simple way of measuring your percentage of body fat; it requires only a tape measure. Generally, the higher your percentage of body fat, the higher your levels of insulin. You're looking for the following numbers:

	Good	Ideal
Males	15%	12%
Females	22%	17%

Although your percentage of body fat will give you a fairly good idea if your insulin levels are too high, your weight won't tell you much about your eicosanoid levels. To get a rough estimate of eicosanoid levels without taking a blood test, I developed my Eicosanoid Status Report. This will give you a pretty good indication of whether your eicosanoid levels are in balance. When you are using my dietary recommendations and your eicosanoids are balanced, the report shows no change from week to week. I recommend taking this test a week after beginning your supplementary fish oil and then taking the test twice a month to help you monitor your progress.

EICOSANOID STATUS REPORT

1. Daily performance

    __ increased   __ no change   __ decreased

2. Appetite for carbohydrates

    __ increased   __ no change   __ decreased

3. Length of time that appetite is suppressed between meals

    __ increased   __ no change   __ decreased

4. Fingernail strength or growth

___ increased   ___ no change   ___ decreased

5. Hair strength and texture

___ increased   ___ no change   ___ decreased

6. Stool density

___ increased   ___ no change   ___ decreased

(sinks or constipation)   (loose or diarrhea)

7. Sleeping time

___ increased   ___ no change   ___ decreased

8. Grogginess on waking

___ increased   ___ no change   ___ decreased

9. Sense of well-being

___ increased   ___ no change   ___ decreased

10. Mental concentration

___ increased   ___ no change   ___ decreased

11. Fatigue

___ increased   ___ no change   ___ decreased

12. Skin condition

___ increased   ___ no change   ___ decreased

13. Flatulence

___ increased   ___ no change   ___ decreased

14. Headaches

___ increased   ___ no change   ___ decreased

Record your dose of pharmaceutical-grade fish oil: _____

At first glance, this collection of external signs looks about as promising as ancient Roman soothsayers' examination of pigeon entrails. Yet from a larger perspective, this report gives a detailed insight into your current eicosanoid status. Let me explain how this seemingly unscientific way of evaluating your eicosanoid status actually provides a unique insight into your physiology.

1. **Daily performance:** Improvements in your daily physical performance (especially increased energy) indicate that your levels of "good" eicosanoids are on the rise. The increase in "good" eicosanoids causes this effect by increasing oxygen transfer from the blood to organs like the brain, heart, and muscles. A decrease in daily performance means a buildup of AA and a corresponding increase in the production of "bad" eicosanoids.

2. **Appetite for carbohydrates:** The craving for carbohydrates will decrease and may disappear altogether with a decrease of "bad" eicosanoids, since they stimulate insulin synthesis.

3. **Lack of hunger between meals:** Since "good" eicosanoids inhibit insulin secretion, blood glucose levels remain stabilized and hunger is suppressed. You should not be hungry for more than four hours after a meal if that last meal was hormonally balanced.

4. **Fingernail strength:** Keratin, the structural protein that determines the strength of your nails, is controlled by eicosanoids. "Good" eicosanoids increase its synthesis, leading to rapid fingernail growth with excellent strength. On the other hand, "bad" eicosanoids decrease keratin synthesis, leading to brittle fingernails that break easily.

5. **Hair strength:** Keratin is also the principal structural component of the hair. Hair texture is an indicator of eicosanoid status similar to fingernail strength.

Thick, shiny, lustrous hair indicates "good" eicosanoids. Dull, brittle hair with split ends indicates an increase in "bad" eicosanoids.

6. **Stool density:** Your stool consistency changes with your eicosanoid levels. An overproduction of "good" eicosanoids will lead to too much water flow into the colon, producing a very loose stool or diarrhea. On the other hand, an overproduction of "bad" eicosanoids will decrease water flow, leading to a very dense stool or constipation. When your stool floats but has a firm consistency, it's likely that you have the right balance of "good" to "bad" eicosanoids.

7. **Sleeping time:** The need for sleep is determined by the amount of time required to reestablish neurotransmitter equilibrium. This process speeds up in the presence of "good" eicosanoids, so that you need less sleep; the process slows down in the presence of "bad" eicosanoids, so that you need more sleep.

8. **Grogginess on waking:** Any increase in tiredness on waking indicates that an overproduction of "bad" eicosanoids is taking place inside the central nervous system.

9. **Sense of well-being:** "Good" eicosanoids give you a happier outlook on life and enable you to feel good about yourself and the world around you. A buildup of "bad" eicosanoids has the opposite effect. You're more likely to feel depressed, anxious, and irritable and to have a negative outlook. This is a very sensitive measure of your current eicosanoid balance. As I will show later, the AA/EPA ratio is an accurate predictor of depression; this may be why clinical studies find that taking fish oil decreases severe depression, as you'll learn in chapter 10.

10. **Mental concentration:** Maintaining your blood

sugar levels will enhance your mental concentration. The way to maintain your blood glucose is to stabilize your insulin levels through an improved eicosanoid balance. "Bad" eicosanoids increase insulin secretion, which causes you to seek out more carbohydrates, causing quick spikes followed by plunges in your blood sugar. A sign of hypoglycemia (chronic low blood sugar) is decreased mental concentration.

11. **Fatigue:** Fatigue can result from an overproduction of "good" eicosanoids, which can deplete electrolytes in your bloodstream through increased urination. On the flip side, fatigue can result from an overproduction of "bad" eicosanoids, which hampers blood flow, preventing an efficient transfer of oxygen. If you experience fatigue, try to determine which type of eicosanoid is being overproduced by checking other indicators such as grogginess on waking and stool density.

12. **Skin condition:** Overproduction of "bad" eicosanoids will lead to dry skin and eczema (caused by increased leukotriene formation). On the other hand, "good" eicosanoids are anti-inflammatory, stimulate collagen synthesis, and improve blood flow to the skin through increased vasodilation.

13. **Flatulence:** Flatulence, or gas, is caused by the metabolism of anaerobic bacteria in the lower intestine. Overproduction of "good" eicosanoids increases the peristaltic action of the intestinal tract, thereby delivering greater amounts of nutrients to these anaerobic bacteria. The result is greater metabolic activity of these bacteria, with increased gas as the end product of their metabolism. If you have this problem, decrease your intake of fish oil.

14. **Headaches:** Headaches are similar to fatigue in that

you can experience them at either end of the eicosanoid spectrum. You might have either a vasodilation headache (too many "good" eicosanoids) or a vasoconstriction headache (too many "bad" eicosanoids). To determine which category you fall into if you suffer from frequent headaches, look at other indicators in this list to gain a clear picture of your eicosanoid status.

By changing the amount of fish oil you consume, you can rapidly alter the physiological indicators in the Eicosanoid Status Report. The better you control your insulin levels, the less variation in the changes from one side to the other of this report. Remember, the Omega Rx Zone is based on controlling two hormonal systems—insulin and eicosanoids—like a linked dynamo, with the result that hormonal communication throughout your body works at peak efficiency.

In summary, wellness can be quantified by the blood values I have described here. These blood tests take diet out of the arena of politics and philosophy and base it on clinical research that defines the Omega Rx Zone. Furthermore, these same blood tests provide the basis of evidence-based wellness. With the help of these blood values and an analysis of how you feel, you can be sure that you are always in the Omega Rx Zone. Since chronic disease starts the day you move out of the Omega Rx Zone, why would you ever want to leave?

Treatment of Chronic Disease in the Omega Rx Zone

Part III deals with specific disease conditions and how you can adapt my dietary program to help reverse these conditions or reduce your risk of getting these problems in the future. At the end of each chapter, I have included a personalized plan that you can use to alleviate symptoms of any chronic disease you may have. All the personalized plans outlined in Part III should be used in conjunction with my basic dietary recommendations outlined in Part II.

If you have more than one medical problem— say, heart disease and depression—following my recommendation and taking more fish oil can help both: the recommendation for depression will also cover you for heart disease, for instance. That said, you should always take the lowest dose of fish oil that meets all your health needs. You can always start with a little less and add more if you're not achieving optimal results. Ultimately your blood values, described in Part II, will tell you the amount of pharmaceutical-grade fish oil you need.

Part III is divided into specific disease conditions that are outlined in the various chapters. You don't need to read all the chapters in Part III; just read those that apply to you. If you're suffering from a chronic medical condition, chances are this part will give you the "drug" you need to feel better. Your biggest challenge will be finding the optimal dose of fish oil that works best for you. I'll tell you how to do that in each of my personalized plans.

chapter 10

When the Brain Goes Wrong

The mind is the next frontier for medical science. Your brain contains thousands of unexplained mysteries. Researchers remain humbled by its complexities as they try to pinpoint the exact areas of the brain responsible for how you speak, feel love, learn to hate, and express creativity. As discussed in chapter 6, you have the potential to improve your brain function simply by giving your brain what it wants and avoiding the things it hates.

If consumption of high-dose fish oil makes your brain more productive, then isn't it possible that a lack of fish oils makes your brain less productive and more prone to neurological disease? If so, my dietary program has the potential to reverse those changes.

Previous population studies have pointed to the fact that people who live in countries where fish consumption is very high (such as Japan) have the lowest rates of depression in the world. Couple this with the fact that the amount of fish oil consumption in the American diet has been steadily decreasing over the past century, and you should be able to figure out why our rates of neurological disease such as depression, attention deficit disorder, and Alzheimer's disease are skyrocketing. The average American's dietary intakes of DHA (which is needed to maintain brain function) and EPA (which is necessary for improved blood flow and decreased inflammation) are now at dangerously low levels compared with what they were early in the twentieth century.

With the recent advent of pharmaceutical-grade fish oil, we can now safely raise our levels of DHA and EPA to the point that we can lower our risk of developing mental disorders. More important, we may finally have the power to reverse the effects of these conditions if they've already debilitated our mental functioning. So this is really the defining moment for pharmaceutical-grade fish oil because there is now finally a product that we can take in high enough amounts to combat the most harrowing diseases known to humankind: those that destroy the mind. Elderly people who work out with weights can dramatically regain their strength; similarly, I believe, both old and young can regain their brain function by following my dietary recommendations. I had an opportunity to explore this hypothesis several years ago when I took a phone call from Florida.

ALZHEIMER'S DISEASE

About three years ago, I received a call from Dan Ward, the founder and owner of the River Oaks Extended Care and Rehabilitation Center in Crystal River, Florida. Dan is a nationally recognized expert in preventing and reversing severe physical and mental disabilities in frail seniors. Furthermore, he is a strong believer in regular exercise for elderly patients, since exercise has been shown to increase brain-derived neurotrophic factor (BDNF), which is necessary to stimulate nerve growth in the brain. Dan usually tackles the most difficult cases that nursing homes can't handle, such as patients with the end-stage dementia of Alzheimer's disease.

Dan's commitment to physical training for seniors comes from being an elite athlete who has kept careful training records over the years. Three years ago some of his athlete friends recommended that he read *The Zone,* and he decided to give it a try. Using his standard routine of aerobic weight training, he would routinely get his heart rate up to 168. After one week on my dietary program using low-dose fish oil (1.3 grams of health-food-grade long-chain omega-3 fatty acids, according to the recommendations I made in *The Zone,* before pharmaceutical-grade fish oils were available), he couldn't get his heart rate over 120. This meant that his heart didn't have to work as hard to pump blood while he was training. He knew that something very beneficial was happening to his body.

Excited by his own success, Dan decided to try my dietary program on four of his elderly patients, all with end-stage dementia of Alzheimer's disease. They were using the USDA diet, but their dementia was continually progressing. Each of these four patients also had Parkinson's disease, and the drugs they were taking were already at the maximum dosage. Even at the highest possible dosage of these drugs, each of them still had severe rigidity in the upper and lower limbs, had no meaningful language skills, needed assistance to be fed, and had very impaired walking ability. In other words, the quality of their lives was bad and getting worse.

Alzheimer's disease is a harrowing illness that robs patients of their mental faculties and eventually kills them. An estimated 5 to 10 percent of Americans have Alzheimer's disease by age sixty-five, and the rate increases to a whopping 50 percent by age eighty-five. Furthermore, it is estimated that by the year 2040 our country will have ten times more beds in nursing homes than in hospitals. If you have ever been to a nursing home, you've seen what happens when the mind begins giving out before the body. Since Dan had nothing to lose with his end-stage Alzheimer's patients, he switched each to my dietary program, using 2.5 grams of health-food-grade long-chain omega-3 fatty acids. Within three weeks they began to show some signs of improvement.

Controlling these patients' diets was the easy part, since Dan could make shakes consisting of the right balance of protein and carbohydrate for each of their meals. More difficult was adding the fish oil. At that time, health-food-grade fish oil was available only in capsule form. Dan's staff had to puncture 32 capsules (8 capsules for each patient) every day and squeeze the smelly liquid out to add to the shakes that Dan was giving his patients. (These patients were too debilitated to swallow whole capsules.)

In an attempt to find a more convenient method of dispensing fish oil, Dan called me to ask if there was anything I could suggest to get around this problem. This was 1999, and I was just beginning to experiment with pharmaceutical-grade fish oils, which had superior taste and smell as well as far lower levels of contaminants. That phone call I received out of the blue from Dan Ward began one of the my most exciting research collaborations to date: understanding the potential role of pharmaceutical-grade fish oil in remodeling the brain.

What happened to those four test patients? First Dan increased their fish oil threefold to about 9 grams of long-chain omega-3 fatty acids per day (1 tablespoon of high-dose pharmaceutical-grade fish oil). Within two weeks, he measured even more dramatic improvements. He told me he saw a continuing improvement in each patient, with no plateaus, as had occurred on the lower doses of fish oil. The patients started to engage in unprompted conversations and began to get their old personalities back. In fact, one of them began speaking in full sentences, could recognize her husband, and started to remember her past.

If increasing the dose of pharmaceutical-grade fish oil to about 9 grams per day could give such significant cognitive improvement to severely debilitated patients with Alzheimer's disease, what benefits would be seen at even higher doses? That's exactly what Dan set out to learn. He began to increase the dosage to 3 tablespoons per day, providing about 25 grams per day of long-chain omega-3 fatty acids. This has become his standard dose, and he continually monitors his patients' progress by measuring the AA/EPA ratios in their blood. Even at these high doses of fish oil, their blood values are routinely between 1.5 and 2, within the optimal range that indicates an appropriate balance between "good" and "bad" eicosanoids.

From these early trials, Dan started splitting his patients up into three groups. One group got only high-dose fish oil (about 25 grams of long-chain omega-3 fatty acids per day); one group got hormonally balanced meals (to control insulin) but no fish oil; and one group got both. Most of the meals his patients consumed consisted of my Big Brain Shakes made with berries, protein powder, and the appropriate oil (fish or olive). This was used to see what role insulin control played in their improvement.

Not surprisingly, the combination of the insulin-controlled meals and the high-dose fish oil was dramatically better than either component alone. This research strongly reinforced my initial belief that achieving the maximum impact of alleviating neurological conditions requires the simultaneous control of *both* eicosanoids and insulin, which could be accomplished using my dietary program.

One of Dan's patients, an eighty-five-year-old man nicknamed the Colonel, had such severe Alzheimer's disease that he couldn't recognize his wife. As his wife said, "He was in and out of every hospital and rehab facility in the Houston area, where we lived at the time. Nobody offered any hope, and my husband was in terrible shape, curled up in a fetal position, unable to walk, talk, or feed himself. I thought he was going to die, and I was feeling desperate." It just happened that the Colonel's niece was a nurse in Dan's rehabilitation center. She called her uncle's virtually hopeless wife and told her to bring him to River Oaks in Florida.

Within five months of going on my dietary program, the Colonel was walking and playing cards with his wife. He had regained his sense of humor and then started going home on weekends. Family members who had not seen him since before he started my program were amazed by his improvement. They are even more amazed now, since is he able to live at home full-time.

Another patient of Dan's had advanced Alzheimer's disease and had been moved in and out of five other facilities because the staff members couldn't handle his highly inappropriate social behavior. He had also broken both of his knees, hips, and shoulders, and the other rehab centers predicted that he would never walk again. When he arrived at Dan's facility, he couldn't raise his arms to feed himself. Also disconcerting was that he would fall asleep in front of his children when they visited. Within six weeks of starting my dietary program, he was able to feed himself and began walking without assistance. As his son says, "My father now greets us with a smile, talks with us for hours, and walks on his own again. Seeing Dad in sneakers again, with healthy skin color replacing the gray, ashen tone we saw for two years . . . it's impressive. And he hasn't fallen since he's been here. We've seen my dad go from a 'man who would never walk again' to enjoying his freedom from the wheelchair in just six weeks. It is by the grace of God that we found Dr. Ward and River Oaks."

Still another of Dan's patients was an independently wealthy man who was formerly an avid fisherman, always going nonstop and constantly looking for new challenges. Since he had been diagnosed with Alzheimer's disease, he had become belligerent and totally bedridden, and he had to be in a locked ward because he was severely confused, even with the extra private nurses his family had hired to aid him at other nursing homes. Within a month of transferring to Dan's facility and starting the Omega Rx Zone program, he was walking without a wheelchair and had become very sociable. In fact, he now dances at social functions in River Oaks and carries on normal conversations. He can be considered to have mild cognitive impairment as opposed to the advanced Alzheimer's disease he had before starting my dietary program.

Alzheimer's disease is highly associated with the development of amyloid plaques in the brain, similar in many ways to the plaques that clog artery walls and eventually lead to heart attacks. In fact, people who have a genetic susceptibility to heart attacks (a variation in the Apo E protein) also have a far higher risk of developing Alzheimer's disease. Thus, a strategy to prevent both heart disease and Alzheimer's disease seems to make sense. In fact, Hippocrates stated this some 2,500 years ago when he said, "Whatever is good for the heart is probably good for the mind."

Since reducing inflammation is good for the heart (remember, aspirin is still the best drug to prevent heart attacks), then reducing inflammation should also be good for the mind (especially to deal with Alzheimer's disease). Perhaps not surprisingly, people who are long-term users of anti-inflammatory drugs have a much lower incidence of Alzheimer's disease than the general population.

Is there an appropriate strategy to reduce the likelihood of developing Alzheimer's disease? Population studies have shown that people over eighty-five years old who eat fish have a 40 percent lower risk of developing Alzheimer's disease than those who don't. Other research has shown that the brains of patients with Alzheimer's disease have 30 percent less DHA than the brains of healthy people. In data from the landmark Framingham Heart Study, patients who had lower levels of long-chain omega-3 fatty acids in their blood had a 67 percent greater likelihood of developing Alzheimer's disease. In fact, supplementation with DHA seems to improve the cognitive function of patients with Alzheimer's disease, according to one intervention study.

An ominous finding is that the people who consume the most omega-6 fatty acids have a 250 percent increase in the development of Alzheimer's disease. Remember, it is the over-consumption of omega-6 fatty acids (such as those found in common vegetable oils) that leads to an increase in arachidonic acid formation. Therefore, we can theorize that making too many "bad" eicosanoids and not enough "good" ones increases your risk of Alzheimer's disease. This hypothesis is confirmed by recent studies that have looked at the AA/EPA ratio in patients with Alzheimer's disease and age-matched controls. Not surprisingly, the AA/EPA ratio was nearly double in the patients with Alzheimer's disease, compared with the healthy controls, as shown on the next page.

AA/EPA Ratio in Alzheimer's Patients and Healthy Age-Matched Controls

	AA/EPA Ratio
Patients with Alzheimer's disease	12
Healthy controls	6

The fact that patients with Alzheimer's disease have double the AA/EPA ratio suggests that they have increased brain inflammation. In fact, Alzheimer's disease is now considered primarily an inflammatory condition. Thus, consumption of high-dose fish oil and control of insulin levels to lessen inflammation are the most effective ways to prevent the development of this disease. On the basis of Dan Ward's experience with my dietary program in his nursing home, it is clear to me that Alzheimer's disease may even be stabilized and possibly reversed with the appropriate dietary intervention. In the final analysis, maintaining yourself in the Omega Rx Zone will be your best defense against Alzheimer's disease, because it reduces brain inflammation (through high-dose fish oil) and maintains a stable supply of oxygen and glucose to your brain (through stabilization of insulin levels). If you have the beginnings of Alzheimer's disease, a family history of the disease, or simply a fear of getting the disease, my dietary plan will be your best medicine, if not your only hope.

OTHER DEMENTIAS

Dementia comes from the death of nerve cells and subsequent loss of brain function. Alzheimer's disease is the primary cause of dementia, but not the only one. The other major form of dementia comes from the continual occurrence of ministrokes (medically known as transient ischemic attacks, or TIAs). These occur when there is insufficient blood flow to the brain, robbing it of the necessary oxygen and glucose to maintain itself. Ministrokes are not as disabling as a full-fledged stroke, but their cumulative effect is the same: loss of brain function. TIAs are caused by blockage of the cerebral arteries. They can be considered brain attacks, similar in nature to heart attacks. The best way to stop them is by preventing the aggregation of platelets, which is caused by an overproduction of "bad" eicosanoids. Drugs such as aspirin can reduce platelet aggregation, but the best long-term "drug" is my dietary plan, because of its ability to alter the levels of "good" and "bad" eicosanoids.

Not surprisingly, when you look at their blood values, patients with dementias other than Alzheimer's disease and those with cognitive impairment also have a higher AA/EPA ratio than age-matched controls, as shown below.

AA/EPA Ratio in Patients with Dementia and Cognitive Impairment

Condition	AA/EPA Ratio
Dementia	11
Cognitive impairment	11
Healthy controls	6

To illustrate this point, Dan Ward told me about another cognitively impaired patient who was put on my dietary program and had a significant improvement in cognitive function. This patient also had a number of other medical conditions that commonly occur in elderly people. He arrived at Dan's center totally wheelchair-bound. He also had a five-inch gangrenous, ulcerated bedsore and chronic diarrhea. At his previous nursing home, the physicians had wanted to do two operations: one to deal with his chronic diarrhea and the other to deal with his gangrenous bedsore. Although these operations were already scheduled, Dan asked that both be postponed so that he could try some nutritional intervention. You can imagine the skepticism of the patient's physicians.

Dan immediately put his new patient on my dietary plan, using 35 grams of long-chain omega-3 fatty acids (4 tablespoons) per day. After three days, the diarrhea disappeared and never came back. By the tenth day, the man was walking independently, and his ulcer had begun to heal. In fact, it healed completely within eight weeks. His daughter was amazed and delighted by the improvement in her father and told Dan, "He is more physically active and more coherent than he was a year ago when he lived in his own home. It's miraculous." But the really miraculous event occurred when her father spent a weekend at Sea World: his friends got tired, so he, with his newfound energy, pushed them in their wheelchairs.

Just a few months ago, Dan had another patient who had been diagnosed with a brain tumor several years earlier. Although the tumor had been removed, he still suffered frequent seizures and had been to five nursing homes before coming to River Oaks. When he was admitted, the director of his most recent nursing home said he probably had only six months to live. This seemed like a realistic estimate, considering that he was wheelchair-bound and couldn't stand or even hold his head up. In fact, he required help to rotate on his bed, to prevent skin ulcers.

By now Dan had extensive experience using my dietary recommendations on disabled patients. He started his new patient on the program using the standard 25 grams of long-chain omega-3 fatty acid per day. Within two weeks the man regained the ability to walk using a walker, though he still needed some help, since he had no control of his left hand.

At the end of one month, the seizures were gone, and he had recovered the use of his left hand. Finally, after two years at River Oaks, he returned home for the first time in years with his memory restored.

STROKES

It has become chic in cardiovascular circles to call a stroke a brain attack in order to make people more aware of this condition, which is the third leading cause of death in this country. Remember, one of the things your brain dearly loves is oxygen. Strokes cut off oxygen to the brain, causing the death of vital nerve cells.

There are two types of strokes. The term *ischemic stroke* is just a fancy way of saying that the blood flow is blocked and not enough oxygen is getting to the brain. The events leading to this type of stroke are similar to those in heart attacks. The other type of stroke is a *hemorrhagatic stroke,* in which the artery supplying blood and oxygen to the brain bursts because of weakness in the vessel wall—usually caused by high blood pressure. This is no different from your garden hose bursting because of a weakness in the lining, and not enough water getting to the plants. In the case of hemorrhagatic stroke, the nerve cells that are normally supplied by the burst artery are deprived of oxygen and begin to die. In either type of stroke, your brain takes a massive hit. The worst strokes (whatever the cause) are the massive strokes that leave you paralyzed. This is why reducing elevated blood pressure has become the first line of defense to avoid a hemorrhagatic stroke.

My friend J. R. best illustrates the potential of my dietary recommendations in treating hypertension. One day he walked into my office, told me his blood pressure was high—a whopping 200/110—and asked me if I had anything to recommend. I knew that he was a stroke waiting to happen; blood pressure shouldn't be higher than 120/80. I tried to remain calm as I told J. R. that his blood pressure was on the high end, even though he had just come back from the local emergency room to get medication. I knew my dietary plan was his last chance, since the medications he was already taking weren't working to reduce his dangerously high blood pressure. I started J. R. on 9 grams of long-chain omega-3 fatty acids per day. Within a week, his blood pressure had dropped to 140/80—still a little high—and within a month it was down to 120/70. With that drop in blood pressure, J. R. has almost certainly reversed the path that was propelling him toward a stroke.

ATTENTION DEFICIT DISORDER

Attention deficit disorder (ADD) has received nationwide attention in recent years, as the condition has taken on epidemic proportions in American children. An estimated 3 to 5 percent of children in this country suffer from ADD. Although there are six types of ADD (characterized by different patterns of blood flow in the brain), I will refer to them all as ADD. A deficiency of the neurotransmitter dopamine appears to be another factor common to all patients with ADD. Drugs such as Ritalin, which increase dopamine production, are commonly prescribed to bring these conditions under control. If decreased levels of dopamine trigger ADD, then naturally increasing dopamine levels using high-dose fish oil should help alleviate ADD—without the need for drugs.

Many of my insights into ADD have come from my association with two colleagues, Rene Espy and Dan Amen. Dan Amen did pioneering work with brain scans to identify the six types of ADD by determining differences in blood flow to the brain using a specialized imaging technique called SPECT. Another even more sophisticated imaging technique called PET, which measures the uptake of glucose (blood sugar) by brain cells, has shown that certain areas of the brain in patients with ADD aren't getting the appropriate amount of glucose. Patients with ADD have brains that are deprived of the two essential things the brain loves: oxygen and glucose. No wonder people with ADD have such a tough time concentrating.

My other collaborator, Rene Espy, who has expertise working with children, has used my program over the years with great success, and therefore has a large pool of potential patients. I knew that previous studies had demonstrated that children with ADD had lower levels of long-chain omega-3 fatty acids in their blood, and that the higher the ratio of AA/EPA in the blood, the more severe their ADD.

Rene and I decided that on the basis of the existing published data, coupled with her own experiences in treating numerous children with ADD, it was time to do an intervention trial with these children. Before I describe the results, let me point out some of the problems that had to be overcome.

We knew we needed to simultaneously control insulin and eicosanoid levels in the kids to provide their brains with a constant supply of glucose (by controlling insulin) and to increase blood flow and oxygen transfer (by controlling eicosanoids). Doing just one but not the other would not give us the best results. We knew how to control insulin: just give them a dietary plan to maintain the same ratio of protein to carbohydrate at *every* meal and snack. The real question was how much fish oil to use.

I determined how much to give on the basis of my previous work with Dan Ward's patients and the published research done at Harvard Medical School in treating depression. I estimated that a range of 10 to 20 grams of long-chain omega-3 fatty acids per day would be safe and effective. Since 2 tablespoons of pharmaceutical-grade fish oil provide 18 grams of long-chain omega-3 fatty acids, I decided that was a good starting point. Since we were dealing with kids, I also insisted that we never let the AA/EPA ratio drop below 1.5; we needed to be cautious, since the original research had been done on adults.

Getting kids to take 2 tablespoons of pharmaceutical-grade fish oil was actually pretty easy, especially when we used my Big Brain Shakes. Getting them to follow the insulin control part of my dietary program was more difficult, because it required strong parental support in the preparation of their meals—small kids aren't very good cooks. Rene and I knew that without insulin control, many of the potential benefits of high-dose fish oil would not be realized.

What were the results? In one word: spectacular. Within a few weeks, these children's ability to concentrate had increased dramatically. Their behavior improved both at home and in school. These behavioral changes were accompanied by a dramatic drop in the AA/EPA ratio in their blood. In fact, all the children had an abnormally high AA/EPA ratio before they began the study. The impact of my dietary program on their AA/EPA ratios is shown below.

	Start	8 Weeks
AA/EPA	23	3

You can see that the AA/EPA ratio was incredibly high before the intervention. In fact, the children's average AA/EPA ratio was twice as high as that in patients with Alzheimer's disease and other mental disorders and 15 times as high as the ratio found in the Japanese population. Within a very short time, the AA/EPA ratio in these children was reduced by nearly 90 percent to a ratio consistent with normal cognitive functioning. More important, the AA/EPA ratio didn't drop below the limit of 1.5 (the ratio found in the Japanese) that I had imposed at the start of the study. Even more important was the dramatic improvement in the children's behavior. We asked both parents and children to assess behavioral changes using a subjective scale. The results are shown below.

Behavior	4.8 (5 = significantly improved, 4 = moderately improved)
Schoolwork	4.8 (5 = significantly improved, 4 = moderately improved)
Hyperactivity	4.6 (5 = significantly improved, 4 = moderately improved)
Dietary changes	3.8 (4 = easy, 3 = difficult)
Response to fish oil	3.5 (4 = easy, 3 = difficult)
Family life	4.3 (5 = significantly improved, 4 = moderately improved)
Time to see improvement	4.0 (5 = first week, 4 = 1 to 3 weeks)

Although blood samples were not taken until eight weeks had elapsed, significant behavioral changes were already evident within the first three weeks of the study. This was important, since another subgroup of children from one family followed my dietary recommendations carefully for four weeks while they were in school. Their behavioral changes were exactly the same as those outlined above.

Interestingly, once these children left school for the summer and went back to their old dietary habits, their behavior rapidly deteriorated. Their follow-up blood test showed that their AA/EPA ratio had returned to the starting level. I wasn't surprised to see this effect, since long-chain omega-3 fatty acids don't remain in the blood for more than a few days. This means that for ADD symptoms to remain under control, supplementation with high-dose fish oil must continue unabated.

What would account for the dramatic improvement in these children with ADD? A likely reason is that high-dose fish oil increases dopamine production—the same effect that drugs like Ritalin have. However, it is also probably due to increased blood flow. Conversations with Dan Amen indicate that fish oil does appear to improve patterns of blood flow as viewed with SPECT scans. A third reason is the maintenance of a steady supply of glucose to the brain. All these effects can be achieved through my dietary program.

We know about the importance of controlling all these factors in the treatment of ADD because of an unsuccessful trial that was recently done at the Mayo Clinic. In that trial, the researchers used only very low doses of DHA (and no EPA) and made no effort to control insulin levels. We used much greater doses of both DHA and EPA, with very strict insulin control. They observed no benefits in four months, whereas we found spectacular changes in three weeks. So unless you combine high-dose fish oil with continual insulin control, you'll never get consistent results in reversing ADD. Either component of my dietary program (insulin control or eicosanoid modulation) will have a benefit, but together they provide an exceptionally strong synergy. This is a relatively small price to pay for your child's improved enjoyment of the world.

DYSLEXIA

Dyslexics often see letters backwards or turned sideways and have a tough time reading printed text. Dyslexia affects about 5 percent of Americans and appears to be a close cousin of attention deficit disorder. Just like people with ADD, dyslexics have a deficiency of long-chain omega-3 fatty acids in their blood lipids. Supplementation with long-chain omega-3 fatty acids should, therefore, reduce this problem. This thinking makes perfect sense, because your retinas, which are responsible for the quality of the visual input to the brain, have the highest concentration of DHA of any cells in the body. Like the children with ADD, those with dyslexia will require the combination of high-dose fish oil and insulin control found in my dietary program.

Rene Espy has found that my dietary program has worked exceptionally well to reverse the visual distortions that occur with dyslexia. Like children with ADD, children with dyslexia initially require between 9 and 18 grams per day of pharmaceutical-grade long-chain omega-3 fatty acids in order to see an improvement in their condition.

DEPRESSION

Clinical depression is a disabling condition in which life becomes a hopeless, joyless morass. In the past, this condition was called melancholy. You lose pleasure in things that once brought you enjoyment. In fact, it becomes difficult even to remember previously happy times. Any motivation for the future—even for the next day—evaporates.

Depression has increased significantly in the past century, and nearly 14 million Americans are now affected by it. This increase correlates very well with our decreasing intake of fish and fish oil over the same time period.

Psychiatric researchers learned several decades ago that depression is often caused by lack of the neurotransmitter serotonin. In fact, drug companies have made billions by developing drugs to boost serotonin levels, such as Prozac, Paxil, and Zoloft, all of which have become household names. More recent research has found that even people who are not depressed experience an improvement in mood when they take one of these drugs. What this indicates to me is that our nation has developed a serotonin deficiency.

Why? I believe the answer lies in our reduced intake of long-chain omega-3 fatty acids. Since one of the benefits of high-dose fish oil is that it increases serotonin levels, it is not unreasonable to think that the decrease in consumption of fish oil over the past century has led to a decrease in the natural levels of serotonin in the brain. Furthermore, using an imaging test known as SPECT, researchers have found that blood flow within a normal brain is uniform, whereas blood flow in depressed patients is scattered with "holes" in which little or no blood flow is observed. Since high-dose fish oil can improve blood flow, we now have another potential clue to explain the molecular basis of depression. Finally, the Eskimos of Greenland have virtually no depression, and they consume more fish oil than anyone else in the world.

Could it be that simply eating a greater amount of fish is the answer to this growing problem of depression? If that is the case, there should be a strong correlation between the amount of fish consumed and the extent of depression.

The rates of depression in Japan are just a fraction of the rates in America and in other countries where low amounts of fish are eaten. In fact, New Zealanders have a rate of depression fifty times greater than that of the Japanese and eat the least fish in the industrialized world. (What's more, they eat very large amounts of harmful omega-6 fatty acids.)

In Greenland, Eskimos (who consume some 7 to 10 grams per day of long-chain omega-3 fatty acids) have virtually no depression, even though their living conditions can be pretty depressing—they get only an hour or two of sunlight a day during the winter months.

Epidemiological studies, however, indicate only association, not causality. Perhaps the Japanese and Eskimos just have good genes, and the amount of fish they consume has nothing to do with it. That's not what I believe, but such confounding factors can come into play with epidemiological studies. In this case, though, the possibility is unlikely, since studies demonstrate a significant increase in the amount of serotonin in the frontal cortex of the brains of test animals if they consume high-dose fish oil, compared with animals that are given a standard diet rich in omega-6 fats.

These animal studies have been verified by recent research with humans that indicates that the AA/EPA ratio is highly elevated in the cerebrospinal fluid of depressed patients, compared with patients who are not depressed. Likewise, Belgian studies indicate that depressed patients have lower levels of total omega-3 fatty acids in their blood and a significantly higher AA/EPA ratio relative to healthy individuals. British researchers have confirmed this observation.

One way that increased consumption of fish oils would improve depression is through a reduction in AA levels. This would, in turn, lead to a reduction in the production of "bad" eicosanoids, such as PGE_2, which is known to be present in much higher levels in the spinal fluid of depressed patients than those found in healthy controls. In addition, researchers have found that the higher the intake of fish oil, the greater the improvement in the AA/EPA ratio. The AA/EPA ratio has also been found to correlate strongly with the severity of the disease.

All these suggestive bits of research called out for an intervention study to determine the impact high-dose fish oil could actually have in treating depression. Andrew Stoll and his colleagues at Harvard Medical School used exactly this approach in tackling the most severe form of depression, called bipolar depression or manic-depression. Patients with bipolar depression cycle from the depths of depression to a manic high and then back again. The most common drugs prescribed for manic-depression, lithium and Valproate, block the release of arachidonic acid in the brain. Unfortunately, both drugs (especially lithium) have significant toxic side effects. So a search for a safer alternative led Andrew to investigate the long-chain omega-3 fatty acids found in fish oil.

In Andrew's experiment, one group of patients with bipolar depression took a pharmaceutical-grade fish oil providing 10 grams per day of long-chain omega-3 fatty acids. The other group of patients took a placebo (olive oil). The trial was supposed to last nine months, but the researchers ended it early—after only four months—because the divergence between the group taking fish oil and the control group was so great that they felt it would be unethical to continue the study. (Another small complicating factor was that the supply of pharmaceutical-grade fish oil provided by the U.S. government had run out.) Even in this shortened trial, the patients taking high-dose fish oil experienced a stabilization of their symptoms, while the controls had a significant worsening of their symptoms.

The question is: What was happening inside the brain to help alleviate depression in the patients who took fish oil? A pretty good assumption is that serotonin levels increased in the brain's frontal cortex, as has already been demonstrated in animal experiments. Increased EPA consumption through supplementary high-dose fish oil also probably decreased the AA/EPA ratio both in the cerebrospinal fluid that bathes the brain and in the blood lipids—which led to a corresponding decrease in depression. Such a decrease in the AA/EPA ratio would also reduce the levels of pro-inflammatory eicosanoids, which would cut off a cycle that leads to the production of "bad" eicosanoids such as PGE_2, which is known to be increased in depressed patients. Finally, high-dose fish oil almost certainly improved blood flow to the depressed patients' brains, providing a more uniform distribution of critical nutrients such as oxygen and glucose.

These are complex and striking consequences for a relatively simple dietary intervention. Yet as dramatic as these results were, I believe they could have been even better if the researchers at Harvard had brought these patients' insulin levels under control (by following my dietary recommendations) while supplementing their diet with even higher levels of fish oil. A lower level of insulin would have further decreased the production of arachidonic acid and thus enhanced the benefits of high-dose fish oil. In addition, lower insulin levels would have maintained a more constant supply of blood sugar to the brain.

PARKINSON'S DISEASE

If depression is the most widespread of all neurological diseases, Parkinson's disease is one of the most feared, because you retain all of your mental faculties inside a body that no longer responds to your commands. In other words, your mind is trapped in an increasingly dysfunctional body. We know that one of the primary causes of Parkinson's disease is the destruction of the cells that produce the neurotransmitter dopamine.

Unfortunately, replacing dopamine in the brain is not easy. Dr. Oliver Sacks's initial exciting results of giving dietary dopamine to his patients (who had extreme

Parkinson-like symptoms, but not true Parkinson's disease) were recounted in the book and movie *Awakenings*. In a matter of weeks, people who had been immobile and unable to speak—trapped within frozen bodies like living tombs—were able to move again and reenter the world. However, the side effects of this drug soon made it an unlikely choice for long-term treatment. Today we hear of potential new treatments like the implantation in the brain of stem cells that, in theory, will grow into new nerve cells. These advances may be decades away, however, even if they are proved to be useful. I believe that a safer and potentially more successful approach is already at hand: the one in this book.

My optimism comes from the results I have seen over the past three years. One of the more striking was another of Dan Ward's patients who had end-stage Parkinson's disease without any sign of dementia. He was extremely immobile because of poor balance that was aggravated by freezing syndrome (the inability to initiate movement), which is common in such patients. His speech volume was also very low, and he drooled constantly because he couldn't control his mouth muscles.

The first thing Dan did was to start him on my dietary program using 25 grams of long-chain omega-3 fatty acids (3 tablespoons). Within two months, the patient was walking on his own and his speech volume and articulation had dramatically improved. Thus, it appears that Parkinson's disease as well as ADD and depression can be significantly alleviated by getting the patient into the Omega Rx Zone.

MULTIPLE SCLEROSIS

Multiple sclerosis is like Parkinson's disease in that it leaves the patient in an unresponsive body but with mental functioning intact. In multiple sclerosis, the insulating membrane that coats nerve cells unravels, making it difficult for the nerve cells to transmit their signals. Although the molecular cause of multiple sclerosis is unknown, scientists have learned that it's primarily driven by inflammation.

Interestingly, multiple sclerosis is virtually unknown among the Eskimos of Greenland. Could their high intake of long-chain omega-3 fatty acids provide a clue to the prevention and treatment of this condition?

Like all inflammatory conditions, multiple sclerosis is characterized by overproduction of "bad" eicosanoids. For inflammatory conditions outside the brain, a variety of drugs ranging from aspirin to nonsteroidal anti-inflammatory drugs like Advil can decrease inflammation and provide temporary relief. Unfortunately, these drugs can't pass through the blood-brain barrier that separates the brain from the bloodstream. One leading treatment for multiple sclerosis is an injectable drug called beta-interferon. The thought behind this drug approach is that it will inhibit the synthesis of pro-inflammatory cytokines like gamma interferon, and that this will slow the progression of the disease. Unfortunately, this extremely expensive drug is successful only about one-third of the time, but it's the only medical intervention that is available to most patients with multiple sclerosis.

High-dose fish oil, however, may hold far more promise as a nonmedical intervention for these patients. Long-chain omega-3 fatty acids are anti-inflammatory agents that *can* cross the blood-brain barrier; what's more, patients with multiple sclerosis are known to have low levels of DHA in the brain. It is also known that long-chain omega-3 fatty acids inhibit the production of pro-inflammatory cytokines like gamma interferon—similar effects that are behind the theory of constant injections with beta-interferon. This may explain why populations that consume the most fish have the lowest rates of multiple sclerosis.

An intervention study, however, is the only way to prove all these theories. Such a study was recently done in Norway. Patients with multiple sclerosis were given 0.9 gram of long-chain omega-3 fatty acids daily for two years. The patients were also told to consume three to four fish meals per week (this would further increase their consumption of fish oil), decrease the consumption of red meat (this would decrease their intake of arachidonic acid), and eat more fruits and vegetables. (This sounds suspiciously like my dietary recommendations to keep you in the Omega Rx Zone.)

By the end of the first year, the patients' AA/EPA ratio had decreased to 1.5, from 6, and it remained there through the following year. The number of multiple sclerosis attacks these patients experienced decreased by 95 percent in the first year. And after two years, their disability index decreased by 25 percent, which means that these patients actually regained a significant measure of mobility. Since patients with multiple sclerosis usually don't get better over time, these published results are quite striking.

However, taking large amounts of omega-3 fatty acids without controlling insulin won't give you the maximum benefits you can achieve if you follow my dietary plan. As I mentioned earlier, elevated levels of insulin can activate the enzyme that produces arachidonic acid, which in turn increases the production of the pro-inflammatory eicosanoids. I believe that the Norwegian researchers could have achieved even better results if their patients had been given higher levels of pharmaceutical-grade fish oil with better stabilization of their insulin levels. This belief comes from seeing the results with another of Dan Ward's patients.

Although Dan Ward deals mainly with elderly patients with Alzheimer's disease and Parkinson's disease, various other neurological conditions often appear at his center. One patient who came to River Oaks had multiple sclerosis. She was only in her early fifties, but she had been in a nursing home for the previous two years because of her disability. She was unable to stand or even bear her own weight, since she had virtually no strength in her upper body, and she needed to use a catheter for urination. For all practical purposes, she was bedridden. Not unexpectedly, she also had severe depression.

Because of her dire condition, Dan started her on 35 grams of long-chain omega-3 fatty acids per day (about 4 tablespoons), then increased the dose to 50 grams per day after the first 30 days. She developed some diarrhea at that higher dose, so Dan reduced her intake to 40 grams and then eventually returned to his standard 25 grams per day.

Within three weeks of starting my plan, with these high doses of fish oil, the woman had regained control over her urination. She had developed enough strength so that she could move herself from the bed to the toilet. By the third month, her depression was gone, and her memory had improved dramatically. Most important, with a walker, she was able to walk around Dan's facility.

SCHIZOPHRENIA

Characterized by hallucinations, delusions, inner voices, and highly abnormal behavior, schizophrenia has been feared through the ages. With the advent of new drugs (really chemical lobotomies), schizophrenia now appears to be a controllable disease. However, the drugs don't work in all patients, and many patients refuse to take their medication because of unpleasant side effects, such as the loss of any creative thought.

The cause of schizophrenia remains unknown, and even the mode of action of the drugs used to treat it is unclear.

What is clear is that the levels of omega-3 fatty acids in the bloodstream are exceptionally low in people with this disease compared with healthy individuals. Early attempts to improve schizophrenia by supplementation with omega-3 fatty acids alone have been mixed. EPA seemed to have an effect, but DHA was relatively ineffective.

Of course, the questions to be addressed are: (1) Was enough omega-3 fatty acid used? (2) Was the right combination of EPA and DHA used? (3) Was any effort made to control insulin levels? These point to the differences between our successful experiments with children with ADD and the failure of those at the Mayo Clinic. On the basis of my research with other forms of neurological disorders, it is likely that my dietary plan would have significant benefits for managing schizophrenia, and it might have altered the outcomes of these initial studies.

VIOLENT BEHAVIOR

Although violence is not officially considered a mental illness some people have a tendency to use violence to try to solve the problems of daily life. Violent behavior may have an underlying biochemical basis that can be corrected by my dietary program. For example, abnormally aggressive animals usually have low levels of DHA in the blood. Studies have also found that violent prison inmates have lower levels of DHA in their blood than nonviolent prison inmates. Other studies have indicated that individuals prone to violence have much lower levels of long-chain omega-3 fatty acids in their blood, and this suggests that the same phenomenon may be occurring in their brains.

It's now well documented that violence (even a violent video game) increases the levels of dopamine in the brain. People may have a tendency to use violence as a form of self-medication to increase depressed levels of dopamine. Other studies have demonstrated that low levels of serotonin may also contribute to violent behavior, since serotonin acts like a morality hormone, stopping us from doing impulsive acts. If low levels of neurotransmitters (such as serotonin and dopamine) play a crucial role in violent behavior, perhaps high-dose fish oil can play a critical role in behavior modification.

Stress is frequently a trigger for violence, and stress also raises cortisol levels. As I will show in chapter 17, one of the best ways to reduce the increased cortisol that comes from stress is supplementation with high-dose fish oil. This has also been found by Japanese researchers, who have shown that students under stress can handle their mental problems better if they take high-dose fish oil before the test, compared with those who take a placebo.

Stress induced by an exam is one thing. Violence produced by constant stress is quite another. The primary difference is that the levels of cortisol can be much higher when there is long-term chronic stress. Higher cortisol levels will increase insulin levels, resulting in lowered blood sugar and increased production of arachidonic acid. This leads to an interesting hypothesis that violent tendencies may be brought under control through dietary intervention. This is especially true using high-dose fish oil that can boost production of both serotonin and dopamine.

So, although you may not be able to alter the stress in your world, you can certainly alter your biological response to that stress by following my dietary recommendations. Although we can't yet prove that high-dose fish oil can reduce violent tendencies, I'd go so far as to venture that instead of building more prisons in this country, we should be devoting more time and resources to building better dietary education.

ALCOHOLISM AND OTHER CHEMICAL DEPENDENCIES

Yes, alcoholism is a disease. In fact, it's a disorder that has a strong genetic component. The way alcoholism and some other chemical addictions develop is that depression results from not using the drug, and so continued self-medication with the abused drug is required in order just to feel normal. Like violent behavior, drug abuse often results in a surge of dopamine (in the case of cocaine) or serotonin (in the case of Ecstasy), or both. However, alcoholism is different. Alcohol is a routinely accepted drug, and new research touts moderate use of alcohol to prevent heart disease. Yet the twenty million alcoholics in this country know they are always just one drink away from social oblivion, no matter what the cardiovascular benefits may be.

Alcoholics often have lower levels of omega-3 fatty acids in their blood than nonalcoholics. This is because alcohol depletes DHA in the brain and results in lower DHA levels in the blood. That is why drinking alcohol during pregnancy can cause fetal alcohol syndrome, leading to irreversible neurological damage because of depletion of DHA in the fetal brain. Animal studies, however, show that increased consumption of fish oil can completely prevent the alcohol-induced depletion of DHA in the fetal brains.

Alcoholics also have lower levels of GLA, the building block of "good" eicosanoids, in their bloodstream. This strongly suggests that supplementation with high-dose fish oil coupled with small amounts of GLA (probably about 10 mg per day) would provide maximum benefits and reduce the craving for alcohol.

As important as high-dose fish oil and GLA are for the treatment of alcoholism, consistent insulin control is just as vital. This is clear if you ever go to an Alcoholics Anonymous meeting, where you see that the addiction to alcohol is often replaced with a new addiction—to cigarettes or doughnuts. It turns out that nicotine increases insulin resistance, which elevates blood sugar levels. Likewise, doughnuts, are another form of self-medication to help maintain blood sugar levels. Without insulin control to stabilize blood sugar, supplementation with high-dose fish oil will have little lasting effect in treating alcoholism. Following all the components of my dietary plan can provide the recovering alcoholic with the hormonal tools necessary to overcome poor genes. This is probably also true of virtually every other type of chemical dependency.

DIETARY GUIDELINES FOR INDIVIDUALS WITH NEUROLOGICAL CONDITIONS

1. Maintain your insulin control by balancing protein and carbohydrate, using the dietary component of my program.
2. Start by supplementing your diet with 10 grams of pharmaceutical-grade long-chain omega-3 fatty acids (equivalent to 1 tablespoon of fish oil or 15 capsules per day).
3. After a month on the plan, have a blood test to check your AA/EPA ratio. This test is vital for anyone taking high doses of fish oil—which I define as anything greater than 5 grams of pharmaceutical-grade long-chain omega-3 fatty acids per day. See chapter 9 for a detailed explanation of this test, and appendix G for a list of labs that do the test.
4. If your AA/EPA ratio is between 1.5 and 3 after a month on my dietary program, you're taking your optimal dose of fish oil. Stay on that dose and have your AA/EPA ratio tested again in six months. If your

AA/EPA ratio is above 3, you should increase your dose of long-chain omega-3 fatty acids to about 15 grams per day. Have a follow-up AA/EPA ratio blood test in another month to see if your ratio is now in the optimal range. If it isn't, increase your dose by another 5 grams. You can safely take up to 25 grams of pharmaceutical-grade long-chain omega-3 fatty acids per day if that's the dose you need to get your AA/EPA ratio into optimal range.

5. If your AA/EPA ratio is below 1.5 on any of your periodic checks, you need to reduce your intake of long-chain omega-3 fatty acids because your body is making too many "good" eicosanoids. For example, if your ratio is low from taking 10 grams a day of long-chain omega-3 fatty acid, cut back to 5 grams a day. The goal is to get your ratio into the optimal range, which indicates a balance between "good" and "bad" eicosanoids.

After you get your AA/EPA ratio into optimal range, continue to monitor your AA/EPA ratio every six months. Your goal is to keep this ratio between 1.5 and 3.

Note: Follow this recommendation for supplementation with long-chain omega-3 fatty acids *only* if you are using pharmaceutical-grade fish oil. You can put your health at risk if you take such high doses of health-food-grade fish oil, because of the high level of contaminants in these products.

In summary, your brain is the key to your humanity. It is without a doubt the most valuable asset you have, so treasure it accordingly. Being in the Omega Rx Zone can have a significant impact in treating a wide range of neurological conditions by simultaneously controlling both insulin and eicosanoids. But it can also have a huge impact on more common killers like heart disease and cancer. My personalized plans for these diseases are found in chapters 11 and 12.

chapter 11

Who Wants to Die of a Heart Attack?

Heart disease is the number one killer of American men and women today—and this is odd, considering that heart disease was an uncommon cause of death at the beginning of the twentieth century. While it's true that more people died of infectious diseases in those days and often didn't live long enough to die of heart disease, they also consumed much greater amounts of long-chain omega-3 fatty acids. As subsequent generations began eating less fish and more beef, their rates of heart disease shot up.

As I noted in chapter 10, Hippocrates said, "Whatever is good for the heart is probably good for the mind." Let's reverse his insight a little and say, "Whatever is good for the mind is probably very good for the heart." As you now know, my dietary program provides excellent benefits for your brain. You can also assume that it's going to provide extraordinary benefits for your heart. In fact, that's the reason I started my research twenty years ago. I wanted to see if I could change the expression of my own genes, which

were programmed for an early death from heart disease—
something that occurred in my father, his brothers, and my
grandfather. This led me to the concept of the Zone and to
my continuing research to evolve and refine that concept.

One of the best ways to live a longer and better life is to
reduce your likelihood of developing heart disease. If we
could eliminate heart disease tomorrow, the average life
expectancy of every American would increase by an estimated ten years. Advances in medical care have cut the
death rate from heart disease, but they haven't touched the
incidence rates. We are getting heart disease more than ever,
and as our population ages, more of us will die from this
condition. We are simply not doing a good enough job of
addressing the underlying cause of heart disease—a
decrease in blood flow to the heart and an increase in
inflammation in the arteries. These both result from an
increased production of "bad" eicosanoids. Rather than putting your faith in the hope that some major surgery or new
drug treatment will save your life after you get heart disease, why not just avoid getting it in the first place?

Protecting yourself against heart disease requires far
more than just simply lowering your cholesterol levels. In
fact, 50 percent of the people who are hospitalized with
heart attacks have normal cholesterol levels, and 25 percent
of people who develop premature heart disease have no traditional risk factors at all. So maybe elevated cholesterol
isn't the real cause of heart disease in the first place.

The best predictors of a future heart attack come from
prospective studies that follow healthy people for a number
of years to determine which ones go on to develop heart disease, and then to figure out why. Because these are expensive trials, very few of them are done. But those that exist
have indicated that cholesterol levels are, in fact, a very poor
predictor of future heart attacks. In fact, the likelihood of

future heart attacks has everything to do with excess levels of "bad" eicosanoids—exactly the hormones that can be modified by my dietary recommendations.

A heart attack is simply the death of muscle cells in the heart from a lack of oxygen. This occurs when blood flow can't reach the heart because of a blockage or clot in the arteries caused by a clumping of blood platelets, or because of inflammation that causes an unstable plaque to break off and block the blood flow in the artery. Sometimes a spasm in the artery blocks the flow to the heart, or the heart goes into electrical chaos and simply stops its synchronized beating on its own.

Causes of Heart Attacks

1. Clot formation
2. Plaque instability
3. Vasospasm
4. Electrical chaos (sudden death)

None of these four causes of heart attacks has much to do with increased cholesterol levels, but all of them have everything to do with excess levels of "bad" eicosanoids.

When I first wrote *The Zone,* I was strongly criticized for asserting that elevated insulin levels were a major factor in heart disease. (This is despite the fact that diabetics are known to be at highly increased risk of heart disease.) People still wanted to believe that the vast majority of heart problems were caused mainly by dietary fat and high cholesterol levels. Now the tide of medical opinion is beginning to turn. During the past several years, more and more research, especially from prospective studies, has shown that elevated insulin puts you at a greatly increased risk of heart disease. The reason why elevated insulin levels increase your risk of heart disease is that excess insulin causes your body to overproduce "bad" eicosanoids. This is why you need to combine insulin control with high-dose fish oil if your goal is treating heart disease. Only this one-two dietary punch can maximally reduce the AA/EPA ratio and thus restrict the formation of "bad" eicosanoids.

"BAD" EICOSANOIDS = BAD HEART

I'm going to get a little more scientific here, but I think it's important for you to understand the how and why behind heart disease and eicosanoid levels. Having a little medical knowledge should motivate you to stick with my plan. If you've ever suffered a heart attack or feel the chest pain or constant fatigue associated with heart disease, you already have a strong motivation to make a change. Still, I want you to know that I'm not selling you a bill of goods. My dietary program works because it's based on sound science.

The link between high "bad" eicosanoid levels and fatal heart attacks involves a variety of factors. First, excessive "bad" eicosanoids increase the likelihood of platelets clumping to form a clot. (Platelets are circulating cells that rush to the site of a wound and clump together, causing your blood to clot so you don't bleed to death.) Excessive production of "bad" eicosanoids trick your platelets into thinking there's a wound in your arteries, so the platelets clump in the wrong places, decreasing the blood flow.

"Bad" eicosanoids are also the primary mediators of inflammation at the molecular level, which increases the likelihood that an unstable atherosclerotic plaque will rupture. When such a plaque bursts, platelets see this as a wound and begin to aggregate in response to released debris. The new clots formed from aggregated platelets may completely plug up the artery, stopping blood flow. Once the blood supply is cut off, heart muscle cells die from lack of oxygen, and this causes a heart attack and the subsequent damage. The reason aspirin is such a powerful weapon against heart attacks is that it reduces the production of "bad" eicosanoids, which cause both increased platelet clotting and the increased inflammation that destabilizes existing atherosclerotic plaques.

These very same "bad" eicosanoids are also the culprit behind vasospasm, a potentially fatal cramp or "charley horse" that prevents blood flow to the heart and is the third cause of fatal heart attacks. "Bad" eicosanoids act as powerful constrictors of your arteries and can lead to a vasospasm. This same type of action occurs during a headache, which occurs as blood flow to the brain is constricted. If you have a headache, what drug do you take? An aspirin, which works by decreasing the production of "bad" eicosanoids and increasing blood flow. My dietary recommendations can serve as your "super-aspirin" against heart disease, because they do an even better job. They improve your overall cardiovascular health by reducing insulin levels and excess body fat and have no side effects like internal bleeding, stomach upset, and ulcers, all while they reduce the levels of "bad" eicosanoids.

Too many "bad" eicosanoids can also lead to a fatal heart attack caused by chaotic electric rhythms in the heart. The heart is a very large muscle that must have all its cells contracting and relaxing in a synchronized manner in order to pump blood effectively. What controls this cardiac symphony is the electrical current that spreads over the heart muscles to maintain the rhythm of the heart. If this electrical network is disturbed by too many "bad" eicosanoids, the muscle cells will start beating in uncoordinated rhythms. Pretty soon, the symphony becomes random noise and the heart stops beating, stopping blood flow. Animal studies have shown that regular doses of long-chain omega-3 fatty acids can prevent this kind of sudden cardiac death.

Of the four ways of dying from a heart attack, none has much to do with elevated cholesterol levels, although our entire cardiovascular establishment has focused on reducing cholesterol as its holy mission. Instead, what all four have in common is a very strong relationship with elevated "bad" eicosanoids. This is why following my dietary program can help you to dramatically reduce your chance of dying from a heart attack.

IT'S NOT TOTAL CHOLESTEROL, IT'S YOUR TG/HDL RATIO THAT'S IMPORTANT

When I first started doing cardiovascular research in the early 1970s, two prevailing theories of heart disease fought for supremacy. One theory held that high cholesterol levels predominantly caused heart disease, and therefore that simply lowering total cholesterol could cure heart disease. The other theory was more complicated and had to do with looking at heart disease as a complex inflammatory process.

Scientists used to think that we had to worry only about our total cholesterol level, but then researchers found that this wasn't a very strong predictor of heart disease. Next came the realization that there was both "good" and "bad" cholesterol. The "good" cholesterol was found in high-density lipoprotein (HDL) particles, and the "bad" cholesterol in low-density lipoprotein (LDL) particles. This launched a war against "bad" cholesterol, which is predominantly elevated by saturated fat.

In more recent years, scientists discovered two types of LDL cholesterol. One type consists of large, fluffy LDL particles that appear to have no potential to cause atherosclerosis or the development of plaques on the large or medium-sized arteries. The other type consists of small, dense LDL particles that are strongly associated with arterial plaques and thus can increase the risk of heart disease. So now you have *good* "bad" cholesterol (large, fluffy LDL particles) and *bad* "bad" cholesterol (small, dense LDL). Getting confused? Well, so is everyone else who is fighting the cholesterol wars, because we now know that the more *bad* "bad" cholesterol you have, the more likely you are to have a heart attack, whereas having a high level of the *good* "bad" cholesterol isn't likely to have any adverse health effects.

How can you tell which type of LDL you have? All you have to do is determine your ratio of triglycerides to HDL cholesterol, which would be found as part of the results of your last cholesterol screening. If your ratio is less than 2, you have predominantly large, fluffy LDL particles that are not going to do you much harm. If your ratio is greater than 4, you have a lot of small, dense LDL particles that can accelerate the development of atherosclerotic plaques—regardless of your total cholesterol levels. The importance of this TG/HDL ratio was confirmed by studies from the Harvard Medical School. This research found that the higher your TG/HDL ratio, the more likely you would be to have a heart attack. How much more likely? In one study, those with the highest ratio had sixteen times the risk of those with the lowest ratio. That's a huge increase in risk for the most common cause of death!

Just to put this into perspective, consider the chart on the next page, which shows how other risk factors for heart attack stack up.

Relative Risk of Having a Heart Attack

Risk Factor	Times Greater Risk
Healthy with no risk factors	1 (no increase in risk)
High total cholesterol level (over 200)	2
Smoking (1 pack per day)	4
Elevated TG/HDL ratio (over 7)	16

In contrast to our national wars on smoking and high cholesterol, you hear nothing of our battle plan for reducing elevated TG/HDL levels. Since a high TG/HDL ratio is a surrogate marker for elevated insulin, you can see why I was making my plea to launch a national war on elevated insulin many years ago.

HOW CAN YOU IMPROVE YOUR TG/HDL RATIO?

You can improve your TG/HDL ratio in two ways. First, decrease your insulin levels. Excess insulin has been shown to increase triglyceride levels; lowering insulin will lower these levels. Another way to decrease the TG/HDL ratio is to supplement your diet with high-dose, pharmaceutical-grade fish oils. Of course, the fastest and most effective way is to do both simultaneously. The speed at which simple changes in the diet can improve your TG/HDL ratio was demonstrated in a study, conducted by Gerald Reaven at Stanford, in which patients were put on diets consisting of the same number of calories but differing in their protein-to-carbohydrate ratio. When these patients consumed a high-carbohydrate diet, they had a much higher TG/HDL ratio than when they were switched to a lower-carbohydrate diet. These changes occurred within four weeks of each dietary change. Likewise, Bruce Holub at the University of Guelph in Canada has shown that postmenopausal women can rapidly reduce their TG/HDL ratio within a month of supplementing their diets with 3.5 grams of pharmaceutical-grade fish oil per day. Now let's say we combine these approaches. This could only result in an enhanced improvement in the ratio. This combined approach is my dietary program.

The importance of the TG/HDL ratio can be seen from the recently published results of the ongoing Copenhagen Male Study, which studied the effect this ratio has on the long-term development of heart disease. The researchers tracked healthy patients who had either a low TG/HDL ratio (less than 1.7) or a high TG/HDL ratio (greater than 6). They were amazed to find that the patients with the low TG/HDL ratio who smoked, didn't exercise, had hypertension, and had elevated levels of LDL cholesterol had a much lower risk of developing heart disease than those who had a far better lifestyle but a higher TG/HDL ratio. This indicates that lowering your TG/HDL ratio may have a far greater impact on whether you develop heart disease than adopting a better lifestyle. Does this mean you should smoke, stay sedentary, and not worry about your blood pressure or cholesterol levels? Not at all, but it does indicate that you need to significantly focus your efforts to lower your TG/HDL ratio if your goal is to reduce heart disease.

If cholesterol levels are not the best way to predict heart disease, what is? The other theory about the molecular cause of heart attacks, put forward in the 1970s, primarily by Russell Ross of the University of Washington, was that atherosclerosis was an inflammatory disease (like Alzheimer's disease). Since inflammation is a very complex process and very difficult to measure in the bloodstream, this theory of heart disease had far fewer advocates.

Cholesterol was still blamed for most cases of heart disease up until the mid-1990s. Through the 1970s and 1980s, drug companies kept rolling more and more cholesterol-lowering drugs into the marketplace, even though these drugs caused only modest reductions in the rate of heart attacks. In 1995, though, a new class of cholesterol-lowering drugs, called statins, came onto the scene. These drugs were found to be far more effective at preventing heart attacks than other cholesterol-lowering drugs. Cardiovascular researchers were certain that those wonder drugs worked their magic by lowering "bad" cholesterol levels. (The fact that lowering insulin did the same was never considered.)

As it turns out, statins were like the great and powerful Oz—just a man behind the curtain. They didn't work their magic by lowering cholesterol levels. They actually had a much broader spectrum of action than anyone ever anticipated: they were also powerful anti-inflammatory agents. At the same time as this discovery was made, researchers at the Harvard Medical School found that certain pro-inflammatory proteins, called C-reactive proteins, were highly predictive markers for an increased risk of heart disease. With this new clinical tool, they and other researchers found that statin drugs lowered the levels of these C-reactive proteins. In fact, it was in the patients with the highest levels of C-reactive protein that the statins had their greatest impact. Thus, statins worked just like aspirin to reduce inflammation and thus reduce heart attacks—only statins cost a lot more and are less effective. (The statins also involve one other small problem: they potentially decrease cholesterol production in the brain. This would lead to decreased production of new synaptic connections and loss of memory, which is one of the known side effects of these drugs.)

HEART DISEASE RX: REDUCE INFLAMMATION

If reducing inflammation is so powerful in reducing our death rate from heart attacks, the solution should be simple: add more fish oil to the diet. This idea was first posed in the 1970s by researchers who found through epidemiological studies that Eskimos in Greenland had virtually no heart disease even though they consumed a high-fat diet. Over the years, additional studies suggested that the more fish you consume, the lower your risk of dying from heart disease.

One of these studies was the DART study, which found that eating one serving of fish per week decreased heart attacks by 29 percent in patients who had had a previous heart attack. The researchers couldn't definitively prove, however, that it was the fish oil in the fish that conferred these protective benefits, or whether there was a confounding factor, such as that people who eat fish have healthier lifestyles in general. More definitive proof of the benefits of fish oil was found in the results of the GISSI trial, in which patients with heart disease who took about 1 gram per day of pharmaceutical-grade long-chain omega-3 fatty acids had a 45 percent reduction in their risk of having a sudden fatal heart attack, a 30 percent reduction in their total risk of cardiovascular mortality, and a 20 percent reduction in overall mortality. Surprisingly, vitamin E (given by itself or in combination with fish oil) had no benefits. Results of this study are summarized below.

Results from the GISSI Study of Taking Pharmaceutical-Grade Fish Oil

Overall mortality	-20 percent
Cardiovascular mortality	-30 percent
Sudden death	-45 percent

The most powerful statement on the role of diet in preventing heart disease, however, comes from the Lyon Diet Heart Study. In this study, survivors of heart attacks were split into two groups. One group was put on a diet that followed the American Heart Association recommendations (basically the USDA Food Pyramid), and the second group was put on a Mediterranean-type diet (rich in fruits, vegetables, and fish; supplemented with short-chain omega-3 fatty acids; and very low in omega-6). At the end of four years, the two groups had the same cholesterol levels. There was, however, a more than 70 percent reduction in both fatal and nonfatal heart attacks in the group on the Mediterranean diet compared with the control group, who were allowed to eat hefty amounts of omega-6 fatty acids. This study was very damaging for the cholesterol theory of heart disease.

More important, during the four years the group on the Mediterranean diet experienced no sudden deaths (a term used to describe electrical chaos in the heart, which makes it stop beating in rhythm and is the primary cause of cardiovascular mortality). The primary difference between the two groups was the ratio of arachidonic acid to eicosapentaenoic acid in the blood. The AA/EPA ratio of the individuals in the active group was 6.1, compared with 9.0 in the group following the American Heart Association diet. Thus, a 30 percent reduction in the AA/EPA ratio resulted in a greater than 70 percent reduction in fatal and nonfatal heart attacks, despite the fact that the TG/HDL ratio didn't change for either group. This is why I believe that the AA/EPA ratio is by far the most powerful predictor of future heart disease.

As dramatic as the results of the Lyon Diet Heart Study were, I believe they could have been even better if the patients had followed my dietary recommendations. The group on the Mediterranean diet never reached an AA/EPA ratio of 1.5, which is similar to that found in the Japanese, who have the lowest rates of heart disease in the world. This is the ideal that I define in my dietary program. Also, the TG/HDL ratio was still elevated in both groups in the study, and this indicates that insulin levels hadn't been lowered and that both groups were still eating diets too rich in carbo-hydrates.

My dietary program represents a considerable improvement over the intervention diets used in both the GISSI study and the Lyon Diet Heart Study. Where the GISSI study provided a little less than 1 gram of pharmaceutical-grade fish oil, I recommend five times as much. (You need at least 3 to 4 grams of long-chain omega-3 fatty acids per day to lower triglycerides and thus lower the TG/HDL ratio.) While the Lyon Diet Heart Study recommended eating more fruits, I recommend 10 to 15 servings of fruits and vegetables per day.

Compared with the Lyon Diet Heart Study, my dietary program would have lowered the TG/HDL ratio through improved insulin control (which reduces the production of "bad" eicosanoids) and would have provided greater eicosanoid control with the increased intake of pharmaceutical-grade fish oil. These differences would have been reflected in the blood by the reduction of the TG/HDL and AA/EPA ratios. On the basis of all the available evidence we have from prospective studies, achieving the clinical goals that define the Omega Rx Zone would bring your risk of heart disease down to almost zero, as seen on the next page.

Comparison of Lyon Diet Heart Study with the Omega Rx Zone Recommendations

	Lyon Diet— American Heart Association Diet Group	Lyon Diet— Mediterranean Group	Omega Rx Zone Recommendations
AA/EPA	9.1	6.1	1.5
TG/HDL	3.4	3.4	1.0
Risk of fatal and nonfatal heart attacks	1.0	0.3	?

Probably my best testimony to the power of high-dose fish oil to prevent almost certain death from a heart attack comes from my friend Yukio, who does much of our computer programming. About a year ago, he started taking about 9 grams a day of pharmaceutical-grade fish oil to treat his gout. Although he could have done a little better on the insulin-control component of my dietary program, I figured the longest journey always starts with the first step.

About six months ago, he was having a pretty good day. He had just sold his condominium and was heading down to Boston to unveil the new computer program he had just finished for me. He had just loaded about half a ton of logs into his SUV to take to a friend, without much effort. Unfortunately, these logs had been sitting in his backyard in upstate New Hampshire and were heavily infested with fecal residues from a variety of his wildlife neighbors. As he was driving along, he started sneezing and having trouble breathing. He thought he was having a severe asthma attack from the infestations in the logs, but his breathing became more labored, so he knew this was not a typical asthma attack. He pulled over on the side of the road, called 911, and then went to lie down alongside his car, even though he had no pain.

He was right; it wasn't an asthma attack—it was a full-fledged heart attack. A volunteer fireman heard the 911 call and raced to Yukio's car. He knew from his previous experience that time was of the essence. He did some CPR and called in a Medivac helicopter to fly Yukio to the nearest hospital, about an hour away. During the flight, Yukio had two more heart attacks, during which his heart stopped beating both times. By the time they got him to the hospital, his prospects looked pretty grim. Even though he had emergency surgery to implant a stent into the only artery that was blocked—all the others were completely clear—it looked unlikely that he would make it through the night, and if he did, he would probably suffer significant damage to all his organs. For the next several days he was heavily sedated and kept on a respirator because he also had developed a severe case of pneumonia and his lungs were clogged.

When he finally regained consciousness ten days later, though still on the respirator, he wrote down three words: more fish oil. Fortunately, all the time he was on the respirator, his wife made sure that Yukio was still getting his tablespoon of pharmaceutical-grade fish oil by tube feeding. The happy ending of the story is that Yukio left the hospital ten days later. In fact, three months later he was skiing in Utah. To this day, the physicians at the hospital still shake their heads in amazement, trying to understand his recovery.

How Yukio could be alive today after three successive heart attacks can be readily understood from the work of Alexander Leaf at the Massachusetts General Hospital, who has demonstrated convincingly that if you induce a heart attack in dogs by tying off one of their arteries, those that have been fed high levels of fish oil survive, whereas those that had normal diets all die. It appears that the long-chain

omega-3 fatty acids in the fish oil prevent the arrhythmias
that characterize sudden death. This is why mortality due to
sudden death was completely eliminated in the Lyon Diet
Heart Study and dramatically reduced in the GISSI study. In
Yukio's case, it is probably why he is alive today.

Intervention diets to treat heart disease, like those used in
the GISSI study and Lyon Diet Heart Study, take a long time
and are costly—that is why so few are done. I would be
remiss, though, if I didn't briefly discuss another dietary intervention study with cardiovascular patients, this time using a
vegetarian, high-carbohydrate diet coupled with exercise and
stress reduction. The Lifestyle Study conducted at the University of California and the University of Texas divided patients
with heart disease into two groups, giving one group a diet that
followed the guidelines of the American Heart Association
and giving the other a plan for a low-fat, high-carbohydrate
vegetarian diet. Below are the results after five years.

Lifestyle Study Five-Year Results

Group	Starting TG/HDL	Ending TG/HDL	Fatal Heart Attacks
Intervention (Vegetarian Group)	5.7	6.7	2
Control (AHA group)	4.3	4.3	1

In this study, unlike the Lyon Diet Heart Study and the
GISSI study, researchers saw an *increase* in the number of
fatal heart attacks. Exercising more and practicing stress
reduction almost certainly wouldn't increase the number of
fatal heart attacks, but an increase in the TG/HDL ratio
would. Time and time again, researchers have found that
people who go on very-low-fat, super-high-carbohydrate

diets often have a dangerous increase in their triglyceride levels. This is probably why the American Heart Association still considers very-low-fat, very-high-carbohydrate diets experimental, even though they've been around for twenty years and have been recommended to tens of thousands of cardiac patients as a "proven" way to fight heart disease. I think the results of the GISSI trial and the Lyon Diet Heart Study would indicate otherwise. In fact, the American Heart Association also tends to agree with me, as shown by these quotations from their nutritional committee which appeared in an issue of *Circulation* in 1998:

> "Very-low-fat diets in the short term increase triglyceride levels and decrease HDL cholesterol levels without yielding additional decreases in LDL cholesterol levels."

> "For certain persons, i.e., those with hypertriglyceridemia or hyperinsulinemia, the elderly, or the very young, the potential for elevated triglycerides, decreased HDL cholesterol levels, or nutrient inadequacy must be considered."

> "Because very low-fat diets represent a radical departure from current prudent dietary guidelines, such diets must be proved both advantageous and safe before national recommendations can be issued."

Not exactly a glowing recommendation of very-low-fat diets. Although I have already discussed my complaints about the American Heart Association's dietary guidelines in general, at least we agree on the potential dangers of very-low-fat, very-high-carbohydrate diets for cardiovascular patients.

CAN'T YOU JUST TAKE AN ASPIRIN A DAY?

Although my dietary program may be your best "drug" for treating and preventing heart disease, what about our old standby drug, aspirin? Most patients with heart disease are told to take a baby aspirin a day. Aspirin, a natural blood thinner, doesn't reduce cholesterol, but it does a great job of reducing heart attacks. Why? For a long time, aspirin was believed to reduce heart attacks by thwarting the production of "bad" eicosanoids, such as thromboxane A_2, which sets into motion the aggregation of platelets leading to a clot. Another possible reason for aspirin's benefits was recently discovered: aspirin appears to reduce inflammation in the arterial wall by triggering the formation of a new type of "good" eicosanoid.

This is where the connection between aspirin and fish oil gets more interesting. This new class of eicosanoids, called aspirin-triggered 15-epi-lipoxins, was discovered by Charlie Serhan at Harvard Medical School. These new eicosanoids are incredibly powerful anti-inflammatory compounds that can reduce the likelihood of a plaque rupture in the artery, which triggers artery-clogging platelet aggregation. What's fascinating, though, is that the best of these 15-epi-lipoxins are made from eicosapentaenoic acids. What this means is that the more fish oil you consume, the greater your potential to make these powerful anti-inflammatory 15-epi-lipoxins. If you take a baby aspirin a day and fish oil at levels recommended on my dietary program, you'll increase the production of those 15-epi-lipoxins, which can, by reducing arterial inflammation, dramatically reduce your risk of having a heart attack caused by a plaque rupture. I truly believe that this

advance will make heart disease as rare as it was at
the beginning of the twentieth century.

YOUR PERSONALIZED PLAN TO COMBAT
HEART DISEASE

1. Before beginning my dietary program, have a fasting
   blood cholesterol screening and find out your ratio of
   triglycerides to high-density lipoprotein.

2. If your TG/HDL ratio is less than 2, supplement
   your diet with 2.5 grams of long-chain omega-3 fatty
   acids per day (1 teaspoon or 4 capsules of
   pharmaceutical-grade fish oil). This is the maintenance dose that I recommended in chapter 7. If your
   TG/HDL is more than 2, supplement your diet with
   5 grams of long-chain omega-3 fatty acids (2 teaspoons or 8 capsules of pharmaceutical-grade fish
   oil) per day for thirty days. Then, reduce the dosage
   to 2.5 grams per day.

3. Maintain your insulin control by following my
   dietary recommendations (balancing protein, carbohydrate, and fat), which I outlined in chapter 7.

4. Check your TG/HDL ratio every six months. Your
   goal is to try to keep it between 1 and 2. If your ratio
   goes above 2, go back to a higher dose of fish oil.

5. Commit yourself to an exercise program to boost
   your HDL levels. The American Heart Association
   recommends getting 30 to 45 minutes of cardiovascular activity (walking, biking, swimming, skating,
   and so on) most days of the week. Even a smaller
   amount of regular exercise can have a positive effect
   on your HDL levels by lowering insulin levels. Make

sure to check with your doctor before beginning an
exercise program.

Note: Follow this recommendation for supplemental long-chain
omega-3 fatty acids *only* if you are using pharmaceutical-
grade fish oil.

chapter 12

Cancer
Your Greatest Fear

Although we have a far greater risk of dying from heart disease than cancer, we're more afraid of cancer, probably because of the harrowing treatments required to manage it. After spending some $30 billion on the war against cancer, however, our government hasn't made any headway in finding a cure or even a way to prevent the disease.

Researchers, though, are now sure of three things. First, the more fruits and vegetables you eat, the less cancer you get. Second, people who take regular doses of aspirin have much lower rates of cancer than people who don't. Finally, high-dose fish oil appears to retard or reverse a wide number of tumors in animal studies. What clues could these observations provide to help in the treatment of cancer? I think the answer lies in their effects on insulin and eicosanoids.

LIVING WELL WITH CANCER IN THE OMEGA RX ZONE

Cancer treatment remains a primitive science. Oncologists treat the disease with deadly interventions (toxic drugs and radiation) in the hope of killing more tumor cells than normal cells. It is a hope that is often not realized, and a patient's health is often sacrificed in the process, but what other choice do we have as patients? Let me give you three examples.

The first is Doreen's story. About two years ago, I found out that she had been diagnosed with a severe form of lymphoma (cancer of the lymph nodes) about a year earlier and had been treated aggressively with chemotherapy. She had all the associated side effects (extreme fatigue, hair loss, nausea, and so on). After a short remission, her cancer had reappeared. Her only remaining option was a bone marrow transplant, a life-threatening treatment that is still highly experimental. After the transplant, her doctors discovered that her previous chemotherapy treatments had caused congestive heart failure. Her future didn't look promising.

I persuaded Doreen to try my dietary program. "What do you have to lose?" I told her. She agreed to give it a shot and followed my plan of balancing her protein-carbohydrate intake at every meal. She also started taking 9 grams of long-chain omega-3 fatty acids in her daily Big Brain Shake. Now, a year later, people who haven't seen Doreen in a while don't recognize her at first. She has dropped from a size 14 to a size 6. Her hairdresser recently asked if she had gotten a face-lift. She continues to spend her summer vacations camping out in the Rockies with her husband—not exactly the kind of vacation most people with congestive heart failure would be able to handle.

Doreen's cancer remains in remission, and she's a great example that living well is the best revenge when it comes to cancer.

Leroy, another friend of mine, who is a limousine driver, recently told me that he had some bad news from his doctor. He had been diagnosed with a massive tumor in his colon. This tumor was so large that it couldn't be surgically removed until it was shrunk with an aggressive combination of highly toxic chemotherapy drugs and radiation. I told Leroy that he needed to prepare himself, because he was soon going to be the sickest dog on the face of the earth. Then I told him the good news: I thought I could give him a dietary program that would help alleviate the toxic side effects of his treatments and, more important, allow him to live longer with his cancer. (Cancer is never "cured," just as you never cure heart disease or diabetes; you learn to live with it.)

First I told Leroy that his days of eating pasta and bagels were over. Then I outlined my dietary recommendations, including the critical need for pharmaceutical-grade fish oil. I told him to take a very high daily dose, 18 grams of long-chain omega-3 fatty acids per day, since he was starting his treatment in a few days. I spoke to Leroy about a week into his chemotherapy, and he told me he felt pretty good. I knew that if he wasn't extremely debilitated after the first few treatments, his outlook would be good. After the third week of treatments, Leroy was still bouncing into the outpatient ward for his radiation treatment and drug infusions. The rest of the people in the outpatients' waiting room looked and felt like death warmed over, but for Leroy it was just another day. Leroy's tumor was finally removed, and he is back working again.

Another example is one of Dan Ward's patients. He had advanced Alzheimer's disease when he came to River Oaks, and upon examination it was found that he also had leukemia. As with all of Dan's patients, he was immediately put on my dietary program, taking 25 grams of long-chain omega-3 fatty acids. Within three months, his white cell count was back to normal.

Why did these patients do so well, while other cancer patients are constantly nauseated, weakened, and exhausted? I believe it's because they had a secret weapon: the Omega Rx Zone. By strict control of both insulin and eicosanoids, they had the key to living well with cancer.

HOW BEING IN THE ZONE ENHANCES CANCER TREATMENTS

Let's look at the science behind why these patients did so well. Cancer is a condition of immune deficiency. A surefire way to depress your immune system is to produce too many "bad" eicosanoids. In particular, overproduction of one "bad" eicosanoid known as PGE_2 appears to be a primary culprit. "Bad" eicosanoids depress the immune system in the local area of the body in which they are overproduced, and tumor cells oversecrete these "bad" eicosanoids. This proves to be a very sophisticated form of stealth technology to trick your body's immune system into thinking that the cancer cells are not foreign invaders.

Aspirin reduces the production of PGE_2, and this may explain why studies have found that taking aspirin lowers the rate of colon cancer. Of course, the most effective way to decrease PGE_2 production is to reduce the levels of its precursor, arachidonic acid. That can best be achieved by my dietary recommendations. Here's why:

1. Lowered levels of insulin will inhibit the activity of the enzyme (delta 5-desaturase) that produces arachidonic acid, the building block for PGE_2.

2. Consuming high doses of pharmaceutical-grade fish oil will increase your levels of eicosapentaenoic acid, a beneficial long-chain fatty acid that inhibits the same enzyme (delta 5-desaturase).

3. The high-dose fish oil improves your AA/EPA ratio. As the AA/EPA ratio decreases, so does your production of PGE_2.

Researchers have known for years that giving animals high levels of omega-6 fatty acids (such as corn oil) significantly increases their death rates from cancer when they have had tumors implanted in their bodies. On the other hand, when these animals were given high-dose fish oil, their implanted tumors dramatically decreased in size, and the animals lived longer. It's pretty easy to understand why. Those getting the corn oil were making more "bad" eicosanoids, while those getting fish oil were making more "good" eicosanoids. In cancer, eicosanoid balance spells the difference between life and death.

LOWERING THE RISK OF METASTASES

A cancer patient's biggest fear is the dreaded words "You have a recurrence." This occurs when cancer spreads or metastasizes from the primary tumor site to another area in the body, where a new tumor begins to grow. Metastases are aided by another group of "bad" eicosanoids, called hydroxylated fatty acids. These eicosanoids are derived from arachidonic acid and allow tumor cells to get a foothold in a distant site in the body. One particular hydroxylated fatty acid, 12-HETE, appears to be the prime suspect. Once again the best way to reduce the production of 12-HETE is simply to lower the levels of arachidonic acid in cells. This can be achieved by lowering your AA/EPA ratio. The best way to lower the AA/EPA ratio and reduce your risk of metastases? You guessed it—my dietary program.

When it comes to thinking about cancer, you have to ask if the glass is half full or half empty. For many years, researchers thought it was half empty—meaning that they thought cancer was a hopeless situation. For instance, they saw it as a wildly uncontrolled division of malignant cells that would live forever. How could they ever stop these immortal cells that reproduced with such reckless abandon? Now researchers are beginning to see that the glass may be half full. They theorize that some tumor cells may simply be healthy cells that have forgotten when to die.

All cells in the human body have an internal time clock programmed for when they're going to die. This programmed cell death is a condition called apoptosis, and it is an essential process in our bodies. If we didn't have programmed cell death, we would have no way to continually remodel our bodies by replacing old cells with new ones. The vital process of apoptosis can be restored by long-chain omega-3 fatty acids, especially DHA. Supplementing your diet with fish oil should help restore the natural balance of life and death of the cells in your body.

In end-stage cancer, one of the biggest threats patients face is wasting. This rapid weight loss usually indicates that the end is near. Cachexia, as wasting is called in medical terminology, is hastened by increased levels in the bloodstream of the pro-inflammatory cytokine known as tumor necrosis factor (TNF). Since fish oil is known to depress the release of TNF, supplementing a patient's diet with high-dose fish oil should reduce, if not reverse, weight loss and extend the patient's life. In fact, that is exactly what happens. When patients with cachexia were given 6 grams of long-chain omega-3 fatty acids per day, they actually gained weight, whereas control patients continued to lose weight. Subsequent studies of patients with advanced pancreatic cancer have used doses as high as 18 grams of pharmaceutical-grade long-chain omega-3 fatty acids per day. In both cases, there was an extension of life compared with what could be historically estimated. Of course, if these researchers had followed my dietary program, it is quite possible that their patients would never have developed cachexia in the first place.

Finally, one of the brightest hopes in cancer treatment was the discovery of antiangiogenesis compounds. A tumor grows by diverting much of the needed nutrients from the body to itself. It does this by increasing angiogenesis, which is the development of new blood vessels to support increased tumor growth. The Holy Grail of cancer research is to find a compound that reduces this tumor-induced angiogenesis. Research has shown that one of the most powerful "bad" eicosanoids, which actually promotes angiogenesis, is a derivative of arachidonic acid.

Reducing the levels of arachidonic acid will decrease levels of this "bad" eicosanoid and thus inhibit angiogenesis. Now you have a powerful antiangiogenesis "drug." It's the Omega Rx Zone. This explains why high-dose fish oil has been shown to be effective in treating and preventing tumor growth in a large number of animal studies. What's more, another component of my dietary program has shown to be effective against angiogenesis: calorie restriction. I believe the Omega Rx Zone may be the breakthrough antiangiogenesis "drug" that the cancer research establishment is looking for.

THE LINK BETWEEN CANCER AND INSULIN

One more benefit of my dietary program in helping to thwart cancer is its ability to reduce insulin levels. Tumors need both insulin and high levels of blood sugar to survive. A growing number of investigators have documented elevated insulin levels as a factor that determines tumor growth. After all, insulin is a growth factor that promotes cell division in both healthy cells and tumor cells. Elevated insulin levels also indicate a condition called insulin resistance in which cells in the pancreas crank out more and more insulin in an effort to get unresponsive cells to take in excess sugar in the bloodstream. Elevated insulin levels (caused by insulin resistance) set up an ideal condition for tumors to grow, since they grow best in an environment where they are fueled by excess blood sugar.

Lowering insulin levels by following my program will alleviate insulin resistance and lead to a decrease in blood sugar levels. As a result, the tumor loses its primary fuel source. In fact, as early as 1919 it was found that blood sugar levels could often indicate the prognosis for a cancer patient. As blood sugar levels increased, the patient's chances of survival diminished.

With a combination of benefits from high-dose fish oil, calorie restriction, and insulin control, the Omega Rx Zone dietary program may represent a major advance in treating all types of cancer. Of course, it's also your best defense against getting cancer in the first place.

So if you take two of the most effective dietary interventions ever tested by the National Cancer Institute—high-dose fish oil and calorie restriction—and combine them with a high consumption of fruits and vegetables plus adequate low-fat protein, you get my dietary program. I can't guarantee you that you'll never get cancer if you can maintain yourself in the Omega Rx Zone, but I can tell you that your chances of surviving cancer will be greatly enhanced. Thus, it's not surprising that researchers at the Harvard Medical School found that women who had the best chance of surviving breast cancer were those who followed a diet with a protein-to-carbohydrate balance similar to what is found in my dietary recommendations.

YOUR PERSONALIZED PLAN FOR MANAGING CANCER

1. Maintain insulin control by following my dietary plan (balancing protein, carbohydrate, and fat), which I outlined in chapter 7.
2. If you are undergoing chemotherapy or radiation, supplement your diet daily with 10 to 15 grams of pharmaceutical-grade long-chain omega-3 fatty acids (4 to 6 teaspoons or 16 to 24 capsules of fish oil). Once you've completed your cancer treatments, decrease your intake of fish oil to 5 to 10 grams of long-chain omega-3 fatty acids per day (2 to 4 teaspoons or 8 to 16 capsules of fish oil).
3. To determine your optimal dose of fish oil, get a blood test to measure your AA/EPA ratio after your first month on my program. If your ratio is greater than 3, increase your dose of fish oil. If it is between 1.5 and 3, you're in your optimal range and should continue taking the dose you're on. If your AA/EPA ratio is less than 1.5, decrease your dose of fish oil.
4. Retest your AA/EPA ratio every three months until you achieve the optimal range for your ratio. Continue to get your blood levels checked every six months, after you reach an optimal range.

Note: Follow this recommendation for supplemental long-chain omega-3 fatty acids *only* if you are using pharmaceutical-grade fish oil.

chapter 13

Obesity and Diabetes
The Twin Epidemics

Up to this point, all the chronic diseases I've discussed are largely caused by an imbalance of eicosanoids. I've told you that you can correct this imbalance primarily by consuming high-dose pharmaceutical-grade fish oil and by stabilizing your insulin levels through the dietary component of my program. When it comes to obesity and diabetes, however, the tables are reversed. Yes, you can take fish oil to help allc-viate these conditions somewhat, but you primarily need to rein in elevated insulin levels. As you may recall from the Optimal Health Matrix in chapter 5, obesity and type 2 diabetes are affected far more by insulin than by eicosanoids. In type 2 diabetes, the impact of eicosanoids is only 30 percent, compared with the 70 percent impact of reducing insulin levels. With obesity, eicosanoids play only a 10 percent role, compared with 90 percent for insulin.

Thus, if you have either of these two conditions—or both, since they often go hand in hand—you need to double your efforts to follow the insulin-control and calorie-conservation elements of the dietary plan I outlined in chapter 7. This plan has been consistently shown to lower excess insulin levels. If you follow my recommendations, I can guarantee you that you'll lose excess body fat. You'll also dramatically decrease the likelihood that you'll ever get type 2 diabetes. More important, you'll be able to reverse the condition if you already have it. The key for both is lowering your levels of insulin. Let's start with obesity, since excess insulin is what makes you fat and keeps you fat.

WINNING THE WAR AGAINST OBESITY

I'll be the first to admit that the power of Hollywood induced many people to try my dietary program, when they saw sleek images of Hollywood celebrities in national magazines saying how easily they lost weight once they were in the Zone. And in Hollywood, if you don't look good, you don't stay a celebrity for long. No wonder the two hottest words in Hollywood are *the Zone*. More important, I've received thousands of testimonials from Zone followers saying that my dietary program was the only thing that worked to help them lose body fat and maintain their weight loss. The reason my dietary plan receives such continual acclaim is that it works. Gaining fat occurs when insulin levels are out of control; losing fat is a matter of regaining control of the same hormone. Insulin is a storage hormone that tells your body to store any excess calories as fat. It also prevents the release of stored fat for energy. Basically, excess insulin is a one-two punch that ensures excess body fat in your future.

Although I'm pleased that people can finally safely lose weight by following my dietary recommendations, I don't think these cosmetic effects should be the main reason for getting yourself there. Rather, you should be trying to shed excess body fat in order to prevent chronic disease, especially diseases that have a strong insulin component. Seeing a protruding stomach when you look in the mirror is a warning sign that you're headed down the road to type 2 diabetes, heart disease, and eventually a shortened life.

THE ILL-WAGED WAR ON FAT

For years, Americans were told that dietary fat is the enemy, even though it has no direct impact on insulin. Unfortunately, our war on fat was led by dietitians and government bureaucrats who had no understanding of the hormonal impact of our food choices. That ignorance has spawned the second greatest public health crisis in the last hundred years. (The other was the dramatic decrease in the consumption of long-chain omega-3 fatty acids.)

How dietary fat came to be declared the enemy in our current obesity epidemic is a tragic tale of what happens when poor science meets politics. Nearly fifty years ago, rates of heart disease started to increase rapidly. Much of this was due to two factors. The first was that more people were living beyond the age of fifty, as premature death from infectious disease and malnutrition decreased. A second reason was that death certificates had new classifications that forced physicians to list a cause of death; a heart attack was often the simplest explanation in lieu of an autopsy. Understanding the statistics behind these first two reasons, Harry Rosenberg, the director of the National Center for Health Statistics, has come to this conclusion: "There is absolutely no evidence that there was an epidemic of heart disease in the 1950s."

What led to our war on fat was not science but politics. It appeared to start in the late 1960s, when Senator George McGovern was chairman of a committee to eliminate malnutrition in America. This was one government program that was truly successful, and by the mid-1970s it had achieved its goals. Rather than disbanding this program, some of his staffers wanted to keep the committee alive by shifting its focus to overnutrition, even though Americans were a lot thinner then. Since McGovern, their boss, had enrolled in the Pritikin Program, which was based on following a very-low-fat, high-carbohydrate diet (and which he eventually quit), the committee members decided that if it was good for their boss, it should be good for all Americans. This marked the beginning of our dietary war against fat. When the committee asked scientists how much money it would take to do the research to verify that a low-fat diet would actually reduce heart disease, the answer was about $1 billion. In the mid-1970s, that was a lot of money, especially after the Vietnam War had drained much of the treasury. Instead, Congress opted to fund shorter, less expensive trials.

One after another, these short trials found virtually no evidence that eating less fat had any impact on heart disease. Never letting scientific facts get in the way of a good political story, a "consensus" for a new war on fat was rapidly growing. To line up scientific support, the government decided to arrange a "consensus" conference of the experts, with most attendees believing the government's position, along with a few token skeptics. Everyone gives his or her viewpoint, and then everyone votes. Majority rules, a consensus report is issued, case closed. Of course, in cases where we have a true dietary consensus, such as the benefits of eating fruits and vegetables, no one ever needs to convene a consensus conference. It's only in the murkier areas of nutrition (like the *fat-is-bad* movement) that consensus conferences are organized by the government to approve its actions.

One of these consensus conferences issued the statement

that if you lowered your intake of dietary cholesterol and fat, you would reduce your risk of having a heart attack. The fact that there was no direct scientific study to support this statement did not stop the massive public health campaign by the government to change the dietary habits of Americans. The USDA used this conference as a basis to develop its famous Food Pyramid. As Walter Willett, chairman of the Department of Public Health at Harvard Medical School, has said about the USDA's dietary recommendations, "You really need a high level of proof to change the recommendations, which is ironic, because they never had a high level of proof to set them."

This war on fat was launched with great fanfare. Little did anyone suspect that the war would unleash a new and frightening epidemic of obesity, an effect exactly the opposite of what the government and the advocates of low-fat (and high-carbohydrate) diets had intended.

In fact, our total fat consumption is probably at the lowest level it's been in the past fifty years, and the percentage of calories of fat in our diet is far lower than it was fifty years ago, yet we've had a massive increase in obesity. If our actual enemy was dietary fat, we should have declared victory over obesity years ago. Experts are finally beginning to realize that dietary fat was never the real enemy—excess insulin is. Remember that insulin is a storage hormone, and it instructs your cells to store incoming nutrients. If you eat more calories (especially those coming from carbohydrates), then you release more insulin, which converts any excess calories into fat that can be easily stored in your fat cells. This is why fat-free foods like bread, potatoes, and pasta get rapidly converted to fat if they are eaten in excess.

What's more, this excess insulin also prevents your fat cells from releasing stored fat for energy. The result is a growing accumulation of excess body fat. In retrospect, the

USDA Food Pyramid was virtually guaranteed to increase insulin levels in Americans. In that regard, it has been an outstanding success. We now have higher insulin levels and an epidemic increase in obesity throughout the country.

THE SOLUTION FOR REDUCING BODY FAT

If you want to reduce excess body fat, you've got to do two things: lower insulin and restrict calories. You can do both effortlessly if you follow my dietary recommendations, because you're balancing protein, carbohydrate, and fat at every meal and snack. David Ludwig at Harvard Medical School found that a single meal with the protein-carbohydrate ratio recommended on my dietary plan will dramatically lower insulin secretion compared with a meal containing the same number of calories but following the protein-carbohydrate ratio recommended by the government. The less insulin you make, the faster you lose weight.

To lose excess body fat effectively, however, you still have to restrict calories. Unfortunately, the thought of restricting calories only brings to mind thoughts of constant hunger and deprivation, which you may recall from the crash diets of your past. However, as I demonstrated earlier, once you begin to replace starchy carbohydrates (bread, pasta, rice, potatoes, and so on) in your diet with low-density fruits and vegetables, you'll find yourself eating a lot more food and a lot fewer carbohydrates and calories. You won't feel hungry; your blood sugar levels are stabilized because your brain is now getting one of the things it wants: adequate blood sugar.

At the molecular level, the reason you become hungry in the first place is that blood sugar levels are lowered below a critical threshold required for brain function. There are only three ways you can address hunger:

1. Severe ketosis
2. Drugs
3. Stabilized blood sugar levels

Let's look first at severe ketosis. This abnormal condition occurs when you consume too much protein and not enough carbohydrate. This is the definition of a high-protein diet. In a short period of time (around 24 hours), the glycogen reserves in your liver are depleted, and without adequate levels of glycogen it is impossible to metabolize fats completely to water and carbon dioxide. This lack of liver glycogen distorts the normal metabolism of fat and causes the liver to begin to produce abnormal ketone bodies. At high enough levels, these ketone bodies can short-circuit the appetite-sensing centers in your brain, decreasing hunger. Unfortunately, at these same high ketone levels, your body works like mad to get rid of these abnormal ketones from the bloodstream by increased urination. This water loss (up to 3 or 4 pounds) accounts for much of the initial weight loss in the first week of such diets.

What's more, your body eventually adapts to continued ketosis by altering the actions of your fat cells; within three to six months, your fat cells become "fat magnets" that are ten times more active in their ability to accumulate fat. Even though you may be following the same high-protein diet, fat loss slows, and then fat begins to reaccumulate. This explains why millions of people have initially lost weight on these high-protein diets over the last thirty years, only to gain it all back—and more—within a short period of time. This is not a long-term solution to the obesity epidemic.

Another approach to controlling hunger is the use of appetite-suppressing drugs. Not surprisingly, this is highly favored by the drug industry. Amphetamines were early candidates, but they were highly addictive. The next generation of drugs, such as phen-fen and Redux, were designed to stimulate serotonin in the brain. The idea behind these drugs was that if you maintained serotonin levels, hunger would be lessened. (Of course, high-dose fish oil also stimulates serotonin.) Unfortunately, these drugs carried the risk of potentially deadly side effects, like weakened heart valves and primary pulmonary hypertension, which causes heart and lung failure. (As a side note, I take some pride in the fact that I was the expert on obesity for the plaintiffs in the class-action suit against the makers of these dangerous drugs.)

Finally, there is the old-fashioned way of controlling hunger: simply maintain stable blood sugar levels. Blood sugar is the fuel the brain needs for optimal functioning. As long as the brain is getting adequate levels of glucose, it has no hunger. The best way to stabilize blood sugar levels is to ensure that your insulin levels do not rise too high (which drives down blood sugar levels) and that you have adequate levels of the hormone glucagon, which is stimulated by the protein content in a meal. Glucagon stimulates the release of stored sugar from the liver, and this release restores blood sugar levels. This is why some low-fat protein at each meal is so important for controlling blood sugar.

My dietary program orchestrates the dynamic balance between insulin and glucagon by giving you the optimal protein-to-carbohydrate ratio at every meal. Eating too many carbohydrates increases your insulin too much, whereas following a high-protein diet increases your glucagon levels too much, leading to a state of ketosis. Either way, you're in trouble. That's why you need to aim for balance. This is the only way to achieve optimal hormonal control of blood sugar and control your appetite on a permanent basis. One warning: the maximum amount of time that an Omega Rx

Zone meal will sustain your blood sugar levels is four to six hours. After that, you will get hungry as your blood sugar levels fall. This is why I always recommend eating a balanced meal or snack every four to five hours. This will maintain your blood sugar levels and control your appetite. Once this is achieved, you'll naturally eat fewer calories without feeling deprived.

IF YOU HAVE A POTBELLY OR SPARE TIRE, READ THIS

Make no mistake about it, losing excess weight is important, but *only* if you reduce your risk factors for heart disease and diabetes, which can be measured by the blood values described earlier. Simply losing weight is not as important as losing abdominal fat, which is far more predictive of future disease complications. In essence, if you lose weight but haven't reduced your waist size, you haven't done much for yourself.

This is why your waist measurement is far more predictive of your health status than your weight on the scale. Men who have a waist circumference larger than forty inches and women who have a waist measurement larger than thirty-five inches are at increased risk of heart disease and type 2 diabetes. A large waist measurement is indicative of increased abdominal fat, which can be more dangerous than excess fat on your hips and thighs. That's because abdominal fat contains visceral fat, which surrounds your organs (liver, intestines, colon, gallbladder, pancreas, and so on). This type of fat is metabolically active, while subcutaneous fat—found mainly on your hips, thighs, and extremities—is primarily used for long-term storage. This metabolically active visceral fat is implicated in the development of insulin resistance, which in turn increases insulin levels in the bloodstream. Thus having too much visceral fat puts you at increased risk of diabetes, heart disease, cancer, and gallbladder disease.

But waist measurement is an inexact science. How can you tell for certain if you have too much visceral body fat? Have a blood test to measure your fasting insulin level or a blood test to measure your fasting lipid levels (which gives you your ratio of triglycerides to HDL). If your insulin level is greater than 15uU/ml, it means you have a lot of visceral fat. If your TG/HDL ratio is greater than 4, it also means you have too much visceral fat.

On the other hand, if you are overweight but your insulin level is under 10 uU/ml and your TG/HDL ratio is less than 2, then your risk of having a heart attack is relatively low. This would indicate that you have more subcutaneous fat around your abdomen, which is far less risky than visceral fat. I've seen many overweight people who are in great physical condition. They swim miles a day or train for marathons. These people have less visceral fat and more subcutaneous fat on the abdomen, and, as a result, their risk of heart disease is no higher—and is often even lower—than that of a person who is thinner but out of shape.

If your goal is to lose fat, then your key to success lies primarily in controlling your insulin levels by maintaining the appropriate protein-to-carbohydrate ratio of my dietary recommendations at each meal. Eicosanoids, on the other hand, will have relatively little role to play in loss of fat (although high-dose fish oil will increase serotonin levels to help decrease your appetite). But as you already know, eicosanoids play a very significant role in preventing heart disease, which is a common outcome of obesity.

REVERSING TYPE 2 DIABETES

As you may already know, people with adult-onset, or type 2, diabetes overproduce insulin because their cells have become resistant to insulin's action of driving nutrients into cells. As a result, the pancreas keeps pumping out more insulin to try to do its job. Eventually, the insulin-producing cells in the pancreas begin to burn out. As a result, they can't secrete enough insulin anymore, and blood sugar levels rise. Elevated insulin levels precede the actual development of type 2 diabetes by five to ten years. (Type 1 diabetics, who account for only about 5 percent of adult diabetics, don't make any insulin and need injections of the hormone to survive.) Several things increase your risk of developing type 2 diabetes: too much visceral fat, a high intake of saturated fat, eating excess carbohydrates, and a family history of the disease.

An estimated sixteen million people are afflicted with type 2 diabetes. In the last decade, the rate has increased by a dramatic 33 percent. This devastating disease puts you at twelve times greater risk of dying from heart disease and also increases the likelihood of kidney failure, blindness, impotence, amputation, and neuropathy (nerve damage) in your extremities.

If fish oil is good for treating heart disease, then, in theory, it should be very good for diabetics—especially since diabetes (like heart disease and depression) is virtually nonexistent among the Eskimos of Greenland. Unfortunately, studies on fish oil and diabetes have had mixed results. A recent analysis of some twenty clinical trials with diabetics came to the conclusion that fish oil won't worsen—or improve—the blood sugar levels of diabetics. Hardly a resounding triumph for fish oil.

These studies, however, didn't look at whether controlling insulin enhances the effects of supplemental fish oil in type 2 diabetes. I had the opportunity to test this hypothesis several years ago with Princeton Medical Resources, an HMO in San Antonio. George Rapier, the owner of the HMO, approached me to see if I could help his HMO make more money. Since patients with type 2 diabetes are the most costly for an HMO because of the prevalence of long-term complications, anything that can reduce those complications goes right to the bottom line of the HMO. The year before George approached me, he had brought in dietary educators trained by the American Diabetes Association (ADA) to counsel 400 of his more than 4,000 diabetic patients. These patients dutifully followed the recommendations outlined in their personalized meal plans provided by these ADA educators. After a year, George found that his costs for these 400 patients had increased by another $1 million!

George called me after he read my first book, *The Zone,* and lost twenty-five pounds on my dietary program. He asked if I would be willing to work with some of his patients—but I had to keep it very simple. Using only the hand-eye method that I described earlier and supplying 1.6 grams a day of health-food-grade fish oil (I didn't have the pharmaceutical-grade oil then), I put together a simple dietary education program for his patients. One of the first groups consisted of sixty-eight patients with type 2 diabetes. After six weeks of following my dietary program, the results were as follows.

Results

Blood Test	Start	6 Weeks	% Change	Significance
Insulin	28	21	−23	< 0.0001
TG/HDL	4.2	3.1	−26	< 0.0001
HbA_{1c}	7.8	7.3	−7	< 0.0001
Fat Mass (lbs.)	72	70	−3	< 0.0001

Not only was every clinical measure associated with type 2 diabetes decreasing, but some of the changes were extraordinary. The two measures that changed the most were the markers (insulin and the TG/HDL ratio) I use to define the Omega Rx Zone. Although the values were still far from optimal after six weeks, the declines were equal to what would be obtained with any drug. Other markers of diabetes were similarly reduced. For example, glycosylated hemoglobin (HbA_{1c}) is one of the best indicators of long-term complications in type 2 diabetics. If it is below 7.3, then many of the adverse consequences, such as kidney failure, amputation, and blindness, just don't occur. Finally, these diabetic patients lost excess body fat, and that is exceptionally difficult if you have high levels of insulin. Equally important was that the declines in each of those blood values had a very high degree of statistical significance. Statistical significance is an indication of how likely it is you will get the same results if you repeat the same experiment. The lower the number, the more likely the results can be repeated again. In this case, the statistics indicated that if the same dietary experiment were done 10,000 times, you would observe the same results 9,999 times.

As I said earlier, insulin resistance (and the resulting rise in insulin levels) is the cause of type 2 diabetes. Although the exact molecular cause of insulin resistance is still unknown, Australian researchers have shown that if type 2 diabetics are put on the same dietary program I used in the San Antonio study, their insulin resistance is totally reversed in three days.

As excited as I was by the results of the San Antonio study, looking back I now know that the results could have been even better if I had used slightly higher levels of pharmaceutical-grade fish oil. I believe that the high-dose fish oil would have enhanced the results, because new research indicates that the insulin resistance found in type 2 diabetes may be mediated by an increase in the hormone known as tumor necrosis factor (TNF), the same hormone that causes wasting in cancer patients. One proven way to decrease the secretion of TNF from fat cells in the body is through the use of high-dose fish oil. This in turn decreases insulin resistance, which in turn reduces insulin levels. Once insulin levels are lowered, your body can access its own stored body fat for energy. In essence, it takes fat to burn fat, especially if that fat can reduce the release of TNF. This is why I now routinely recommend about 5 grams of pharmaceutical-grade fish oil to type 2 diabetic patients.

Like the heart disease epidemic, the obesity and diabetes epidemics may be a result of our misguided advice to decrease dietary fat and increase the consumption of fat-free carbohydrate. I believe that if we aimed for an optimal protein-to-carbohydrate balance at every meal and got adequate levels of pharmaceutical-grade fish oil, our epidemics of heart disease, type 2 diabetes, and obesity would be history within a few short years.

Bottom line: If you want to lose excess body fat, you need to double your efforts to follow my dietary recommendations. If you want to reverse or prevent type 2 diabetes, you need to follow the insulin-control diet and incorporate more eicosanoid control by taking higher doses of pharmaceutical-grade fish oil.

YOUR PERSONALIZED PLAN FOR MANAGING OBESITY

1. Maintain your insulin control by following my dietary recommendations (balancing protein, carbohydrate, and fat), which I outlined in chapter 7.

2. Have a fasting blood cholesterol screening to measure your TG/HDL ratio. Supplement your diet with 2.5 grams of long-chain omega-3 fatty acids per day (1 teaspoon or 4 capsules of pharmaceutical-grade fish oil) if your TG/HDL ratio is less than 2. If your TG/HDL ratio is greater than 2, supplement your diet with 5 grams of long-chain omega-3 fatty acids per day (2 teaspoons or 8 capsules) for thirty days, then reduce your intake back to 2.5 grams per day.

3. Check your TG/HDL ratio every six months. Your goal is to try to maintain the TG/HDL ratio between 1 and 2.

4. Commit yourself to an exercise program to help lower your insulin levels. The American Heart Association recommends getting 30 to 45 minutes of cardiovascular activity (walking, biking, swimming, skating, and so on) most days of the week. Make sure to check with your doctor before beginning an exercise program.

Note: Follow this recommendation for supplemental long-chain omega-3 fatty acids *only* if you are using pharmaceutical-grade fish oil.

YOUR PERSONALIZED PLAN FOR MANAGING TYPE 2 DIABETES

1. Maintain your insulin control by following my dietary recommendations (balancing protein, carbohydrate, and fat), which I outlined in chapter 7.

2. Have a fasting blood cholesterol screening to measure your TG/HDL ratio. Supplement your diet with 5 grams of long-chain omega-3 fatty acids per day (2 teaspoons or 8 capsules of pharmaceutical-grade fish oil) if your TG/HDL ratio is less than 2. If your TG/HDL ratio is greater than 2, supplement your diet with 8 grams of long-chain omega-3 fatty acids per day (3 teaspoons or 12 capsules) for thirty days, then reduce your intake back to 5 grams per day.

3. Check your TG/HDL ratio every six months. Your goal is to try to maintain the TG/HDL ratio between 1 and 2.

4. Commit yourself to an exercise program to help lower your insulin levels. The American Heart Association recommends getting 30 to 45 minutes of cardiovascular activity (walking, biking, swimming, skating, and so on) most days of the week. Make sure to check with your doctor before beginning an exercise program.

Note: Follow this recommendation for supplemental long-chain omega-3 fatty acids *only* if you are using pharmaceutical-grade fish oil.

chapter 14

Why It Hurts
Pain and Inflammation

Pain is often the hallmark of disease. Chronic pain is itself not a defined medical condition, but rather a symptom that something in the body has gone awry. Pain usually stems from inflammation of the body's tissues. Although there is no blood test for pain, the patient is acutely aware of its existence.

Throughout the centuries, one of the most pressing goals for medical researchers has been to find more effective ways to diminish pain. As medicine enters the twenty-first century, we are still seeking a perfect pain reliever with no side effects. After all, end-stage cancer patients are still given morphine, a narcotic drug that was used during the Civil War, to dull their excruciating pain. And experts on pain are sizing up the benefits of marijuana for their patients. Somehow, we haven't been able to develop a pain reliever that's truly effective and doesn't cause a drug-induced high.

Sometimes physicians can't make a definitive medical diagnosis to explain the underlying cause of chronic pain.

They may shrug their shoulders or use a term like fibromyalgia, a diagnosis made to describe intense, diffuse pain of unknown origin. Regardless of whether a definitive cause of chronic pain can be found, every patient knows that the pain is very, very real.

Take the case of Linn, the wife of my chief programming consultant, Yukio, whom I described in the chapter on heart disease. Linn had suffered for years with fibromyalgia and had found little relief in the painkillers her doctor had prescribed. Yukio, an avid user of high-dose fish oil for treatment of his gout (and now an even more avid user for his heart), was convinced that fish oil was a powerful anti-inflammatory "drug." After listening to him rave about the way high-dose fish oil made him feel, Linn decided to give it a try. She started with a tablespoon a day of pharmaceutical-grade fish oil, containing 9 grams of long-chain omega-3 fatty acids (the amount Yukio had also been taking). On the very first day, her pain was dramatically reduced for the next eight hours; then it started to reappear.

Yukio called and asked me what he should do next. I told him to give her 2 tablespoons of fish oil containing 18 grams of long-chain omega-3 fatty acids (the same amount given to children with ADD). Now Linn's pain was reduced continually throughout the day.

Okay, this is just one person, and her experience hardly qualifies as a clinical trial. But two months after Linn started taking the high-dose fish oil, Yukio was skiing in Utah and staying at a spa where he had known the head of maintenance for years. One night, this friend told Yukio about his own wife's chronic pain and her diagnosis of severe fibromyalgia. His wife's pain was so severe that she had been taking three different narcotic drugs at one time to control it and was spending her days in a mental fog. She had finally decided that she'd rather endure the pain than live like a zombie. But for a year now her pain had virtually immobilized her.

Yukio thought the woman's condition sounded a lot like his wife's. He decided to give his friend some of his high-dose fish oil and suggested that his wife take 2 tablespoons that night. After taking the fish oil, his friend's wife slept through the night for the first time in a year. The next morning, she did something truly remarkable: she got out of bed, dressed herself, and made breakfast for everyone. But Yukio had given them only enough oil for the next three days. Four days later, he got a phone call from her husband saying that his wife's pain was returning, since she had used up all the oil. Yukio sent another bottle of fish oil to them by overnight mail, and to this day, her fibromyalgia remains under control.

You might be thinking that this sounds suspiciously like the stories of snake-oil salesmen at the turn of the twentieth century. Yet once you understand what causes pain (an over-production of "bad" eicosanoids), you understand that anything that decreases their production will have the rapid effect of reducing pain. In fact, the wonder drugs of the twentieth century were compounds that reduced pain—the most famous of which was aspirin.

The most powerful pain relievers, however, are corticosteroids. They have an immediate effect, but they knock out all eicosanoids—"good" and "bad"—indiscriminately. This can lead to severe side effects, such as immune depression, cognitive impairment, and diabetes. Aspirin, on the other hand, affects a more limited number of eicosanoids (only prostaglandins and thromboxanes), but at least it knocks out the "bad" eicosanoids at a slightly faster rate than it knocks out the "good" ones. Nonsteroidal anti-inflammatory drugs (such as Advil) also work like aspirin. In recent years, new and very expensive medications called COX-2 inhibitors were added to the stockpile of pain relievers. These have a little more selectivity than aspirin, but not as much power as corticosteroids.

Corticosteroids, aspirin, and other anti-inflammatory drugs inhibit the actions of enzymes that make "bad" eicosanoids, whereas high-dose fish oil reduces the actual building block (arachidonic acid) necessary to make the same "bad" eicosanoids. The medications won't reduce the building blocks of "bad" eicosanoids, so it's almost as if you're fighting an uphill battle against pain. High-dose fish oil, on the other hand, reduces the materials necessary to make these weapons of pain. Thus, you're able to charge downhill to conquer your enemy. This explains why high-dose pharmaceutical-grade fish oil can so effectively keep inflammatory pain under control.

While medicine has a variety of blood tests to check for heart disease and diabetes, it has virtually none to test for pain. The primary way your doctor determines the extent of your pain is by your own reporting of symptoms. Medical science has coined a lot of terms to describe the various parts of your body that hurt. Many end in—*itis,* a Greek root meaning inflammation. Below are some of the common forms of inflammatory pain.

Inflammatory Pain

Name	Body Part That Hurts
Arthritis	Joints
Encephalitis	Brain
Pancreatitis	Pancreas
Hepatitis	Liver
Meningitis	Brain
Bronchitis	Lungs

Colitis	Colon
Gastritis	Stomach
Tendonitis	Muscle tendon

I think you get the picture. Virtually wherever your pain is, it comes from the overproduction of "bad" eicosanoids like prostaglandins or leukotrienes. Always striving for balance, your body also produces an equally impressive number of "good" eicosanoids that decrease pain. The trick is to achieve the right level of the "good" and the "bad." As you now know, our lifestyles favor an overproduction of "bad" eicosanoids. That's why you need to reach the Omega Rx Zone: to shift the scales the other way in order to strike an appropriate balance of eicosanoids.

In the Optimal Health Matrix on page 44, I told you that eicosanoid control has 90 percent of the impact on the pain you feel—compared with a 10 percent impact by insulin (and thereby diet). This means that you need to focus most of your efforts on consuming high-dose pharmaceutical-grade fish oil if your aim is to decrease chronic pain.

Besides fibromyalgia, a wide number of painful conditions caused by chronic inflammation can be alleviated once you are in the Omega Rx Zone.

ARTHRITIS

The first published journal article on the benefits of high-dose fish oil as a treatment for arthritis appeared in 1775. The oil used in that study was a very crude form of cod liver oil. (Remember that I said people used to let the oil from the cod's liver ooze out into the streets?) Patients who could stomach the horrific-tasting oil (estimated to be a daily dose of 7 grams of long-chain omega-3 fatty acids) enjoyed spectacular relief of pain. But the taste of the oil was so putrid that they soon abandoned the fish oil for other, more pleasant-tasting elixirs, like alcohol.

Some two hundred years later, fish oil finally returned to the arthritis scene. In the 1980s, positive research findings ushered in claims that fish oil was a "new" miracle cure for arthritis. Since fish oil was now more refined and could be consumed in soft gelatin capsules, the taste was not so bad. Early studies used only about 3.6 grams of long-chain omega-3 fatty acids, so although the results were positive, they were not spectacular. Also, this fish oil was health-food grade, so higher doses wouldn't have been tolerable. Because such a low dose of long-chain omega-3 fatty acids was used, it isn't too surprising that the benefits were not dramatic.

On the basis of my experience using high-dose pharmaceutical-grade fish oil for patients with severe pain (such as from fibromyalgia and gout), I'm confident that high-dose pharmaceutical-grade fish oils, especially when coupled with improved insulin control, will have a significant role to play in the treatment of chronic pain, including arthritis.

AUTOIMMUNE DISORDERS

Arthritis isn't the only inflammatory condition that can be relieved by high-dose fish oil. Autoimmune disorders, in which the immune system begins attacking the body as if it were a foreign invader, can also be alleviated with fish oil.

Multiple sclerosis is one autoimmune disorder that can be positively affected by high-dose fish oil, as I described in chapter 10. Lupus, a life-threatening autoimmune disorder that causes kidney failure, has also been shown to be positively affected by high-dose fish oil. In animal studies using rats that were bred to develop lupus, significant increases in their life spans are observed if their standard diet is supplemented by high-dose fish oil. However, injections of "good" eicosanoids (like PGE_1)—which fish oil is known to boost—have a spectacular effect on the life spans of the same types of inbred animals. In fact, at the end of thirteen months (a very long life for a rat), all the control rats had died, whereas all the rats injected with "good" eicosanoids were still living, even though the injections of the "good" eicosanoids started well after lupus had been established in the animals.

IgA nephropathy is another inflammatory condition that attacks the kidneys. This disease, which is a major cause of kidney failure, has been found to be alleviated with fish oil. Long-term studies with fish oil indicate a dramatic reduction in the development of kidney failure in these patients compared with those taking a placebo. Here high-dose fish oil is acting not only as a modulator of eicosanoids but also probably as an inhibitor of the release of various inflammatory cytokines such as IL-1, IL-6, and TNF.

As you can see, high-dose pharmaceutical-grade fish oil has a remarkable ability to decrease a broad spectrum of inflammatory mediators, resulting in a reduction in pain associated with seemingly hopeless chronic conditions.

REDUCE INFLAMMATION, LOOK YOUNGER

No one wants to look older than his or her age. But if your skin is full of premature sags and wrinkles, you can't avoid it. Although you may not think of your skin as an organ, it's actually the largest organ in your body, and one of the most critical. Your skin has an extremely critical role to play, as it has to provide a barrier against a very hostile external environment that includes bacteria, fungi, and perpetual oxidation caused by the sun. Furthermore, unlike other organs, your skin is constantly renewing itself to maintain that protective barrier. With new layers of skin cells forming all the time, your skin is even more sensitive than your other organs to changes in eicosanoid levels.

Your skin's visual appearance gives you a window into the internal state of your body. Let's face it: you know when you look good, and usually it's when you're feeling strong and healthy. When your skin has a rosy glow, this means you've got good blood circulation within the skin, and probably through the rest of your body. On the other hand, you often know you're getting sick when you see a pallor to your skin, indicative of poor blood flow. You can bet that the rest of your body is not too far behind.

One unmistakable sign of aging is the formation of wrinkles. Scientifically speaking, wrinkles are caused by the cross-linking of collagen fibers in the skin, and this cross-linking can be accelerated by inflammation caused by constant exposure to the sun. The most effective way to reduce wrinkle formation (other than staying completely out of the sun) is to reduce arachidonic acid levels in the skin, thus decreasing the potential for the production of pro-inflammatory "bad" eicosanoids.

An even more powerful approach to preventing wrinkles is to increase the levels of "good" eicosanoids in your body, because of their powerful anti-inflammatory actions. These "good" eicosanoids will do far more to reduce the inflammatory process that leads to wrinkles than all the fruit acids and vitamin E creams you can possibly rub on your skin. This is because "good" eicosanoids are both very powerful vasodilators (which increase blood flow) and very powerful anti-inflammatory agents. With improved blood flow and decreased inflammation, your skin will look years younger.

Skin diseases, especially conditions that cause dry,

scaly skin like eczema and psoriasis, often result from excessive levels of "bad" eicosanoids. While neither eczema nor psoriasis is life-threatening, both conditions are cause for concern, because they indicate that a significant inflammatory process is already taking place in the skin. Research shows that both of these conditions stem from the overproduction of "bad" eicosanoids called leukotrienes. Reducing arachidonic acid levels by using high-dose fish oil chokes off the production of leukotrienes while simultaneously increasing the levels of "good" eicosanoids. Dermatologists usually prescribe corticosteroid creams to reduce inflammation, but these drugs also unfortunately knock out "good" eicosanoids, and that leads to a thinning of the skin. Various studies have indicated that high-dose fish oil, without the use of corticosteroids, can contribute to some improvement in psoriasis. Other inflammatory skin conditions, such as eczema, also respond well to high-dose fish oil.

Another key to improving your skin's appearance is to increase your production of the key structural proteins of the skin—collagen and elastin—as you age. These structural proteins give your skin its firmness and elasticity. As the production of collagen and elastin decreases with aging, your skin starts to droop and sag. In order to keep collagen and elastin at increased levels, you need to increase blood flow to your skin, since that stimulates the enzymes that produce these structural proteins. Using techniques such as laser resurfacing, dermabrasion, and chemical peels, plastic surgeons not only remove cross-linked proteins from the top layer of skin but also stimulate the blood flow to your skin. This increased blood flow enhances the new production of both collagen and elastin, but unfortunately with significant increase in inflammation and pain in the process.

Just as my dietary program stimulates blood flow in your heart and brain, it can also stimulate blood flow to your skin, which will increase the production of collagen and elastin to give aging skin new body and elasticity without a need for laser resurfacing and other tools of the plastic surgeon. At the same time, it will reduce the likelihood of wrinkles by reducing inflammation in the skin because of the increased production of anti-inflammatory "good" eicosanoids.

Since beautiful skin ultimately begins with what you eat, the Omega Rx Zone diet may represent the best cosmetic product you can use.

LUNG DISEASES CAUSED BY INFLAMMATION

You may think your skin is the only protection you have from the outside world. But you also have an internal "skin" that is in constant contact with your surrounding environment. Just think of your lungs. Every time you inhale oxygen, you suck in whatever pollutants and potential allergens are floating in the air surrounding you. It would be nice if you could extract the oxygen without its fellow travelers. I consider your lungs to be part of your internal skin because they're barriers against toxic agents that assault your body from the outside world. These barriers can be subject to the same inflammatory insults as your skin.

Three distinct lung conditions all stem from inflammation: asthma, bronchitis, and emphysema. Together they are known as chronic obstructive pulmonary disease (COPD). My dietary program can provide benefits to help bring each of these three conditions under control.

Asthma

Asthma is a condition in which your bronchial passages constrict so much that you can barely breathe. Asthma attacks can be triggered by a number of offenders, including pollen, molds, animal furs, and even exercise. The initial trigger may vary from person to person, but the lungs respond in a universal way: they overproduce "bad" eicosanoids. The primary mediators of asthma are leukotrienes. Production of these eicosanoids will not be affected by drugs such as aspirin or other nonsteroidal anti-inflammatory drugs (NSAIDs). This is because leukotrienes are produced by enzymes that are not inhibited by aspirin or NSAIDs. Corticosteroids, on the other hand, do inhibit the formation of leukotrienes. For years they were the primary drug defense for severe asthma.

As I have mentioned, corticosteroids have an impressive number of very adverse side effects, including immune suppression and cognitive impairment. A far better way to reduce an overproduction of leukotrienes without any side effects is simply to reduce the amount of arachidonic acid in the lungs. This can be achieved most effectively through high-dose fish oil. The question is how much you need. I have found that 5 to 10 grams per day of long-chain pharmaceutical-grade omega-3 fatty acids provide an effective dose. This would be equivalent to 2 to 4 teaspoons or 8 to 16 capsules of pharmaceutical-grade fish oil. This represents a higher dose than I recommend for treating heart disease, but that's because of the greater impact of eicosanoids on inflammatory diseases, as shown by the Optimal Health Matrix on page 44.

Bronchitis

As the ending *-itis* implies, bronchitis is an inflammatory condition of the lungs. By now you can probably surmise the best way to control lung inflammation: cut off the over-production of pro-inflammatory eicosanoids (primarily leukotrienes). You can either use steroids (with their side effects—loss of cognitive function, depressed immune system, weight gain, and so on) or try a different approach that alters the same molecular mechanism but without the side effects: my dietary program. Once again, you can use high-dose fish oil as a powerful and elegant way to decrease the formation of arachidonic acid without side effects. While steroids treat the symptoms of bronchitis, my program goes after the underlying cause of the problem: excess arachidonic acid. As with asthma, you will need to take significant levels of high-dose fish oil (5 to 10 grams per day) to receive the full benefits.

Emphysema

Of the three lung conditions caused by inflammation, emphysema is the most difficult to treat, because it is like "heart failure" of the lungs. Your lungs really do begin to wither and fail, and the structural damage is often irreversible. Although there's not much you can do to gain renewed function in your lungs, you can make your remaining lung tissue more efficient at extracting oxygen by increasing the vasodilatation of the capillaries that line the bronchial passages, which increases blood flow to these tissues. What increases blood flow and decreases inflammation? You guessed it—my dietary program.

It is often stated that emphysema cannot be reversed because of the structural damage it does to the lungs. If so, how could my dietary plan be of any benefit? Let me use another of Dan Ward's patients who had emphysema to answer that question. When this patient came to Dan's facility, she was on oxygen twenty-four hours a day. Even though she was taking high-dose prednisone (a synthetic corticosteroid that decreases the formation of "bad" eicosanoids, especially leukotrienes), she still was experiencing significant daily pain and had been housebound with constant fatigue and depression.

As with all Dan's patients, she was put on my dietary program, taking 25 grams per day of long-chain omega-3 fatty acids coming from pharmaceutical-grade fish oil. Within four weeks, she was pain-free and off the oxygen and prednisone. Instead of being confined to her room, she was walking all around Dan's facility, and her depression was completely gone. Maybe emphysema is not quite as irreversible as we are led to believe.

GASTROINTESTINAL DISEASES CAUSED BY INFLAMMATION

Like your lungs, your gastrointestinal (GI) tract also meets my definition of an "internal skin." Every morsel you put into your mouth has both nutrients and potentially noxious agents like pesticides and other potentially cancer-causing agents. Considering the length of your gastrointestinal tract (about twenty feet) and the number of toxic things that enter your body when you swallow, it's surprising that we don't all have overwhelming inflammation in our GI tract.

Those who do suffer from inflammation know that the pain can be intense. Two of the most common inflammatory conditions that occur in the gut are Crohn's disease (inflammation localized in the small intestine) and ulcerative colitis (inflammation that can occur throughout the GI tract).

Research suggests that supplemental fish oil can benefit patients with either Crohn's disease or ulcerative colitis.

One study of patients with Crohn's disease, published in the *New England Journal of Medicine,* found that using pharmaceutical-grade fish oil decreased pain significantly. This study used relatively low levels (1 gram of long-chain omega-3 fatty acids per day), so one can only imagine the impact that would have been measured at the higher levels of 5 to 10 grams per day that I recommend for this inflammatory condition.

Ulcerative colitis also responds well to fish oil. Researchers found that patients who took 1.4 grams per day of long-chain omega-3 fatty acids (though it was the lower-quality health-food grade) had a statistically significant improvement in their pain levels. As with Crohn's disease, I feel that a higher dose of fish oil (5 to 10 grams of long-chain pharmaceutical-grade omega-3 fatty acids per day), especially if it was coupled with improved insulin control, would have given these patients a more dramatic improvement in their inflammatory pain.

If you have either Crohn's disease or colitis, you should realize that you may need one to two weeks on my program before you experience a significant anti-inflammatory response that brings some measure of relief. During your initial few weeks on my dietary program, you should continue to follow a diet that is low in fiber, especially insoluble fiber (a diet that physicians usually recommend for these two conditions). This will keep you from having any physical irritation of the GI lining as it heals. But you still need to maintain the appropriate protein-to-carbohydrate ratio to control insulin (and thus reduce the production of arachidonic acid).

I realize that it can be particularly challenging to get 10 to 15 servings of fruits and vegetables a day without getting a lot of fiber. I think you can best meet this goal by consuming as your primary carbohydrate source moderate amounts of fruit and vegetable juice, from which the fiber has been extracted. I'm normally not a fan of juices, since soluble fiber and pectin are so valuable in helping to control your insulin response. However, for your gut's sake, you can do fine without fiber for the one to two weeks as your intestines are beginning to heal from the inflammation. After two weeks, inflammation should be reduced enough so that you can go back to eating fresh fruits and vegetables and getting all the fiber that nature intended.

Pain is an unfortunate hallmark of nearly every chronic disease. But the fact is that we can control pain much more than we think. All we have to do is get our "bad" eicosanoids under control. We can do this by using powerful drugs like corticosteroids, which have some serious side effects, or by choosing my dietary recommendations as the "drug" of choice. I know what I would choose: the option that hurts the least.

YOUR PERSONALIZED PLAN FOR ALLEVIATING PAIN

1. Maintain insulin control by following my dietary recommendations (balancing protein, carbohydrate, and fat), which I outlined in chapter 7.
2. Supplement your diet with 5 to 10 grams of long-chain omega-3 fatty acids per day (equivalent to 2 to 4 teaspoons or 8 to 16 capsules of pharmaceutical-grade fish oil) for the first few weeks, or until you see a reduction in your pain.
3. Once you've felt a reduction in pain, decrease your dosage in small increments until your pain reappears.

This will help you find the minimum dose of fish oil you need to relieve your pain.

4. As a verification that the plan is working, have a blood test to measure your AA/EPA ratio a month after beginning my program. Your goal is to reach an optimal range between 1.5 and 3. If your ratio is too high, increase your dose of fish oil. If your ratio is too low, decrease your dose of fish oil. Check your AA/EPA ratio every six months to ensure that you're staying within the optimal range. A sudden increase in your pain level is an indication that you've moved out of this optimal range.

Note: Follow this recommendation for supplemental long-chain omega-3 fatty acids *only* if you are using pharmaceutical-grade fish oil.

chapter 15

Women's Health Concerns
Infertility, Menopause, and Beyond

One question I am often asked is, "Does your dietary plan work the same for women as it does for men?" After all, my dietary recommendations are based on controlling your hormone levels, and aren't men and women supposed to be hormonally different? The answers are yes. Yes, both men and women can reach the Omega Rx Zone through my dietary plan. And yes, the sexes are hormonally different.

From a hormonal standpoint, women are far more complex creatures. (My wife would argue that women are more complex from an emotional and intellectual standpoint as well.) Women's hormones must speak a language that prepares their body for pregnancy, deals with the complexities of pregnancy, and ushers the body through menopause. As a result, throughout their lives women travel on a hormonal roller coaster much more than men. That's also why I think women understand the power of hormones to a far greater extent than men do. Yes, women get the same hormonal-based health problems as men, like heart disease, diabetes, obesity, and depression, all of which can be mitigated by my dietary program. And they also have an expanded list of health problems, like premenstrual syndrome, menopause, osteoporosis, and breast cancer, that can be addressed by the same dietary technology, with a few small adjustments.

An adult female's hormonal life can be divided into three distinct time periods: premenopause (menstruation and pregnancy), menopause, and postmenopause. Let's see how my dietary program can help alleviate conditions that may occur through each of these phases of her life.

PREMENOPAUSE

Pregnancy and Infertility

During the 1960s, many premenopausal women would have identified their main health concern as *not* becoming pregnant. In the 1990s, women have a far larger array of contraceptive options, but they face a growing problem of *how* to become pregnant. While it's true that women who choose to delay childbearing until their thirties or forties have increased the rate of infertility, I also believe that a dietary component may be involved. Americans are eating far more carbohydrates today than they ate in the 1960s, and this has caused a dramatic surge in our insulin levels. Another clue to the growing amount of female infertility may lie in an imbalance of eicosanoids, since research has indicated that low-dose aspirin significantly improves the success rates in women undergoing in vitro fertilization. This would suggest that my dietary recommendations might provide a unique intervention to improve fertility. Let me discuss why.

A primary cause of female infertility is polycystic ovary syndrome (PCOS). This condition is linked to increased insulin levels. In women with PCOS, the ovaries release an egg from a follicle only sporadically, if at all, instead of every twenty-eight days as usual. Once women with PCOS lower their elevated insulin levels, their fertility almost magically reappears. Unfortunately, even after women with PCOS become pregnant, they still have higher rates of miscarriages. Thus, simply reducing insulin levels alone is not the total answer. The other important factor appears to be an imbalance of eicosanoids, which can be treated with increased consumption of fish oil. According to epidemiological studies, pregnant women who consume large amounts of long-chain omega-3 fatty acids tend to carry their babies for a longer time and have a correspondingly lower rate of premature births (which can cause physical and neurological problems such as learning disabilities). Of all births in America, 6 to 10 percent are premature, and I think it is quite likely that this unfortunate fact may be linked to our decreasing consumption of long-chain omega-3 fatty acids.

The question is: Can women with problems in conceiving children dramatically improve their outcome just by following my dietary program? Although there are no direct clinical trials, a great number of women have reported that once they begin to follow my program, their previous difficulties in achieving successful pregnancies seem to recede dramatically.

My former employee Wendy followed my dietary recommendations to treat her PMS (see page 230). When she became pregnant, she left the office to become a full-time mother. Her first pregnancy was totally uneventful, and she never complained of nausea or morning sickness. I saw her several years later and asked her if she had any more children. The answer was no. It turned out after she left, she had been unable to conceive again, and she and her husband had been to every fertility specialist in Boston.

I asked whether all these experts thought it was unusual that she would have an incredibly easy first pregnancy and then be unable to conceive again. She said they all thought it odd. Then I asked her if her PMS had returned, and she admitted that it had. Finally, I asked her if she was still following my program. Not unexpectedly, her answer was no. I advised her to resume balancing protein, carbohydrate, and fat and gave her some pharmaceutical-grade fish oil (and a little GLA for her PMS), and six months later she was pregnant with twins.

I consider my dietary program to be ideal both to raise the likelihood of overcoming infertility and achieving a successful pregnancy (by lowering insulin) and to increase the likelihood of carrying a fetus to full term (through increased intake of omega-3 fatty acid).

There are many reasons why high-dose fish oil is the most important supplement you can take during pregnancy, but the most important is the optimum development of the child's brain. Long-chain omega-3 fatty acids are critical for fetal brain development and give your child the best possible mental advantage when he or she comes into this world. The fetus's need for DHA is greatest in the last trimester of the pregnancy, when fetal brain cells are being created at a prodigious rate (more than 250,000 nerve cells per minute). If you don't have adequate supplies of DHA in your body, your fetus's brain is going to have trouble keeping up with the growing demand for DHA building blocks. Thus, pregnancy is a critical time to take supplementary fish oil.

As if this weren't enough, fish oil can also help women avoid two serious conditions that can occur during pregnancy: pregnancy-induced hypertension (preeclampsia) and gestational diabetes. Gestational diabetes can be treated by lowering insulin levels, and preeclampsia by decreasing the levels of "bad" eicosanoids. To accomplish the first goal,

pregnant women need to consume an optimal ratio of carbohydrates to protein. To accomplish the second, they need to
take supplementary fish oil.

Thus, the best way to reduce pregnancy-related complications and also provide adequate levels of DHA for the
developing child is to follow my dietary recommendations.
The only proviso I recommend if you are pregnant is that
you should be consuming extra calories beyond a typical
woman's nutritional needs—on the order of about 300 calories more a day. This simply means using a slightly larger
plate at each meal, but still balanced as I described in chapter 7. (Alternatively, you can consume an extra two or three
glasses of low-fat milk every day, since milk has the appropriate balance of carbohydrates to protein.) Following my
dietary plan during pregnancy will ensure adequate protein
for both you and your fetus, and the increased consumption
of fruits and vegetables will supply the necessary micronu-
trients for both. It's never too late in your pregnancy to go
on my dietary program, because your fetus actually gets the
biggest benefits during the last trimester.

One of the best examples of how my program can
improve the outcome of pregnancy is the case of Silvia, a
physician in Mexico, with whom I have worked for the past
few years. Silvia became pregnant with her third child at
age thirty-eight. During her second pregnancy, six years earlier, she had developed preeclampsia. She knew there was a
high probability that the preeclampsia would recur with this
new pregnancy, and she wanted to take measures to avoid
this condition. Silvia was already following my dietary recommendations to control insulin, and I told her to increase
her intake of pharmaceutical-grade fish oil to about 1 tablespoon per day (about 9 grams of long-chain omega-3 fatty
acids). I told her this would not only prevent the recurrence
of the preeclampsia but would probably make her newborn

the smartest child in Mexico, because the high levels of DHA in the fish oil would accelerate neural development of the baby *in utero*. Therefore I was not surprised when Silvia called and told me that she had had no complications with her pregnancy. In fact, she said this birth was far easier than her earlier two births, and she agrees with me (although what mother wouldn't agree?) that her new son seems to have an intelligence far beyond his age.

After giving birth, new mothers should keep supplementing their diet with high-dose fish oil to lower their risk of postpartum depression. After birth, the levels of long-chain omega-3 fatty acids (especially DHA) in the mother's blood drop dramatically. This is similar to the decreased levels of long-chain omega-3 fatty acids that are observed in depressed patients. By supplementing her diet with adequate levels of high-dose fish oil, a new mother can avoid that drop in long-chain omega-3 fatty acids, and thus will probably not experience any resulting depression. Supplementation with high-dose fish oil is also important for the mother who is breast-feeding her child, in order to maintain the DHA levels in her breast milk, which are crucial for the development of a young baby's rapidly growing brain.

Premenstrual Syndrome

Premenstrual syndrome (PMS) affects about one-third of all premenopausal women, and about 5 to 10 percent of these women have significant impairment, including severe depression that lasts for two weeks of the menstrual cycle. Although theories about the cause of PMS abound, the most likely explanation is that it is caused by disturbances in the balance of "good" and "bad" eicosanoids. My own experience in treating women with PMS confirms that thinking. Previous research suggests that women with PMS have a defect in the ability to make gamma linolenic acid (GLA). Like alcoholics, women with PMS appear to have a blockage of the enzyme that makes this key fatty acid, which is the building block of "good" eicosanoids. Supplying extra GLA in combination with my dietary recommendations can have a dramatic effect in boosting "good" eicosanoid levels in women with PMS.

There is one caveat: taking too much GLA can cause a harmful buildup of arachidonic acid, which can make PMS worse. Thus, you need a little but not too much GLA if you have symptoms of PMS. What is the right amount of GLA? My experience suggests that if a woman is following my dietary plan and supplementing her diet with 40 mg of GLA per week, this should be sufficient to reduce the symptoms of PMS dramatically. This amount of GLA can be obtained from one capsule of evening primrose oil per week.

MENOPAUSE

During menopause, your ovaries completely shut down, reducing your body's production of estrogen by about two-thirds (your adrenal glands and fat cells make the remaining amount). During this time of rapid hormonal changes, your body's eicosanoid balance gets thrown off, giving rise to hot flashes and other discomforts. New evidence suggests that hot flashes may stem from rapidly changing levels of eicosanoids and may be due in part to overproduction of the "bad" eicosanoid PGE_2. One reason may be that the plunge in estrogen levels during menopause also leads to a corresponding increase in the production of insulin. This increase in insulin leads to increased production of arachidonic acid, the building block of "bad" eicosanoids such as PGE_2. High-dose fish oil will reduce the production of this eicosanoid by lowering the level of arachidonic acid, and this may explain why your grandmother rarely complained of hot flashes. Her daily dose of cod liver oil would have reduced or even eliminated this symptom.

Moreover, Japanese women who consume large amounts of seafood and soy rarely suffer from hot flashes. As I pointed out in my book *The Soy Zone,* soy is rich in chemicals called phytoestrogens, which mimic the effects of estrogen in your body. Researchers have found that eating 20 grams of soy protein per day (in the form of soybeans, tofu, tempeh, or soy milk) provides a modest decrease in the severity of menopausal symptoms. However, phytoestrogens are not the cure-all that they were hoped to be, because without adequate levels of long-chain omega-3 fatty acids, there won't be the full inhibition of excess PGE_2 production.

POSTMENOPAUSE

The rise in insulin that begins after menopause helps explain why women's rates of heart disease catch up to men's within ten years of menopause. For many years, experts on heart disease blamed the rise in heart disease following menopause on a drop in estrogen levels, and they held out the hope that estrogen replacement therapy would prevent heart attacks in postmenopausal women. Millions of women taking hormone therapy still believe that they'll avoid heart disease, despite the fact that scientific studies haven't confirmed this. The recent HERS study demonstrated that postmenopausal women who received hormone replacement therapy (HRT) experienced no reduction in heart disease compared with their counterparts who took a placebo. This is because HRT doesn't lower insulin levels; in fact, it may actually increase them, as well as increase the levels of inflammatory cytokines, which increase the level of C-reactive protein (a significant risk factor for heart disease).

The American Heart Association finally acknowledged this fact by stating that women should not consider HRT if their only goal is to reduce the risk of heart attack. If heart disease is your concern—as it should be, since it is the number one cause of death in women and men—following my dietary program to lower your insulin levels and reduce the AA/EPA ratio will give you a far better defense against heart attacks than HRT. What's more, Bruce Holub at the University of Guelph in Canada has shown that high-dose fish oil can decrease the TG/HDL ratio (an indirect marker for decreased insulin levels) and change the AA/EPA ratio in postmenopausal women within thirty days.

Although heart disease is the number one cause of death in women, breast cancer is the disease that's most feared. As I discussed in chapter 12, controlling insulin and decreasing the AA/EPA ratio in the blood will reduce the likelihood of breast cancer. Following my dietary program is your best bet for maintaining an appropriate AA/EPA ratio and for decreasing your risk of breast cancer, as well as any other type of cancer.

Another major health problem seen in postmenopausal women is osteoporosis. Although HRT can slow the loss of bone that leads to debilitating spine curvatures and hip fractures, hormones only delay the process and can't reverse it. Just as with heart disease, the underlying rise in osteoporosis after menopause may not be primarily due to a lack of estrogen. Physicians have long known that corticosteroids will induce rapid bone loss. It turns out that another mediator of the development of osteoporosis is overproduction of "bad" eicosanoids, in particular PGE_2. Bruce Wadkins at Purdue University has demonstrated that high-dose fish oil has the ability to significantly reduce bone loss by decreasing PGE_2 levels. Therefore, reducing excess production of both cortisol and "bad" eicosanoids may be the optimal treatment for osteoporosis. As I discussed earlier, two of the best ways to reduce cortisol output are taking high-dose fish oil (to reduce inflammation) and stabilizing insulin levels (since stable blood sugar levels lower your body's production of excess cortisol). Thus, my dietary recommendations can be your best dietary weapon to reduce the likelihood of developing osteoporosis or even to reverse osteoporosis once it has developed.

An example of the ability of my dietary program to reverse osteoporosis was one case in which a sixty-six-year-old woman followed my dietary program on the advice of her daughter for about three years but had not been taking any supplemental fish oil. She then began to take 3 grams of long-chain omega-3 fatty acids every day, and within a year the loss of bone mass in her backbone had ceased, and her overall bone density had gone from well below average to 10 percent greater than normal for a women of her age.

I find it interesting that our grandmothers rarely had menopausal problems, heart disease, or osteoporosis. We know their bones didn't turn to dust, nor did their hearts stop beating before their time, probably because their diet was similar to my current dietary recommendations—except that they took a tablespoon of cod liver oil each day instead of a teaspoon of high-dose pharmaceutical-grade fish oil.

Yes, the hormonal communication system is vastly more complex in a woman's body than in a man's. My dietary program, however, can see a woman through those phases of life when her hormones are likely to go haywire. My dietary plan gives you the advantage of maintaining hormonal communication within your body throughout pregnancy, menopause, and the postmenopausal years. It's a "drug" that's far superior to fertility shots or hormone replacement therapy. And unlike these pharmaceuticals, my dietary recommendations will help you improve your overall health as well as the fidelity of your hormonal system.

YOUR PERSONALIZED PLAN FOR PREGNANCY AND NURSING

1. Before beginning my dietary program, have a fasting blood cholesterol screening and find out your ratio of triglycerides (TG) to high-density lipoprotein (HDL).

2. If your TG/HDL ratio is less than 2, supplement your diet with 2.5 grams of long-chain omega-3 fatty acids per day. If TG/HDL is more than 2, supplement your diet with 5 grams of long-chain omega-3 fatty acids per day for thirty days, then reduce the dosage to 2.5 grams per day.

3. Maintain insulin control by following my dietary recommendations (balancing protein, carbohydrate, and fat), which I outlined in chapter 7.

4. Adjust the plan for pregnancy by giving yourself larger portions during every meal or snack or by adding an extra two snacks per day. You should be eating 300 extra calories a day, compared with what the average woman would normally eat on my dietary program.

5. If you have a history of infertility or pregnancy-related problems, begin using 5 grams of long-chain omega-3 fatty acids per day.

6. Check your TG/HDL ratio every six months. Your goal is to try to keep it between 1 and 2.

Note: Follow this recommendation for supplementary long-chain omega-3 fatty acids *only* if you are using pharmaceutical-grade fish oil.

YOUR PERSONALIZED PLAN FOR PMS

1. Before beginning my dietary plan, have a fasting blood cholesterol screening and find out your ratio of triglycerides (TG) to high-density lipoprotein (HDL).
2. If your TG/HDL is less than 2, supplement your diet with 2.5 grams of long-chain omega-3 fatty acids per day. If TG/HDL is more than 2, supplement your diet with 5 grams of long-chain omega-3 fatty acids per day for thirty days, then reduce the dosage to 2.5 grams per day.
3. Maintain insulin control by following my dietary plan (balancing protein, carbohydrate, and fat), which I outlined in chapter 7.
4. Take 40 milligrams of GLA per week. *Caution:* Don't take more than 40 milligrams of GLA a week, because too much GLA may cause an increase in your levels of arachidonic acid.
5. Check your TG/HDL ratio every six months. Your goal is to try to keep it between 1 and 2.

Note: Follow this recommendation for supplementary long-chain omega-3 fatty acids *only* if you are using pharmaceutical-grade fish oil.

YOUR PERSONALIZED PLAN FOR MENOPAUSE AND BEYOND

1. Before beginning my dietary program, have a fasting blood cholesterol screening and find out your ratio of triglycerides (TG) to high-density lipoprotein (HDL).
2. If your TG/HDL is less than 2, supplement your diet with 2.5 grams of long-chain omega-3 fatty acids per

day. If TG/HDL is more than 2, supplement your diet with 5 grams of long-chain omega-3 fatty acids per day for thirty days, then reduce the dosage to 2.5 grams per day.

3. Maintain insulin control by following my dietary program (balancing protein, carbohydrate, and fat), which I outlined in chapter 7. Consume one serving a day of soy protein, which has phytoestrogens that combat the symptoms of menopause if your levels of long-chain omega-3 fatty acids are adequate. You can simply replace some of your animal protein sources—meat, chicken, fish, or cheese—with a soy protein product like tofu, tempeh, or soy milk.

4. Check your TG/HDL ratio every six months. Your goal is to try to keep it between 1 and 2.

Note: Follow this recommendation for supplementary long-chain omega-3 fatty acids *only* if you are using pharmaceutical-grade fish oil.

part IV

Reaching Your Full Potential in the Omega Rx Zone

If you want to reach your full potential, then you want to be in the Omega Rx Zone. Perhaps you're in training for a marathon or embarking on a rigorous weight-lifting program. Or maybe you're in a high-pressure job, like an air traffic controller or a stockbroker, that requires unfaltering mental concentration. My personalized plan in each of these chapters will map out a way to get bigger benefits from my dietary plan. Like the personalized plans in Part III, these plans should be used as a supplement to the basic plan included in Part II. In fact, I recommend following the basic plan in Part II for at least two weeks to set a baseline for yourself. Then you can fine-tune your program with one of the plans in Part IV.

Once you are in the Omega Rx Zone, the changes will be quite obvious, and your blood values will validate the perceived changes. You'll feel good about yourself as you accomplish the goals you set—without feeling overwhelmed or incapable—because you know that you have done everything possible with your diet to maximize your full genetic potential, the essence of being human.

chapter 16

Building a Better Brain

Throughout this book, I've discussed brain wellness and emphasized that you have to keep your brain healthy in order to decrease your chances of getting mental illness. I've also told you that you can help alleviate brain disorders that you may already have, such as depression, attention deficit disorder, multiple sclerosis, and Alzheimer's disease. Let's say, though, that you would like to bring your normal, healthy brain to a higher state of functioning. Let's say you want a supernormal brain, so to speak. Can my dietary plan fulfill this expectation?

The answer is yes; otherwise you wouldn't be reading a chapter called "Building a Better Brain." Just what is a supernormal brain? It's a brain that processes information at a faster rate. It's a brain that can more efficiently make new neural connections, which are the basis for learning. It's a brain that can better orchestrate the complex hormonal symphony that is constantly operating within your body. In other words, a supernormal brain lets you achieve your brain's full genetic potential. A supernormal brain also gives you an unfair advantage over everyone else.

As you may recall from chapter 6, the key to improved neurological functioning is giving your brain what it loves and avoiding the things it hates. This can best be achieved by following my dietary recommendations. If you have a neurological problem, your goal is to restore normal functioning to your brain. If your brain already functions normally, your goal is to become supernormal. The pathways for both goals are exactly the same.

By following my dietary plan, you can remodel your brain function to fulfill the potential that your brain was meant to give you. In essence, you're getting your brain to operate at maximum efficiency. To do so, you have to provide the brain the things it loves (oxygen, glucose, and long-chain omega-3 fatty acids) and avoid the things it hates (inflammation, loss of neurotransmitters, and excess cortisol). If you have a normal brain to begin with, what can you expect by following my dietary recommendations? Within a few weeks, if not within a few days, you will start to feel the effects of a supernormal brain. You'll have:

- Greater concentration
- Improved memory
- Better management of stress
- Increased calmness
- Increased creativity

Greater concentration comes from an increase in dopamine levels induced by high-dose fish oil. Dopamine is your brain's action hormone as well as your reward hormone. The more dopamine you produce, the greater your ability to focus on immediate tasks and the more pleasure you gain from their completion. Children with ADD have very low dopamine levels, and I have already described how my dietary program has a dramatic impact on their ability to concentrate. Many of us have a less than optimal level of dopamine, and therefore any increase will provide an immediate mental boost. It's not that we're dopamine-deficient; rather, our diet has significantly reduced the natural production of the dopamine that we would be genetically capable of producing if we had adequate fish oil in our diet.

Impaired memory and feelings of stress both result from overproduction of the hormone cortisol, which is released to stop the overproduction of "bad" eicosanoids. Excess cortisol not only disrupts short-term memory but also can destroy the nerve cells in the brain that are responsible for memory. One of the best ways to reduce excess cortisol is to reduce your body's levels of "bad" eicosanoids. One of the primary reasons that cortisol is secreted is to lower the overproduction of "bad" eicosanoids. High-dose fish oil will do exactly that, thereby decreasing the need to deliver more cortisol into your body.

Another way to control cortisol is to stabilize blood sugar levels. If blood sugar in the brain is inadequate, the brain sends hormonal signals to the adrenal glands to increase cortisol levels, which in turn will cause the release of stored blood sugar from the liver. The excess cortisol is bad enough for the brain, but it also increases insulin levels so that the cycle of low blood sugar is guaranteed to continue. This is why in stressful situations you tend to reach for carbohydrate-rich foods as a form of self-medication to increase blood sugar levels.

High-dose fish oil also increases serotonin, which increases your threshold to stress. As I discussed earlier in this book, Prozac has been shown in studies to improve the mood of normal individuals by increasing serotonin levels. As with dopamine, I think these results indicate that we've chosen diets that have profoundly reduced the normal levels of serotonin that we are genetically capable of producing.

Increasing serotonin and dopamine will lead to increased calmness as you adapt to stress levels with greater ease and develop an increased ability to cope with difficult problems. The result is that you have greater creativity, which comes from getting rid of all the mental clutter that normally hampers it. The ability to think clearly, with greater concentration, improved memory, and increased calmness, is the key to creativity, and my dietary recommendations improve your likelihood of reaching that goal.

TO INCREASE YOUR INTELLIGENCE, THINK DHA

If you were to drain all the fluid out of your brain, you'd find that 60 percent of its mass is fat, and a good chunk of that fat is composed of DHA. As you'll recall, DHA is one of two beneficial long-chain omega-3 fatty acids found in fish oil. EPA is the other one, but it's found in very low concentrations in the brain. The tissues that have the highest concentrations of DHA are the retina of the eye (essential for taking in visual information), the synapses that control the flow of neurotransmitters between nerve cells in the brain, and the mitochondria in each brain nerve cell that provide the energy to keep those cells alive. If DHA is deficient in any of these three critical brain components, your mental functioning suffers and your intelligence begins to fall.

Much of the knowledge about the role of long-chain omega-3 fatty acids in intelligence comes from animal studies in which researchers carefully manipulated dietary intakes to see what effect they had on the animals' learning. The data are quite clear. Remove long-chain omega-3 fatty acids from an animal's diet, and the animal's learning ability will be severely diminished. Researchers didn't have to remove all these fatty acids completely to see a progressive loss of learning ability; they only had to significantly reduce the animal's intake. Conversely, supplementing an animal's diet with long-chain omega-3 fatty acids increases its learning ability.

To understand the implications of the need for long-chain omega-3 fatty acids, let's look at the importance of DHA for the developing fetus. A baby is born with more than 100 billion nerve cells in the brain. To synthesize this enormous number of nerve cells, the fetal brain makes nearly 250,000 nerve cells every minute. In fact, six weeks after conception the fetal brain accounts for half the size of the fetus. By the last trimester of the pregnancy, nearly 70 percent of all fetal energy is dedicated to brain cell development. This requires huge amounts of DHA. This DHA comes from only one place: the mother's body. Lovable as it is, the developing fetus is like a parasite, sucking from the mother all the DHA it needs for its brain development. In fact, the DHA extracted from the mother normally takes four years to replace, assuming that the mother is consuming adequate levels of long-chain omega-3 fatty acids both during and after pregnancy.

What happens if the mother is not consuming adequate amounts of fats that are rich in DHA? Animal studies are very clear on this point: she produces less intelligent offspring. For example, the brain weight of offspring in each successive litter of dogs becomes smaller. This lends credence to the old wives' tale that the firstborn child is usually the smartest—that may be the case because the firstborn gets first crack at the mother's limited store of DHA. In fact, when omega-3 fatty acid intake is highly restricted in animals for three generations, the third-generation offspring have significantly fewer brain cells than the previous generations. There is also a significant decrease in the number of nerve endings (synapses), with a corresponding decrease in learning abilities.

This is an ominous signal for our current generation of children, since the intake of long-chain omega-3 fatty acids in America has decreased by nearly 80 percent in the past century. This decrease in DHA in the American diet can be reflected in the composition of breast milk of nursing mothers throughout the world, as shown here.

DHA Levels of Human Breast Milk

Country	Percent DHA
Canada (Eskimos)	1.40
Malaysia	0.90
China (urban)	0.84
Japan	0.63
Netherlands	0.35
France	0.32
Australia	0.32
United States	0.23
China (rural)	0.18
Vegans (European)	0.14
Sudan	0.07

As you can see from this chart, the breast milk of American mothers has one of the lowest levels of DHA in the world, and this is a reflection of Americans' extremely low intake of long-chain omega-3 fatty acids. These differences in DHA levels in breast milk are also reflected in the blood of both infant and mother. Also, the higher the DHA level in the mother's blood, the higher the DHA level in the infant's blood. We also know that DHA levels in the brain will correspond closely to levels of DHA in the red blood cells. Therefore, the low levels of DHA in the breast milk of

Americans strongly suggest that the next generation of our children will get a less than optimal start in life, and that adults are running dangerously low in this critical brain nutrient.

These biochemical facts become even more important after birth, since the primary way a newborn child can meet his or her continuing needs for more DHA is by breast-feeding. There is no question of the importance of the early intake of DHA for a child's future intelligence; children who were born preterm have IQs 5 to 12 points greater if they are breast-fed than if they are fed formulas. Among full-term infants, breast-fed children have IQs 2 to 5 points higher than those of nonbreast-fed children. Furthermore, the longer a full-term child is breast-fed, the greater the differences in IQ.

What if breast-feeding isn't possible? Even though American breast milk doesn't appear to be a great source of DHA, it does contain more than infant formulas sold in the United States, which have no DHA. However, infant formulas from Europe and Japan are fortified with this key long-chain omega-3 fatty acid. Most infant formulas sold in the United States have only short-chain omega-3 fatty acids derived from soybean oil that contain alpha linolenic acid (ALA). In one recent study, babies were either given infant formula that contained DHA or formula that contained only ALA. After ten months, the babies who consumed the infant formula fortified with DHA had better problem-solving abilities than those whose infant formula contained ALA. This shows why consuming DHA (as opposed to ALA) was so important in our evolutionary leap toward becoming human.

What about adults? It turns out that their need for DHA is just as great. Even though the number of neurons will not appreciably increase in adults (and in fact neurons are often lost), the number of connections that neurons make will increase. During its lifetime, any one neuron will make more than 20,000 connections with other neurons. These new connections constitute learning. Each new connection requires DHA, which must ultimately be supplied by the diet. Obviously, without enough DHA in the diet, the brain will not have enough DHA for building, let alone maintaining, its ability to learn new information and retrieve stored memories.

The precipitous drop in the intake of long-chain omega-3 fatty acid in America (which is confirmed by the low levels in the breast milk of American women) may represent the greatest public health disaster of the past century in our country. Without adequate levels of DHA in the diet, do we run the risk of regressing as a species? I'm afraid the answer may be yes.

You might say, "But we are smarter today than at any other time in our history." You might point to our use of the computer and all the knowledge it offers at our fingertips. My response is that there is a great difference between accessing knowledge and being able to filter and manipulate knowledge. Technology is cumulative, whereas intelligence is not. Do you really think that the latest Internet guru is actually more intelligent than Socrates, Plato, or Aristotle? (In fact, our brain size has decreased some 10 percent in the past 10,000 years.) If you are intelligent, you can master technology very quickly. Unfortunately, the converse is not true. Having more technology doesn't make you more intelligent.

The good news is that we can reverse any decline in intelligence in a matter of weeks by increasing our consumption of high-dose fish oil. It seems amazingly simple that something as common as fish oil can increase our ability to think. However, it was true 150,000 years ago, and it is just as true today. All you need to do is follow my personalized plan on page 254 for building a supernormal brain.

WHAT'S GOING ON AT THE MOLECULAR LEVEL?

The secret to building a more functional brain is having the appropriate bricks and a good mason for building new neural networks. You have to have adequate levels of DHA to make the neural connections. DHA represents the bricks for the brain. The mason is a hormone called brain-derived neurotrophic factor, or BDNF. BDNF is a growth factor found only in the brain, and its specific function is to cause the sprouting of new dendrites between nerves.

For many years it has been known that existing nerves can generate new connections between themselves to enhance learning. Only recently has it been discovered that new nerve growth is also possible in adults. In both cases, BDNF is the critical linkage. One of the best ways to increase BDNF levels is through calorie restriction, which occurs without hunger or deprivation if you follow my dietary recommendations. In addition, it has been shown that calorie restriction minimizes any neurological damage if the brain is exposed to neurological toxins.

Interestingly, another critical component has recently emerged that may be important in maximizing neural development: cholesterol. It turns out that the ability of neurons to form the new synaptic connections that are necessary for learning new information depends on an adequate supply of cholesterol in the brain. This raises some very interesting questions about our growing national obsession with reducing cholesterol levels by taking various statin drugs. If these same drugs are reducing cholesterol synthesis in the brain, that might explain one of their side effects: loss of memory. Frankly, what is the good of lowering the risk of heart disease if in the process the brain is being destroyed? But as you know from chapter 11, you can have the best of both worlds. High-dose fish oil not only will improve the brain's functioning but also is the best way to reduce cardiovascular mortality.

WHAT ELSE CAN YOU DO?

Controlling insulin and eicosanoid levels by following my dietary recommendations will help you achieve a supernormal brain. Other lifestyle factors, however, can also have a significant impact on your mental abilities and will enhance the effects of my program. Here's what I recommend.

Exercise

Exercise is an important component of ultimate brain performance because it can increase the production of BDNF needed for new neural growth. Actually you have two kinds of exercise to work with: aerobic and anaerobic. Aerobic exercise is steady exercise that makes you breathe harder because your body requires more oxygen. It includes jogging, walking, biking, swimming, and skating. Aerobic exercise decreases insulin levels and increases your heart's capacity to pump blood, especially to the brain. A reduction in elevated insulin levels will help stabilize your blood sugar levels, and increased blood flow to the brain will improve oxygen transfer (by decreasing the production of "bad" eicosanoids). Carl Cotman of the University of California at Irvine has shown that animals that exercise have significantly improved brain function and learning capacity relative to their sedentary brothers and sisters. More important, Fred Gage at the Salk Institute has shown that exercise appears to stimulate the growth of neurons (nerve cells in the brain). In both cases, it is likely that increased BDNF production is a primary mediator. Of course, even with increased BDNF production, you still need to have enough DHA for the formation of new nerve cells.

Anaerobic exercise includes such activities as lifting weights and other short bursts of exercise like running short sprints. This is the type of exercise that most people don't enjoy, because discomfort or even pain is often associated with the high levels of lactic acid that are produced in the muscle cells. This is the "burn" you often read about in fitness magazines.

Of course, one of the things that make anaerobic exercise more enjoyable is the druglike effect often known as a "runner's high" or "second wind." It turns out that your body has a unique system to dull pain by releasing neuropeptides called endorphins. These natural compounds have an effect on your brain like that of opiates. They are usually released after a bout of intense training, and this means that they are far more likely to be released during anaerobic training than aerobic exercise. However, if you run long enough (an hour or more), they are also released. In a sense, "no pain, no endorphin release" is true. This is why you see many people exercising to an extreme or even why exercise becomes an addiction—they are looking for the endorphin high. This is also why extreme exercisers may quickly become depressed when they cease regular training and fail to get their endorphin release. Overtraining, however, can lead to excess cortisol production, since your body is under so much stress that it increases the production of cortisol. And as I have already pointed out, excess cortisol may be one of the worst nightmares for your brain.

Meditation

Whereas exercise is an effective way to increase BDNF production, meditation is a highly effective way to reduce excess cortisol output. The key is to learn how to develop a *relaxation response,* a term coined by Herbert Benson, a professor of medicine at Harvard Medical School.

The secret to meditating effectively is to try to think of nothing at all (which is a lot more difficult than you think). It's easier if you follow the technique I outlined in *The Anti-Aging Zone:*

1. Pick a word or phrase that you can continue to repeat to yourself.
2. Sit in a comfortable chair.
3. Close your eyes.
4. Breathe slowly and deeply, and when you exhale, repeat the word or phrase.
5. When other thoughts come into your mind, simply let them pass and return to focusing on the repetition of the word or phrase.
6. Meditate for twenty minutes.

If you can meditate only once a day, do it in the evening. High cortisol levels can impede your sleep, and meditating lowers your cortisol levels naturally and puts you in a restful state for getting a good night's sleep—not to mention decreasing the likelihood of consumption of carbohydrate-rich late-night snacks.

PUTTING IT ALL TOGETHER

Now you can put together a total lifestyle program to make your brain supernormal, as shown on the next page.

Supernormal Brain Lifestyle Program

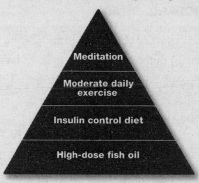

Meditation

Moderate daily exercise

Insulin control diet

High-dose fish oil

The most important factor in developing a supernormal brain is adequate dietary supplementation with high-dose pharmaceutical-grade fish oil, providing at least 5 to 10 grams of long-chain omega-3 fats per day. Without that foundation, it will be virtually impossible to improve your brain functioning. Next in importance is following my dietary guidelines to control your insulin levels. You should also incorporate moderate exercise; I recommend 30 to 45 minutes a day. You should do aerobic exercise every day and anaerobic strength training two or three days a week. Do your workouts early in the day, since exercise temporarily increases cortisol, which can keep you from getting a good night's sleep. Meditate for 15 to 20 minutes every evening to reduce elevated cortisol levels and induce a more restful sleep. If you follow this comprehensive program, you will achieve this result: a supernormal brain with enhanced cognitive functions that gives you an unfair advantage in the world around you.

YOUR PERSONALIZED PLAN FOR DEVELOPING A SUPERNORMAL BRAIN

1. Maintain insulin control by following my dietary recommendations (balancing protein, carbohydrate, and fat), which I outlined in chapter 7.

2. Start by supplementing your diet with 5 grams of long-chain omega-3 fatty acids per day (equivalent to 2 teaspoons of fish oil or 8 capsules).

3. After a month, have a blood test to check your AA/EPA ratio. If it is between 1.5 and 3, you're taking an optimal dose of fish oil. If the AA/EPA ratio is below 1.5, decrease your intake of the fish oil to 2.5 grams a day (equivalent to 1 teaspoon or 4 capsules). If your ratio is greater than 3, increase your fish oil dose to 8 grams a day (equivalent to 1 tablespoon or 12 capsules).

4. Test your AA/EPA ratio every three months until you've reached your optimal range, between 1.5 and 3. After that, check your ratio every six months.

5. Do 30 to 45 minutes of aerobic or anaerobic exercise every day, avoiding late-evening workouts.

6. Do 20 minutes of meditation every day, especially at night, before bed.

Note: Follow this recommendation for supplementary long-chain omega-3 fatty acids *only* if you are using pharmaceutical-grade fish oil.

chapter 17

Emotions
The Mind-Body-Diet Connection

For years, the medical establishment laughed at the notion that our emotions could influence the way our bodies work. They viewed the mind-body connection as simply New Age gobbledygook unsubstantiated by hard evidence. One reason for their skepticism was the complex biochemistry underlying our emotional states, which no one fully understands. Today, biochemists are on the verge of understanding how emotions, mediated by hormones, affect the physiological function of the body. If hormones do play a central role in our psychological well-being, then my dietary recommendations should, in theory, lead us to a healthier emotional as well as physiological state.

Just in case you've never taken a college-level neurology course, here's a quick review of the emotional map of your brain. Your brain stores and generates emotions in the limbic system, the most primitive portion of the brain. The limbic system contains two other structures, the hypothalamus and the hippocampus. The hippocampus stores dry, unemotional facts, such as where you live and your spouse's telephone number at work. The hypothalamus acts as the commander in chief of your hormonal communication system, deciding which gland should release what amounts of hormones at what particular time.

The central processing facility for your emotional memories is called the amygdala. If you're, say, having a heated argument with a driver who has just rear-ended your car, the incoming words are filtered through your hippocampus, amygdala, and frontal cortex (the thinking part of the brain) to determine whether or not an appropriate hormonal response needs to be generated by the hypothalamus. Ultimately, your limbic system forms the basis of the mind-body connection. As you argue with the other driver, your heart rate speeds up and you begin to sweat. All these physiological reactions result from the hormone flow that was initiated by your hypothalamus as a result of emotional distress perceived by your limbic system. This is an extremely simplified explanation of what's really happening in your brain, so you can imagine how much more complex your emotional system really is.

Although the emotions that your brain processes and stores are complex, the chemicals that mediate these emotions are not. The two primary mediators of emotions are cytokines (hormones that are involved in inflammation) and eicosanoids. High-dose fish oil gives you the ability to control both cytokines and eicosanoids and thus helps you deal with the wide variety of emotional issues that arise in your life.

HOW STRESS AFFECTS THE IMMUNE SYSTEM

Hans Seyle put forward the concept of adaptation to stress in the 1930s. Stress can be viewed as anything that causes a disequilibrium in the body. It could be an injury, emotional trauma, overtraining in a sport, or even taking a test. At the molecular level, any type of stress induces changes in the eicosanoid output at the cellular level. The higher the concentrations of arachidonic acid in the cell, the greater the number of pro-inflammatory "bad" eicosanoids produced in response to a stressor. The body's response to stress is to increase the secretion of cortisol to dampen down the overproduction of "bad" eicosanoids, but if too much cortisol is secreted, the immune system is turned down too much, making your body more susceptible to infection and illness. The body responds to illness by increasing inflammation through the production of more "bad" eicosanoids, and the cycle continues. These "bad" eicosanoids also stimulate the production of pro-inflammatory cytokines. Cytokines are a class of immune-system chemicals that cause you to feel woozy, have a fever, and feel tired and down in the dumps when you're sick. They also cause the loss of appetite, cause the loss of desire, and can even provoke sadness. Your body releases cytokines when you have an infection, in an effort to get you to conserve energy and stay in bed as it tries to fight off the illness. If your immune system has been depressed by too much stress, this overproduction of cytokines happens with increasing frequency, generating a continuing downward spiral of physical illness through increased inflammation. This explains how emotions, especially stressful ones, can make us more prone to illness. But how can illness affect emotions?

HOW THE IMMUNE SYSTEM AFFECTS EMOTIONS

It is clear that when you are ill, more pro-inflammatory cytokines will be released by your immune cells to fight infections. The cytokines produced by your immune cells are too big to cross the blood-brain barrier, but they can interact with receptors on the surface of this barrier to make pro-inflammatory "bad" eicosanoids that *can* easily cross into the brain. Once inside the brain, these pro-inflammatory eicosanoids can stimulate the production of pro-inflammatory cytokines there. The brain responds to this new round of inflammation inside its boundaries by sending out for more cortisol to be secreted by the adrenal glands. Now the emotion-inflammatory cycle is complete, from the initial stress response perceived by the brain to an immune response and back to an increased stress response within the brain. To control your emotions and your immune system, you have to have some means to break this inflammatory cycle. High-dose fish oil gives you that tool.

I discussed in chapter 10 how high-dose fish oil can be successfully used in the treatment of depression and help you more readily adapt to stress by increasing serotonin levels. Also, we know that depression is highly associated with increased levels of "bad" eicosanoids in the brain and an increased AA/EPA ratio in the blood. Both observations strongly suggest the underlying role of pro-inflammatory eicosanoids in depression. Furthermore, the increased AA/EPA ratio in depressed patients may help explain why depression seems to accelerate the development of both cancer and heart disease, two diseases that have strong inflammatory components. The ancient Roman physician Galen recognized this fact when he commented that depressed women were more prone to breast cancer than their more cheerful counterparts. This also explains why depressed individuals have depressed immune systems with abnormally low levels of natural killer cells, lymphocytes, and T-helper cells. This same immune-system depression has been observed in people who report being chronically stressed and in people who have been given a single injection of corticosteroids.

At the opposite extreme of the emotional spectrum is laughter, which is associated with decreased cortisol production and increased production of two types of immune cells: natural killer cells and activated T cells. This is the molecular reason behind Norman Cousins's famous book on laughter as the best medicine against cancer. His theories make perfect sense if you understand the role of eicosanoids and cytokines in cancer.

To visualize all the links between your brain and your hormonal and immune systems, take a look at this diagram:

Hormonal Links Betwen the Nervous and Immune Systems

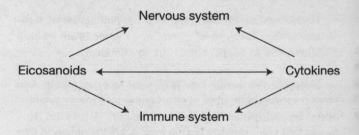

Hormonal messengers such as cytokines and eicosanoids mediate the communication between the brain and immune system. The complexity of these interactions is increased because eicosanoids and cytokines can influence each other. Think of cytokines and eicosanoids as the grammar of the very complex language of emotions. Without the right grammar, any language would be difficult to understand.

IMPROVING YOUR EMOTIONAL STATE

If your emotions affect your physiological health, can your diet affect your emotions? I believe that it can, and that you can enhance your emotional well-being with the foods you choose to eat—provided you make the correct choices. My dietary recommendations have the potential to improve your emotional state in three ways:

- Supplementation with high-dose fish oil reduces your levels of both pro-inflammatory cytokines and eicosanoids.

- Stabilizing insulin levels will reduce the output of cortisol (which is often released in response to decreased blood sugar levels).

- High-dose fish oil also increases the production of serotonin, the "feel-good" hormone in your brain, which allows you to adapt to stress more effectively.

Now that you understand how your diet can manipulate your emotions, you also need to consider how your emotions can manipulate your diet. If you are depressed (this means that you probably have a high AA/EPA ratio and low serotonin levels) or are physically or mentally stressed (this increases cortisol levels), you are likely to crave carbohydrate-rich comfort foods like mashed potatoes, candy bars, and pizza. These foods provide temporary emotional comfort by increasing blood sugar levels and serotonin levels in your brain. Two or three hours after eating these foods, however, your insulin levels will soar, causing your blood sugar levels to plunge. This forces your body to increase cortisol production to maintain adequate blood sugar levels to the brain. Thus, you'll wind up increasing your production of cortisol, which will in turn generate more depression and require another cycle of self-medication with carbohydrates.

You might try to end these mood swings with more comfort food, but all you're doing is setting off a cascade of hormonal events that will continue to thwart your efforts to lift your spirits. In fact, you're also giving yourself a surefire prescription for accelerated aging and continued emotional lows. On the other hand, using high-dose fish oil will improve your control of insulin and, correspondingly, improve your eicosanoid balance. This will lead to far better emotional health. I'm not saying that my dietary recommendations can totally control your emotions, but they will give you significantly more control than you probably have now.

In the final analysis, your emotions and your immune system are intertwined in a complex orchestration. As you begin to understand how emotions stem from hormonal communication, you will have a starting point from which to develop dietary strategies to improve emotional control. The "mind-body" connection really becomes the "mind-body-diet" connection, and my dietary recommendations should become your primary tool for emotional control. Conversely, the wrong diet (especially one deficient in high-dose fish oil and rich in carbohydrates) is your passport to emotional chaos. The choice is yours.

YOUR PERSONALIZED PLAN FOR BETTER EMOTIONAL CONTROL

1. Maintain insulin control by following my dietary recommendations (balancing protein, carbohydrate, and fat), which I outlined in chapter 7.
2. To determine how much fish oil to take, check the results of your last cholesterol screening if you had it within the past six months. If you haven't had a

recent test, get a fasting cholesterol blood test to find out your TG/HDL ratio. If the TG/HDL ratio is less than 2, supplement your diet with a maintenance dose of 2.5 grams of long-chain omega-3 fatty acids per day (equivalent to 1 teaspoon or 4 capsules of pharmaceutical-grade fish oil). If your TG/HDL ratio is more than 2, supplement your diet with 5 grams of long-chain omega-3 fatty acids per day for thirty days and then reduce the dosage to 2.5 grams per day.

3. Check your TG/HDL ratio every six months. Your goal is to try to keep it between 1 and 2.

Note: Follow this recommendation for supplementary long-chain omega-3 fatty acids *only* if you are using pharmaceutical-grade fish oil.

chapter 18

How to Build a Better Athlete

If my dietary recommendations can help prevent heart disease and strengthen your heart, can they also improve athletic performance? The answer is a resounding yes.

Though I initially developed my dietary plan to treat patients with cardiovascular disease, I did much of my early field-testing of supplemental fish oil with world-class athletes. I decided to start with athletes because I've found that they are generally more motivated to stick with a dietary program than patients with cardiovascular disease.

My first interaction with world-class athletes came more than a decade ago with the then Los Angeles Rams. A friend, Marv Marinovich, who is a top trainer of elite athletes, introduced me to their strength coach, Garrett Giemont. Garrett, like most professional coaches, was always looking for safe new ways to give his athletes a performance edge. I told him about my theories on hormonal control for improved athletic performance. He listened politely, then said, "OK, I'll do the flip test." He told me that every Tom, Dick, and Harry would walk into his weight room with some new magic elixir for improved athletic performance. To weed out the snake oils, Garrett devised the "flip test": He read all the supporting medical literature (if there is any), and if it made sense to him, he used the product himself for two weeks. If he didn't see any significant benefits, he would flip the product back to the sender. He told me that more than 99 percent of all products brought to him were flipped back.

I thought Garrett's flip test made sense, and I provided him with my earliest prototypes of fish oils containing small amounts of gamma linolenic acid (GLA). I described in detail how the fish oil plus GLA would increase the body's production of "good" eicosanoids. The increase in these eicosanoids causes the enhanced release of growth hormone from the pituitary gland, and this increases muscle mass. These same "good" eicosanoids will increase blood flow and oxygen transfer to improve endurance. And, I told Garrett, "good" eicosanoids are superb anti-inflammatory agents that work like aspirin to relieve pain. Finally, the combination of increased growth hormone (to repair damaged tissue) and faster recovery from pain would allow the athlete to recover quicker from an intense workout or a game.

In essence, I promised Garrett four things that all athletes—regardless of their sport—can benefit from:

1. Increased strength
2. Increased endurance
3. Decreased pain
4. Faster recovery

Garrett called me two weeks later and wanted to talk. I had passed his flip test—everything I had predicted (better endurance, improved strength, less pain after a workout, and decreased recovery time between workouts) had occurred. Now that I had Garrett's attention, he told me his goal wasn't to improve his football players' endurance as much as it was to maintain their strength during the season. NFL players train during the off-season to build up their muscle mass because they know they'll suffer numerous muscle injuries during the season. The players are pretty beat-up by the end of the season, and their strength is usually significantly lower. Garrett figured that if his players could maintain their strength during the season, they would have a competitive edge.

Although he was convinced of the benefits of fish oil plus GLA from his own experience, Garrett experimented further on a few of his players. One of them was Doug Smith, an All-Pro center for the Rams. After a few weeks of taking the combination of fish oil and GLA, Doug came back to Garrett and said, "Coach, I've got to quit taking this stuff, because I am getting stronger in the middle of the season, and that just doesn't happen." Garrett told Doug that there were no steroids or other illegal performance enhancers in these products, and persuaded him to keep using them.

Over time, Garrett and I added some improvements to the program. First we started experimenting with cycling different ratios of fish oil and GLA, and Garrett found that he could produce extraordinary strength in his players. (The cycling was necessary to prevent a buildup of arachidonic acid, which may result from too high a level of GLA in the tissues.) Second, we tried to get the players to maintain a more consistent protein-to-carbohydrate balance. This is easier to do with NFL players than other elite athletes, since they didn't have any problem with eating protein, but they had to cut back on some of their carbohydrate intake.

Garrett wanted to keep his new "secret weapon" to himself, and I just wanted to see if elite athletes would comply with my dietary program. I figured that if this program was too difficult for athletes, who are used to following the advice of their coaches, I could not really expect the average patient with heart disease to comply. And even with disciplined athletes, I found that getting them to be consistent with regard to their meals was a constant challenge.

Soon after I met Garrett, I was introduced to Stanford University's swimming coaches Skip Kenney and Richard Quick. I told them about the potential of using my diet and fish oil (coupled with the right amount of GLA) to improve athletic performance. I discussed the results Garrett and I were getting with the Los Angeles Rams, and said I believed their swimmers could also benefit greatly from this approach. But before trying out the program with the Stanford swimmers, I suggested that Skip and Richard both do Garrett's "flip test." Two weeks later, both of them called me and said, "Let's get going."

To be frank, not all their swimmers agreed with my dietary recommendations, since in this sport a high-carbohydrate diet was considered the norm. However, 1992 was an Olympic year, and every swimmer had the ultimate goal of making the Olympic team. Several of the swimmers decided to listen to their coaches about changing their diet. One said, "Coach, if you think this will help me make the Olympic team and maybe even win a gold medal, then count me in." The rest—as they say in Hollywood—is history. Those Stanford University swimmers who followed my dietary recommendations and supplemented their diet with the fish oil plus GLA combinations won seven gold medals at the 1992 Barcelona Olympics. Not bad for the United States, and truly amazing for a single university.

In the last three Olympics, athletes I have personally worked with have taken home twenty-one gold medals. You might say that those athletes were already in their prime, and any dietary program really wouldn't have made much of a difference. That's why I love the story of Dara Torres, who won two gold medals at the Olympics in Sydney in 2000. At age thirty-four, Dara was well past her prime when she competed in this Olympics. Dara had been an Olympic swimmer in 1992, but for the next eight years she developed a successful modeling and television career. Then, in 1999, she got the urge to go back to the pool and give it one more try.

Swimming is a sport for young athletes. Most world-class swimmers hit their prime during their early twenties. Competing at the world-class level in swimming at thirty-four is like playing NBA basketball at sixty-five. It just doesn't happen. The bottom line is that Dara decided to give my dietary program a try, and she applied the same dedication to it that she did with her training in the pool. As a result of her discipline both in the pool and at the dinner table, Dara became the oldest gold medal winner in swimming in Olympic history.

PHYSICAL INTELLIGENCE

To understand how these stories of improved athletic performance were achieved through the application of my dietary recommendations, you need to understand how your muscles respond to your brain. This is what I refer to as "physical intelligence."

Just what is physical intelligence? Simply stated, it is the ability to command your muscles to move according to your desires. There are 236 muscles in the body, each composed of numerous bundles of muscle cells. Each muscle cell has neural connections to the brain so that the complex symphony of contractions and relaxations can be orchestrated to achieve movement. We all move our muscles in this way. Great athletes just do it better than the rest of us.

World-class athletes have a grace of movement that is simply impossible for us mere mortals to re-create. Their physical intelligence is probably genetically greater than the average person's, but it is also honed through constant practice that reinforces those neural networks that make their majestic movement possible. And as I described above, this natural talent can be taken to an even higher level by using my dietary recommendations to orchestrate an improved hormonal harmony that results in greater physical intelligence.

THE MYTH OF HIGH-CARBOHYDRATE DIETS

For years, coaches, trainers, and nutritionists have told American athletes that the more carbohydrates they eat, the better they will perform, especially in endurance running. (In fact, it's very much the same thing that most of us were told to do to lose weight.) Considering all the sports energy drinks and pasta that American runners consume, it isn't hard to understand why the last American male to win the Boston marathon was Greg Meyer in 1983. The fact is that winners of the Boston marathon don't attend the typical carbohydrate-loading dinners on the day before the race. These winners know intuitively that excess insulin from too many carbohydrates is an athlete's worst nightmare.

Here are the three greatest fears of an athlete during competition:

- Low blood sugar ("bonking") for the brain
- Decreased access to body fat for energy
- Decreased oxygen transfer to the muscle cells

Let's see how my dietary program helps athletes to avoid these three killers of physical performance. First, my plan stabilizes insulin levels. High levels of insulin increase the likelihood that all three performance problems will occur at the same time:

- Excess insulin lowers blood sugar levels and simultaneously prevents the release of stored glycogen from the liver to restore blood sugar.
- Excess insulin prevents the fat cells from releasing stored fat for energy.
- Excess insulin decreases blood flow by increasing the production of arachidonic acid and ultimately "bad" eicosanoids, which reduce oxygen transfer to muscle cells.

What is the best way to increase insulin levels and induce these adverse performance effects? Eat lots of pasta or drink "sports energy" drinks composed of sugar water.

How did this myth arise about the benefits of carbohydrate loading? More than thirty years ago, the following experiment was done. For several days, well-trained athletes were put on a high-protein diet that was virtually free of carbohydrates. Within a few days, virtually all the stored carbohydrate in their muscles was depleted. They were then tested on a treadmill, and—not surprisingly—their performance was below par. Then the athletes were loaded up with high-carbohydrate meals for the next three days and again tested on the treadmill. Now their performance was enhanced.

The researchers concluded that a high-carbohydrate diet improves athletic performance. Was this the right conclusion? Or should the conclusion have been that if you don't eat any carbohydrates at all, you are going to feel bad and perform poorly? I think the data are very clear that it is the latter, since not a single study in the past thirty years has proved that consuming a high-carbohydrate diet for more than seven days improves performance. I am still waiting for just one experiment to prove the hypothesis that consuming a high-carbohydrate diet for an extended period of time improves performance.

On the other hand, numerous studies with elite athletes demonstrate that eating an adequate amount of carbohydrates (but not too much) combined with higher levels of fat for seven days will dramatically increase their performance. In addition, the extra dietary fat (and lower carbohydrate intake) also improves the lipid profile of elite athletes, thus lowering their risk of cardiovascular disease. How is it possible that fat-loading instead of carbohydrate-loading can dramatically improve athletic performance and improve cardiovascular health? I'll answer that question below.

THE IMPORTANCE OF DIETARY FAT

Fat can be an athlete's greatest ally. Simply increasing the levels of fat in the diet can enhance performance in endurance athletes. This is because muscle tissue contains far more calories of stored fat than stored carbohydrate as an energy source. In fact, it contains nearly twice as many. By increasing the fat content of your diet, you can increase the levels of intramuscular fat, thereby giving yourself an unfair advantage over your competitors in a long-distance race. This is especially true in ultramarathons (distances greater than fifty miles), for which high-fat diets are the norm.

To get the most enhanced athletic performance, however, you need to consume the right type of fat. The fat you consume should help increase the production of "good" eicosanoids or at least should not cause any increase in "bad" eicosanoids. The long-chain omega-3 fatty acids found in fish oil will boost your production of "good" eicosanoids and can therefore become your primary dietary tool (especially when combined with small amounts of GLA). Monounsaturated fats (found in olive oil, avocados, and nuts) come in second. They won't improve your levels of "good" eicosanoids, but they won't increase your "bad" eicosanoids either. On the other hand, a high intake of omega-6 fats will increase your production of arachidonic acid. The result is an increase in "bad" eicosanoid production and decreased physical performance. "Good" eicosanoids, on the other hand, increase athletic performance in the same ways that they increase brain and cardiovascular performance: they increase blood flow and decrease inflammation. When you increase blood flow, more oxygen is delivered to your muscle cells so that greater endurance is maintained at a higher energy output. The "good" eicosanoids also decrease inflammation, improving recovery rates after a workout; this allows you to train harder the next day. The combination gives you an edge over your competitors.

YOUR OWN SECRET WEAPON

The first written reports of my work with the Stanford swimming team appeared in 1993, in an issue of the magazine *Swimming World*. The article was titled "Stanford's Secret Weapon." It described my dietary recommendations, but it never disclosed the real "secret weapon": my Eicosanoid Status Report (yes, it's the same one that appears on page 123). Each week, every Stanford swimmer filled out an Eicosanoid Status Report, and the coaches faxed the reports to me. On the basis of their individual physiological changes during the previous week, I would individually alter each swimmer's essential supplementary fatty acid pattern by changing the ratio of fish oil to GLA, just as I had done with the Los Angeles Rams. This ensured that by the time the national championships, the Olympic trials, or even the Olympic Games rolled around, the athletes would be in the optimal hormonal zone.

I knew that controlling insulin was important, but controlling eicosanoids would be the real key to success. That was Stanford's real secret weapon, just as it was for Garrett Giemont and the then Los Angeles Rams.

Sometimes things go in strange cycles. Several months ago, Marv Marinovich (who initially introduced me to Garrett) called and asked if I was working on anything new for athletic performance. Marv already had all his athletes following my earlier dietary program, as they had been doing for the past ten years. I told Marv about the new pharmaceutical-grade fish oil I had developed. I suggested that he start some of his athletes with 2 tablespoons per day, which would provide about 16 grams of long-chain omega-3 fatty acids, plus a trace of GLA. Two days after he got the oil, he called me and said, "Doc, this is amazing. My athletes can go through longer training sessions and recover faster. Is there some type of drug in this oil?" My reply was, "Only good science."

You don't have to be a world-class athlete to gain improved strength and endurance from my dietary recommendations. Regardless of your level of physical activity, performance will be increased because of improved blood flow and stabilization of insulin levels. You might not have the genetics, training, or discipline of a world-class athlete, but you can at least eat like one.

DIETARY GUIDELINES FOR ENHANCED ATHLETIC PERFORMANCE

1. Maintain insulin control by following my dietary recommendations (balancing protein, carbohydrate, and fat), which I outlined in chapter 7.

2. To determine how much fish oil to take, get a fasting cholesterol blood test to find out your TG/HDL ratio. If the TG/HDL ratio is less than 2, supplement your diet with a maintenance dose of 2.5 grams of long-chain omega-3 fatty acids per day (equivalent to 1 teaspoon or 4 capsules of pharmaceutical-grade fish oil). If your TG/HDL ratio is more than 2, supplement your diet with 5 grams of long-chain omega-3 fatty acids per day for thirty days, and then reduce the dosage to 2.5 grams per day.

3. Take a supplement containing about 10 milligrams of GLA every day.

4. Check your Eicosanoid Status Report (page 123) every week. If you are making too many "bad" eicosanoids, decrease your GLA intake.

5. Check your TG/HDL ratio every six months. Your goal is to try to keep it between 1 and 2.

Note: Follow this recommendation for supplementary long-chain omega-3 fatty acids *only* if you are using pharmaceutical-grade fish oil.

chapter 19

At the Crossroads of the Future

As we settle into the unsettling twenty-first century, we stand at a crossroads, both in terms of our health care and our future potential as a species.

With regard to our future health care, we can continue on the path we've been on, which is to develop new, more expensive drugs to treat the symptoms of chronic disease. This means we'll continue to treat the symptoms of a chronic disease decades after it first started developing. Wouldn't it make more sense to prevent the disease in the first place? After all, most chronic diseases result from reduced blood flow and increased inflammation—two physiological problems that my dietary program can reverse. Why not focus your efforts on maintaining yourself in the Omega Rx Zone instead of leaving yourself in the hands of the drug companies?

I don't want you to think of the Omega Rx Zone as a form of alternative medicine. Keeping yourself in the Omega Rx Zone should be your primary goal with regard to health care, and you should use only pharmaceuticals as a backup. Once you move out of the Omega Rx Zone, the first signs that you're heading toward chronic disease will be reflected in your blood values. It is only years later that the signs of chronic disease will make their appearance. However, you don't have to wait for a chronic disease to develop to know that you are moving out of the Omega Rx Zone. It often takes only one high-carbohydrate meal to drive you out, because of the sudden rise in insulin secretion. And if you stop taking a maintenance dose of fish oil for two weeks, your other blood values will reflect that you have already moved out of the Omega Rx Zone and into the area of subchronic illness. Almost suddenly, you are getting fatigued more often and dragging yourself through the day in a type of brain fog. I wouldn't want to live in this state, and I'm sure you wouldn't either.

As with any drug, however, you have to use my dietary plan correctly if you want to prevent premature chronic disease. This means monitoring your blood profile and adjusting your dose of fish oil until you get the blood values that indicate you've reached the Omega Rx Zone.

If you can do only one thing in your life to improve your health, take a daily dose of pharmaceutical-grade fish oil. This type of fish oil can at least partially compensate for a wide variety of lifestyle sins, like eating too many carbohydrates, not exercising enough, not reducing stress, or being overweight. I'm not saying that lifestyle interventions are not important in improving your health. They will indeed help you stabilize your insulin and cortisol levels and, indirectly, your eicosanoids. But high-dose fish oil has an immediate and direct impact on your eicosanoid levels, and there lies the key to long-term wellness.

Unfortunately, the growing time constraints in our society make it increasingly difficult to do all the lifestyle modifications you need to do consistently to maintain your health.

High-dose fish oil goes right to the foundation of health, since it directly affects your eicosanoid balance. Eicosanoids are the true mediators of your health, so having these hormones in balance will ensure that you're doing everything possible to avoid chronic disease. Thus, I invite you to enter the Omega Rx Zone. I've incorporated all the components of my program in my Omega Rx Zone Lifestyle Pyramid:

Omega Rx Zone Lifestyle Pyramid

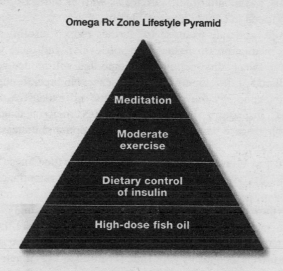

The base of my Omega Rx Zone Lifestyle Pyramid contains the most important element of my program, the one that will have the greatest hormonal impact, and the top of the pyramid contains the element that has the least hormonal impact. So if you need to set your priorities regarding what lifestyle modifications you have time to make, I recommend first taking your high-dose fish oil. Whatever other lifestyle modification you undertake, supplementing your diet with high-dose pharmaceutical-grade fish oil will dramatically improve the outcome. The next level of the pyramid is your diet, specifically one in which you balance your protein and carbohydrate consumption to control your insulin levels. You should be consuming primarily fruits and vegetables, adequate amounts of low-fat protein, and small amounts of heart-healthy monounsaturated fat. At the same time, you should be minimizing your consumption of breads, pasta, and other starches as well as omega-6 fatty acids found in common vegetable oils.

Add moderate exercise (to further reduce insulin) and daily meditation (to reduce cortisol levels), and there you have it: twenty-first-century medicine that will reduce your likelihood of developing chronic disease. No breakthroughs in biotechnology, no gene transplants, no expensive new drugs, just going back to the basics: macromanaging chronic disease by decreasing inflammation and increasing blood flow.

Just as I have ranked the interventions in the Omega Rx Zone Lifestyle Pyramid by order of hormonal importance, I can also rank these interventions on the basis of how much time they'll require from your busy life. Interestingly, the most important hormonal changes you can make are those that require the least time. Taking fish oil every day requires only fifteen seconds of your time (or three to five minutes if you are making a Big Brain Shake), compared with the twenty minutes required for daily meditation. Yet high-dose fish oil has a far greater hormonal impact. I created the Time Expenditure Pyramid on the next page to illustrate amount of hormonal benefits for time expended:

Time Expenditure Pyramid

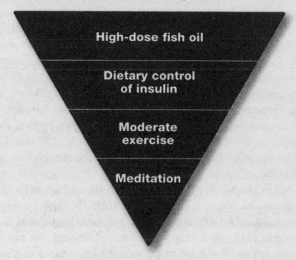

If you have only a few minutes (or seconds) a day to devote to a lifestyle change, then taking your high-dose fish oil will give you the maximum hormonal cluck for the buck. The other lifestyle interventions are good, but they are going to take more time to get the same level of hormonal benefits. This means that you would have to spend an extraordinary amount of time doing a lifestyle intervention like meditation to get the same hormonal benefits that you would get supplementing your diet with high-dose fish oil. Of course, the more lifestyle interventions you make, the better your overall health results. The choice is yours: how much time do you want to devote in order to control your future health?

WILL WE SURVIVE AS A SPECIES?

More ominously, I believe we're standing at the crossroads for our future as a species. Evolution is punctuated by abrupt starts and stops. Our own history as a species is no different. Some 150,000 years ago, modern humans suddenly emerged, after the some three million years that our rather puny ancestors had spent roaming in the African savanna. In fact, the archeological data strongly suggest that the precursors of modern humans may have been hanging by their fingertips over the precipice of extinction. Something earth-shattering happened that ensured the survival of our ancestors.

All available evidence points to the decision by our ancestors to begin to consume shellfish, rich in long-chain omega-3 fatty acids, as the defining moment that moved us forward in leaps and bounds through the evolutionary chain. If we are to ensure the long-term survival of our species, then we can't walk away from our nutritional heritage. If we do, we may disappear as quickly as we ascended.

We have to consider the possibility that human evolution is stalled because our current technology has negated the need for new biological adaptations to our environment. For example, we are not going to develop X-ray vision, since we have X-ray machines that do a better job than any genetic mutation ever could. Furthermore, there would be no survival advantage for those types of mutations. So if we are not evolving any more, is it possible that we may be in the process of de-evolution? I believe that as a species we're not currently anywhere close to realizing our potential intelligence, and that we're squandering our potential brain power by not consuming adequate levels of long-chain omega-3 fatty acids.

How many of us can say that our minds truly operate at peak efficiency? That we think with clarity, appreciate the world around us, feel joy in associating with others, and have a sense of spirituality that unifies us with all humankind? We all demand that our computers, cell phones, and cars operate at peak efficiency. Why do we demand less of our brains, our bodies, and our emotions?

As we move rapidly through the information era, we are beginning to lose sight of those very qualities that make us human. We've become more disjointed as a society and have weaker social bonds with our friends, coworkers, and families than previous generations had. People might say that we are evolving into a new society that doesn't need the support mechanisms of the past, but I doubt it. We've chosen to neglect our diets and shun the commonsense approach to life that our grandmothers advocated. Is it any wonder that we've seen a rise in violence, depression, and behavioral problems?

Politicians call this the breakdown of family values. I think it is more accurate to say that many of our social problems may be strongly linked to the dramatic depletion of long-chain omega-3 fatty acids in our diet. At the beginning of the twentieth century, the amount of omega-3 fatty acids in the American diet was relatively high. During the past hundred years, we've steadily decreased the long-chain omega-3 fatty acids in our diet and simultaneously increased the omega-6 fatty acids. I consider this to be the single greatest public health disaster in America over the past century because of its adverse impact on eicosanoid levels. I believe this one dietary change has caused more deaths than all the epidemics of infectious disease of the past century combined.

Don't despair, because within an incredibly short time, we can reverse the "de-evolution" of our society and get it going on a course to bring our species to a new higher level. Just start with yourself to get your mind and body in optimal working condition in a matter of weeks. And if it works for you, then tell your friends and family. After all, that is how all revolutions get started.

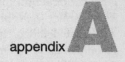

Continuing Support

By now, I hope you realize that reaching the Omega Rx Zone by following my dietary recommendations may be your most powerful "drug" for improving daily performance (both mental and physical), losing excess body fat, and living a longer and healthier life. This program isn't a short-term diet but a lifelong food management system for better health. You'll be able to achieve enhanced hormonal control with foods you already enjoy eating.

This is the ninth book I have written on the Zone. My first book, *The Zone,* was written primarily for cardiovascular physicians' patients to educate them about the power that food has to alter hormone levels. I specifically discussed how the levels of the hormones insulin, glucagon, and eicosanoids vary with the macronutrient composition of each meal. However, *The Zone* is not the best introduction for a beginner to understand how simple the dietary control of insulin can be. That's why I strongly recommend reading my mass-market paperback book, *A Week in the Zone,* as a great introduction to the basics. Two of my other books, *Zone-Perfect Meals in Minutes* and *Mastering the Zone,* provide more detailed "how-to" information about my dietary recommendations. Once you understand the basic logic of the Zone, you can refer back to *The Zone* to better understand the biochemistry behind it.

If you really want to learn how to reverse aging and extend your life, I strongly recommend reading *The Anti-Aging Zone.* This is a detailed discussion of the hormonal control that is the basis of my entire Zone technology. *The Anti-Aging Zone* provides the information and motivation to make your diet your lifelong ally to increase and enhance your longevity by reversing the aging process. This book completes the foundation of my Zone technology by providing the biochemical basis into the need for high-dose fish oil.

Although each of my books represents the latest research on the complex relationship between diet and hormonal response, the field is constantly changing. Access to up-to-the-minute information can be found on my website, *www.drsears.com,* which reviews the latest developments in this rapidly evolving field. In addition, I am constantly updating this site with new recipes (many of them vegetarian), new information about research, and simple tips on how to maintain yourself in the Omega Rx Zone on a lifelong basis.

Omega Rx Zone
Meals and Snacks

Since I didn't have space in this book to include hundreds of recipes for meals and snacks, I'd like to refer you to my previous books, including *Mastering the Zone,* which contains 150 classic recipes modified to meet my dietary recommendations; *Zone-Perfect Meals in Minutes,* which contains some 150 meals designed for type 2 diabetics; *The Soy Zone,* which has more than 100 meals designed for vegetarians; and *The Top 100 Zone Foods,* which contains 100 dishes designed around the primary food ingredients used to make Omega Rx Zone meals.

You can also log on to my website, *www.drsears.com,* which has dozens of recipes and is constantly being updated with new meal suggestions.

Your Biological Internet

Until recently, we thought of hormones mainly in terms of how wild they become during puberty. Now we see advertisements in every magazine referring to estrogen, testosterone, or growth hormone as the new elixirs of youth for an aging population.

While some hormones, like estrogen and testosterone, decrease with age, other hormones, such as insulin and "bad" eicosanoids, increase with age. These are the hormones that can be rapidly modified by my dietary recommendations. Ultimately, by controlling both insulin and eicosanoids, you will find the fountain of youth that so many are seeking.

What exactly is a hormone? A hormone can be considered any chemical that can transmit information. Essentially, hormones are messengers. Think of the computer-based Internet. What actually transmits the information through that system? It's electrons, but only if they travel through the right pathways. Hormones play the same role in your body, but they are far more complex in their interactions, thereby allowing information of greater texture and sophistication to be communicated.

The word *hormone* is derived from the Greek word meaning impelling, exciting, or setting into motion. Make no mistake about it: hormones are exciting because they hold the key to twenty-first-century medicine. They are hundreds of times more powerful than any drug. I believe that the most important hormones for the peak efficiency of your biological Internet are the ones controlled by the Omega Rx Zone diet: insulin and eicosanoids. This makes food potentially the most powerful drug of the twenty-first century.

The key to the Omega Rx Zone lies in understanding how hormones communicate to maintain equilibrium within your body. This is why I use the term *biological Internet* to describe that interaction.

WHAT IS YOUR BIOLOGICAL INTERNET?

Many people believe that the Internet is the wave of the future for humankind. It allows you to transmit great amounts of information almost instantaneously. We marvel at the technological brilliance that made the Internet possible. Yet within our bodies lies a biological Internet that is vastly more complex. Some sixty trillion cells need to maintain constant communication with one another. This communication system is controlled by hormones, in particular hormones that can be modified by my dietary program.

When your biological Internet is working well, you're in a state of *wellness*. But when it is giving garbled information, you're heading toward *chronic disease*. As I stated earlier in this book, the way to move from a state of chronic disease to a state of improved wellness is simply to reduce inflammation and increase blood flow, both of which are controlled by eicosanoids. This is why eicosanoid control is the core of your biological Internet.

HORMONES

The key players in the biological Internet are your hormones. Within your biological Internet there is a considerable subdivision of tasks, giving rise to three distinct classes of hormones called endocrine, paracrine, and autocrine. The differences between these types of hormones are best explained by an analogy to your telephone. Consider *endocrine* hormones to be like the microwave towers that send your telephone conversation into the air when you speak. Once the telephone signal is transmitted, it hopes to find the location it is being directed to. Likewise, endocrine hormones are sent from a secreting gland into the bloodstream with the eventual aim of finding the right cell (out of some sixty trillion other cells) to communicate its message. Just as the telephone conversation relies upon the microwave tower, a hormone needs to lock onto the right cell. That is done by receptors on the cell surface. The hormone attaches onto the cell receptor like a spacecraft docking at a space station.

Unlike endocrine hormones, *paracrine* hormones don't travel randomly in the bloodstream. They are cell-to-cell regulators that have very defined constraints on how far they can travel. In this respect, paracrine hormones are more like the physical telephone wires that come directly into your house after the signal is received by the microwave tower. From an evolutionary view, paracrine hormones are older than endocrine hormones, since they don't need a supporting system like a bloodstream to carry them. All they need is either a nerve or very short pathway from the secreting cell to the target cell. Neurotransmitters (like serotonin and dopamine) that control the information flow in your brain are paracrine hormones. These hormones can be increased by high-dose fish oil. Paracrine hormones also work by binding to receptors.

Predating the paracrine hormones in evolutionary time are the *autocrine* hormones. These hormones are a type of molecular scout: they are sent from a cell to test the immediate environment, and then come back to report to that cell what lies just outside its perimeter. These hormones also use receptors to report that information back to the cell. Taking our analogy one step further, autocrine hormones are similar to the receiver of your telephone. No matter how good the microwave towers (endocrine hormones) might be or what the fidelity of the information transmitted via the telephone wires (paracrine hormones) to your home might be, unless the receiver (autocrine hormones) works properly you are not going to have a telephone conversation. The most important autocrine hormones are the eicosanoids, because they ultimately drive your biological Internet just as electrons drive the Internet you access by your computer.

SECOND MESSENGERS

Second messengers are the ultimate key to hormonal action. Once a hormone, like insulin, docks onto a cell receptor, the receptor (which spans the membrane of the cell) undergoes a change that is transmitted to the interior of the cell. Depending on the receptor and the hormone that has activated it, another molecule is synthesized within the cell that completes the message. These new molecules are called second messengers. There are two primary second messengers for all cells. In essence, the complexity of hormonal interaction becomes reduced to a biochemical traffic signal with either a green or a red light.

Among the most important of these molecular traffic lights is cyclic AMP. (The Nobel Prize in medicine of 1971 was awarded for the discovery of this molecule.) Cyclic AMP can be considered the green light for the cell, and it starts a cascade of new molecule synthesis that tells the cell what to do. "Good" eicosanoids interact with receptors that produce this second messenger.

The other major second messenger system is called the inositol triphosphate/diacylglyccrol (IP_3/DAG) pathway. This is equivalent to a red light in the cell, since it usually has a physiological action opposite to that of cyclic AMP. Both insulin and "bad" eicosanoids use this pathway. Think of these second messengers as the internal traffic signals in each of your sixty trillion cells, as shown below.

Internal Traffic Signals

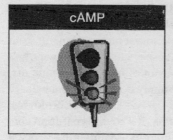
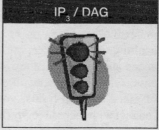

If the green and red lights are balanced and working smoothly, the result is wellness. If you have an excess of red lights, then your traffic signals are out of balance, then the result is the development of chronic disease. In the final analysis, the great complexity of your biological Internet comes down to maintaining the appropriate balance of green and red lights in each of the trillions of cells throughout your body.

If you simply took high-dose fish oil, you would automatically alter the balance of the traffic signals, since you would be making more "good" and fewer "bad" eicosanoids (see appendix D), thereby increasing the number of green lights. However, if your insulin level remains elevated, you will be constantly turning on more red lights. This is why controlling the production of both insulin and "bad" eicosanoids is so important in optimizing your biological Internet. By changing the levels of these second messengers, you can ultimately control cellular function moment by moment. It does little good to increase the number of green lights unless you are simultaneously reducing the number of red lights.

SUMMARY

Each of your sixty trillion cells is controlled by a traffic signal giving either a green or a red light that switches complex molecular functions on or off moment by moment. Your health depends on keeping these second messengers balanced and in sync. If they are out of balance, chronic disease is the consequence. By simply controlling the balance of green and red lights, you can control your biological Internet with incredible precision. It's no different from controlling traffic flow in any major city. Maintaining yourself in the Omega Rx Zone gives you that control, since you can now manipulate both insulin and eicosanoid levels. You can't completely control one without the other if your overall goal is maximizing your health.

Eicosanoids

Strange, mysterious, and almost mystical, eicosanoids are the key to our health because they control the flow of information in our biological Internet (see appendix C). Why are eicosanoids so important? They were the first hormones developed by living organisms, more than 500 million years ago. As such they can be considered "superhormones" because they control the actions of other hormones. Furthermore, you don't have an eicosanoid gland, since every one of your sixty trillion cells can make eicosanoids.

Even though they are the earliest hormones, eicosanoids were not identified until the twentieth century, starting with the discovery of essential fatty acids in 1929. It was found that if fat in the diet of rats was totally removed, the rats would soon die. Restoring certain essential fats (then called vitamin F) was found to enable fat-deprived rats to live. Eventually, as technology advanced, researchers realized that essential fats are composed of both omega-6 and omega-3 fatty acids that both need to be obtained in the diet because the body cannot synthesize them. The word *eicosanoids* is derived from the Greek word for twenty, *eicosa,* since all these hormones are synthesized from essential fatty acids that are twenty carbon atoms in length.

The first actual eicosanoids were discovered in 1936 by Ulf von Euler. These were isolated from the prostate gland (an exceptionally rich source of eicosanoids) and were called prostaglandins (a small subset of the much larger family of eicosanoids). Since it was thought at that time that all hormones had to originate from a discrete gland, it made perfect sense to call this new hormone a prostaglandin. With time it became clear that every living cell in the body could make eicosanoids, and that no discrete organ or gland was the center of eicosanoid synthesis.

To date, biochemists have identified more than a hundred eicosanoids and are finding more each year. The breakthrough in research on eicosanoids occurred in 1971, when John Vane finally discovered how aspirin (the wonder drug of the twentieth century) actually works: it changes the levels of eicosanoids. The Nobel Prize in medicine for 1982 was awarded to Vane and his colleagues Bengt Samuelsson and Sune Bergstrom for their discovery of how eicosanoids play a role in human disease.

MY JOURNEY INTO EICOSANOID RESEARCH

This is where my journey with eicosanoids first started twenty years ago. It was apparent to me that if certain "bad" eicosanoids were associated with chronic disease conditions (heart disease, cancer, arthritis, and so on), the key to wellness would be to induce the body to make more "good" eicosanoids and fewer "bad" eicosanoids. Rather than using drugs to achieve that goal, I reasoned that I could use food *as if* it were a drug. All I needed to do was figure out the right balance of protein, carbohydrate, and fat that would turn food into this beneficial "drug." After more than twenty years, I think I've come pretty close to that "drug" with the Omega Rx Zone.

Of course, my colleagues in academic medicine didn't quite share my initial enthusiasm. Almost overnight, I went from being a respected research scientist with numerous patents in intravenous delivery systems for cancer drugs to being called a snake-oil salesman because of my constant refrain that the appropriate diet could change the balance of eicosanoids throughout the body. Part of the problem was that very few of my colleagues even knew what an eicosanoid was.

I believe that the foundation of twenty-first-century medicine will be the manipulation of eicosanoids. Yet ask most physicians and medical researchers what an eicosanoid is, and you will usually get a blank stare. I guess they're not familiar with the Nobel Prize–winning research. As unknown as they are to the medical community, eicosanoids are the hormones that maintain the information fidelity of your biological Internet, and this means that they become the key to health and longevity.

If eicosanoids are so important, why are they so unknown? First, they are made, act, and self-destruct within seconds and thus are very difficult to study. Second, they don't circulate in the bloodstream and thus are extremely difficult to sample. Finally, they work at vanishingly low concentrations and thus are almost impossible to detect. Despite these difficulties, more than 87,000 articles on eicosanoids have been published in peer-reviewed journals. So the basic research community is interested in eicosanoids, even if your doctor never learned about them in medical school.

Eicosanoids encompass a wide array of hormones, many

of which endocrinologists have never heard of. They are derived from a unique group of polyunsaturated essential fatty acids containing twenty carbon atoms. The classes of eicosanoids are shown below

Subgroups of Eicosanoids

- Prostaglandins
- Thromboxanes
- Leukotrienes
- Lipoxins
- Hydroxylated fatty acids
- Aspirin-triggered epi-lipoxins
- Isoprostanoids
- Epoxyeicosatrienoic acids
- Endocannabinoids

If you mention the word *prostaglandins* to physicians, they are likely to have heard of those hormones. However, prostaglandins are only a small subgroup of the eicosanoid family. Some of the other subgroups have been discovered only recently. For example, aspirin-triggered epi-lipoxins, which give rise to the powerful anti-inflammatory properties described in the chapter on heart disease, were discovered only a few years ago.

The glory days of eicosanoid research lie ahead, with continual discoveries of new eicosanoids and a growing realization of the vast role these hormones play in controlling other hormonal systems. This fact has not been lost on pharmaceutical companies, which have already spent billions of dollars trying to develop eicosanoid-based drugs. Eicosanoids as drugs, however, have a very limited role in the world of pharmaceuticals. They are not only difficult to work with but also too powerful to be used as a drug.

However, there does remain one way to manipulate eicosanoids directly: the Omega Rx Zone diet. The reason the Omega Rx Zone diet can be successful when the largest drug companies have been unsuccessful is based on evolution. Eicosanoids were the first hormonal control system that living organisms developed. You can't have organized life unless you have cell membranes separating the internal workings of the cell from its environment. Since all cell membranes contain fatty acids (including the building blocks of eicosanoids, which are known as essential fatty acids), the cell's own membrane became the ideal reservoir for eicosanoid·synthesis—you could always be certain that the raw materials for making these hormones were close by.

As autocrine hormones, eicosanoids have a mission: to be secreted by the cell to test the external environment and then report back to the cell what was just outside by interacting with its receptor on the cell surface. On the basis of that information, the cell could take the appropriate biological action (via the appropriate second messenger) to respond to any change in its environment.

In biotechnology, one of the hot research areas today is biological response modifiers. Eicosanoids represent the first (and probably the most powerful) biological response modifiers developed by living organisms. In fact, many of the eicosanoids that we make in our bodies today are identical to ones made by sponges beginning hundreds of millions of years ago.

Eicosanoids play such a central role in our physiology because of second messengers that certain eicosanoids generate. There are various eicosanoid receptors on the surface of the cell, and depending on which eicosanoid interacts with a particular receptor, a specific second messenger is synthesized by the cell. Sometimes a second messenger, such as cyclic AMP, is generated; sometimes a totally different second messenger, such as the DAG and IP_3 system, is generated. If one second messenger goes up, the other goes down. In essence, the complexity of your biological Internet is reduced to a digital system consisting of green and red lights.

The eicosanoids that generate increased production of cyclic AMP are your key to maintaining wellness. Why? Cyclic AMP is the second messenger used by a number of endocrine hormones in the body to translate their biological information to the appropriate target cell. By maintaining adequate cellular levels of eicosanoids that increase cyclic AMP levels, you ensure that a certain baseline level of cyclic AMP is always present in a cell. Thus, it's far more likely that the overall cyclic AMP level in the cell will be high enough to guarantee an appropriate biological response, and therefore, better hormonal communication.

HOW CAN YOU TELL A "GOOD" EICOSANOID FROM A "BAD" EICOSANOID?

An eicosanoid's effect on second messengers becomes the definition of a "good" or "bad" eicosanoid. A "good" eicosanoid will increase the levels of cyclic AMP in a cell, whereas a "bad" eicosanoid will decrease the levels of cyclic AMP by elevating the IP_3/DAG second messengers. The table on the next page lists "good" and "bad" eicosanoids and the receptors with which they interact.

Receptors for "Good" and "Bad" Eicosanoids

	Receptor	Effect on Cyclic AMP
"Good" Eicosanoids		
PGE_1	EP2, EP4	increase
PGI_2	IP	increase
PGD_2	DP	increase
"Bad" Eicosanoids		
TXA_2	TP	decrease
PGE_2	EP1, EP3	decrease
PGF_{2a}	FP	decrease
LTB_4	BLT	decrease
LTC_4	Cys-LT1	decrease
LTD_4, LTE_4	Cys-LT2	decrease

Once an eicosanoid interacts with its unique receptor, a second messenger is synthesized inside in the target cell. If a "good" eicosanoid interacts with the right receptor, cyclic AMP is the second messenger that is formed. On the other hand, if a "bad" eicosanoid interacts with its receptor, then cyclic AMP levels are decreased. Adding to this complexity is the fact that some eicosanoids, such as PGA and PGJ, are cyclopentenone eicosanoids. These eicosanoids don't have cell receptors on the surface, as they can directly enter into the cell, where they can interact with the cell's nucleus to affect cellular growth and differentiation.

Since there is no discrete eicosanoid "gland," there is no central site that turns eicosanoid action "on" or "off." Nature solved this problem by developing different types of eicosanoids that have diametrically opposed physiological actions. The balance of these opposing actions of different eicosanoids creates an equilibrium of biological activity. These differences in biological actions are the foundation for the eicosanoid "axis."

This eicosanoid "axis" is composed of "good" eicosanoids on one side and "bad" eicosanoids on the other. Before the evolutionary development of more advanced hormonal systems (like corticosteroids) to help control this eicosanoid activity, the balance of "good" and "bad" eicosanoids was the best solution available. Obviously, there is no such thing as an absolutely "good" eicosanoid or an absolutely "bad" eicosanoid, since both are required for optimal health.

Most chronic diseases, however, are a consequence of an imbalance of "good" and "bad" eicosanoids. I have already discussed in this book the role of eicosanoids in heart disease, cancer, diabetes, arthritis, and depression, among other disorders. The Nobel Prize in medicine of 1982 gave me an insight into the molecular nature of chronic disease, since it could be viewed as an imbalance in eicosanoid levels. It became apparent to me at the same time that the appropriate balance of eicosanoids could provide a molecular definition of wellness. In essence, the more the balance of eicosanoids is tilted toward "bad" eicosanoids, the more likely you are to develop chronic disease. Conversely, the more the balance is tilted toward "good" eicosanoids, the greater the chance that you'll achieve wellness and longevity. The AA/EPA ratio in the blood will indicate where you stand in terms of such a balance.

If you are skeptical about the statement that eicosanoids play a fundamental role in such a number of diverse disease conditions, ask any physician what happens when a high dose of corticosteroids is given to a patient for more than thirty days. The answer will be physiological devastation, if not death. This occurs because corticosteroids have only one mode of action: they knock out all eicosanoid production—"good" and "bad"—by inhibiting the release of essential fatty acids from the cell membrane. This chokes off any supply of precursors to make any type of eicosanoid. Without eicosanoids, you can't survive.

HOW EICOSANOIDS ARE SYNTHESIZED

Since eicosanoids are produced in every cell—not one specific gland—it's as if you had sixty trillion separate eicosanoid glands capable of making these exceptionally powerful hormones. The endocrine hormones are under the control of the hypothalamus in the brain, but there is no such central control site for eicosanoids. Rather than responding to some master signal, each cell responds to changes in its immediate environment. The first step in generating a cellular response is the actual release of an essential fatty acid from the phospholipids in the cell membrane. The enzyme responsible for the release of the essential fatty acid is called phospholipase A_2.

Since there is no feedback loop to stop the production of eicosanoids, the only way to inhibit their release from the membrane is by the production of corticosteroids (such as cortisol) from the adrenal gland, which causes the synthesis of a protein (lipocortin) that inhibits the action of phospholipase A_2. By inhibiting this enzyme, which releases essential fatty acids from the cell membranes, you choke off the supply of a substrate required for all eicosanoid synthesis. Obviously, if you are overproducing cortisol (or taking corticosteroid drugs), you will bring all eicosanoid synthesis to a crashing halt, which can cause the shutdown of your immune system.

The most powerful eicosanoid-modulating drugs are corticosteroids. As I mentioned above, they inhibit the release of any essential fatty acid so that no eicosanoids can be synthesized. Obviously, if you have intense pain or inflammation, this may be your only course of action on a short-term basis. Over the long term, corticosteroid therapy lowers the response of your immune system, decreases cognitive function, increases fat stores, thins the skin, and accelerates osteoporosis. In fact, if you give a single injection of corticosteroids to healthy individuals, within twenty-four hours their lymphocytes will show a pattern very similar to that in AIDS patients.

ENZYMES THAT MAKE EICOSANOIDS

There are three primary pathways a long-chained essential fatty acid (composed of a string of twenty carbon atoms), once released from the cell membrane, can follow. The first is the cyclo-oxygenase system (COX) that makes prostaglandins and thromboxanes. In this pathway the highly contorted essential fatty acid is closed in on itself to form a prostanoid ring. The second is the 5-lipoxygenase (5-LIPO) pathway that makes leukotrienes. There is a third pathway in which a 20-carbon essential fatty acid is simply modified via either the 12- or the 15-lipoxygenase (12- or 15-LIPO) enzymes as in the case of hydroxylated essential fatty acids and lipoxins. It is on this third pathway that many of the newly discovered eicosanoids are made. The pathways are shown on the next page.

Certain drugs can inhibit the cyclo-oxygenase pathway of eicosanoid formation. The best-known is aspirin, which literally destroys a cyclo-oxygenase enzyme on a one-on-one basis. This is what is known as a suicide inhibitor. When you are suffering from a headache or arthritic pain, you are overproducing "bad" eicosanoids, in particular "bad" prostaglandins. Aspirin temporarily shuts down all prostaglandin formation (but not leukotriene formation), until the cell can make more of the cyclo-oxygenase enzyme to replace the ones destroyed by the aspirin. However, you can't be using these suicidal soldiers forever, as aspirin also

Types of Eicosanoid-Synthesizing Enzymes

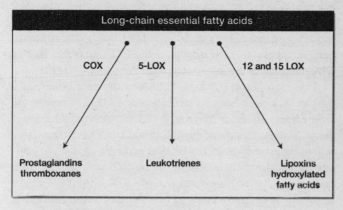

shuts down the synthesis of "good" prostaglandins, especially those that protect the stomach from dissolving itself. When that happens, you get internal bleeding. This is why there are more than 10,000 deaths per year associated with the overuse of aspirin. Other drugs known as nonsteroidal anti-inflammatory drugs (NSAIDs) also inhibit the cyclo-oxygenase enzyme but not the lipo-oxygenase enzyme that makes leukotrienes. Common names for these NSAIDs are Motrin, Advil, Aleve, and others. Continued use of these NSAIDs generates the same problems as long-term use of aspirin.

COX Enzymes

The most common types of anti-inflammatory drugs are those that can affect only those eicosanoids synthesized by the cyclo-oxygenase enzymes or COX. It was recently discovered that there are two forms of this enzyme; they are known as COX-1 and COX-2. COX-1 enzymes are a constant fixture of the vascular cells that line the bloodstream or in stomach cells that secrete bicarbonate to neutralize stomach acid. COX-2 appears to be an enzyme that is synthesized only in response to inflammation. Standard drugs like aspirin and NSAIDs (such as Advil) don't discriminate between these specific forms of the COX enzyme; that is why side effects are associated with their long-term use.

For example, it appears that the anticancer benefits of aspirin may stem from its inhibition of COX-2, whereas the side effects (like an increased risk of internal bleeding) come from its simultaneous inhibition of COX-1. However, this same inhibition of the COX-1 enzyme appears to convey the cardiovascular benefits associated with aspirin. This may explain why long-term use of COX-2 inhibitors may not work to decrease rates of heart attack: these inhibitors don't target the COX-1 enzyme. Weighing the risks against the benefits presents a dilemma associated with all drugs that affect eicosanoid synthesis.

LOX Enzymes

Unlike inhibitors of the COX enzymes, inhibitors of the LOX enzymes are few in number. Since leukotrienes (particularly LTB_4) represent a primary mediator of pain, the only way to affect their production is to use corticosteroids, with all their associated side effects. However, the leukotrienes synthesized from EPA are physiologically neuter compared with those derived from arachidonic acid. This is why the AA/EPA ratio is a very good indicator of the body's potential to prevent the overproduction of leukotrienes without resorting to corticosteroids.

Overlooked in this frantic search by drug companies seeking new and more expensive drugs to go downstream to modify eicosanoid synthesis is the fact that an existing "drug" can achieve all these benefits without any side effects. This is because it goes upstream to modify eicosanoid production by reducing levels of arachidonic acid. That "drug" is high-dose fish oil, since the elevated levels of EPA will reduce the production of "bad" eicosanoids (such as PGE_2 and LTB_4) derived from arachidonic acid.

SYNTHESIS OF ESSENTIAL FATTY ACIDS

To understand the importance of diet in controlling these eicosanoids and reestablishing an appropriate eicosanoid balance, we have to understand how the actual precursors of eicosanoids are made. To begin with, all eicosanoids ultimately are produced from essential fatty acids that the body cannot make and that therefore must be part of the diet. These essential fatty acids are classified as either omega-3 or omega-6 depending on the position of the double bonds within them. Typical essential fatty acids are only eighteen carbons in length and must be elongated to twenty-carbon fatty acids by the body before eicosanoids can be made. Remember that all eicosanoids come from essential fatty acids twenty carbon atoms in length. It is not just the number of carbon atoms that counts but also their configuration. Eicosanoid precursors must have a certain spatial configuration with at least three double bonds in order to be converted into an eicosanoid. How your diet controls the formation of dietary essential fatty acids into the actual twenty-carbon atom precursors of eicosanoids is a complex story.

The discovery of essential fatty acids was first reported in 1929. At that time essential fatty acids were called vitamin F. But vitamin F was useless unless transformed into an eicosanoid. Thus began a seventy-year attempt to understand how your diet does three things: controls eicosanoid formation, alters eicosanoid balance in the body, and determines how eicosanoids become central players in your health.

The differences between the two classes of essential fatty acids, omega-6 and omega-3, are based on the position of the double bonds within the fatty acid molecule. This is important, since the positioning of these double bonds dictates their three-dimensional structure in space, which ultimately determines how they interact with their appropriate receptors. Although the synthesis of essential fatty acids involves the same enzymes, the metabolic pathways are quite different. The metabolism of long-chain omega-3 fatty acids is more complex, so let's start with the simpler pathway to make omega-6 fatty acids.

Omega-6 Fatty Acids

There are two steps in this process, which ultimately determine the amount of eicosanoid building blocks that will be made. These are known in biochemistry as rate-limiting steps. The first rate-limiting step is controlled by the enzyme delta 6-desaturase. This enzyme inserts a necessary third double bond in the essential fatty acid in just the right position to begin bending inward and forms gamma linolenic acid (GLA) from linoleic acid, as shown in the figure on the next page.

(The number after the C tells how many carbon atoms the essential fatty acid contains, and the number after the colon tells how many double bonds there are in the essential fatty acid.)

I define an activated essential fatty acid as any essential fatty acid that has this new double bond inserted by the delta 6-desaturase enzyme. This is because the new double bond starts bending the essential fatty acid to get the appropriate spatial configuration required to make an eicosanoid. Once

Synthesis of Long-Chain Omega-6 Essential Fatty Acids

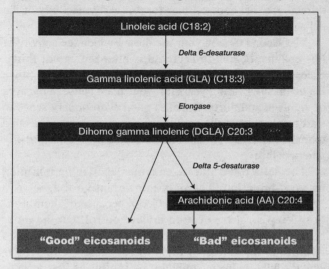

this new double bond has been inserted into a short-chain essential fatty acid, very small amounts of these activated essential fatty acids can profoundly affect the eicosanoid balance in your body.

However, there are many factors that can decrease the activity of delta 6-desaturase enzyme. The most important factor is age itself. There are two times in your life during which this enzyme is relatively inactive. The first is at birth. For the first six months of life, the activity of this key enzyme is relatively low. But this is also the time when maximum amounts of long-chain essential fatty acids are required, since the brain is growing at the fastest possible rate, and these long-chain essential fatty acids are the building blocks for the brain. Nature has developed a unique solution to this problem: breast milk. Breast milk is very rich in GLA and other long-chain essential fatty acids such as EPA and DHA. Supplying these activated essential fatty acids through the diet compensates for this early inactivity of the delta 6-desaturase enzyme.

The second time in your life during which the activity of this enzyme begins to decrease is after the age of thirty. Eicosanoids are critical for successful reproduction. Since the main childbearing years for women are between the ages of eighteen and thirty, it makes good evolutionary sense to start turning down the activity of a critical enzyme needed to make the precursors of eicosanoids required for fertility after age thirty.

The delta 6-desaturase enzyme can also be inhibited by viral infection. The only known antiviral agent is a "good" eicosanoid (such as PGA_1), because of their ability to keep viral replication under control. On the other hand, if you are a virus, then your number one goal is to inhibit the formation of this type of eicosanoid. This is exactly what many viruses do, by inhibiting the delta 6-desaturase enzyme. The virus has thus devised an incredibly clever way to circumvent the body's primary antiviral drug (PGA_1).

The final factor that can decrease the activity of delta 6-desaturase is the presence of two types of fatty acids in your diet; trans fats and omega-3 fats. Trans fatty acids don't exist naturally but are produced by food manufacturers. They are essential omega-6 fatty acids that have been transformed by a commercial process (known as hydrogenation) into a new spatial configuration that is more stable to prevent oxidation. The increased stability of trans fatty acids makes them ideal for processed foods but also makes them strong inhibitors of the delta 6-desaturase enzyme. Trans fatty acids occupy the active site of the delta 6-desaturase enzyme, thus preventing the formation of the activated essential fatty acids required for eicosanoid synthesis. In

essence, trans fatty acids can be viewed as anti–essential
fatty acids because of their inhibition of eicosanoid synthesis. This may be the reason why they are strongly implicated in the development of heart disease. How do you know
if a food product you're consuming contains trans fatty
acids? Look for the words *partially hydrogenated vegetable
oil* on the label. Surprisingly, omega-3 fats can also inhibit
the delta 6-desaturase enzyme activity in producing GLA,
as the short-chain omega-3 fatty acids such as alpha
linolenic acid (ALA) preferentially bind to the enzyme,
thus decreasing GLA synthesis, and the long-chain omega-
3 fatty acids such as DHA acts as feedback inhibitors of the
enzyme.

The journey toward becoming an eicosanoid is still far
from over after the first hurdle—making GLA—has been
passed. Once GLA is formed, it is rapidly elongated into
dihomo gamma linolenic acid (DGLA), which is the precursor of many "good" eicosanoids. However, DGLA is also
the substrate for the other rate-limiting enzyme in the essential fatty acid cascade in the chart on page 307. That enzyme
is called delta 5-desaturase. Its activity ultimately controls
the balance of "good" and "bad" eicosanoids, and so altering its activity by the Omega Rx Zone diet is your primary
concern if your goal is to treat chronic disease and promote
wellness.

This is because the end product that the delta 5-
desaturase enzyme creates from DGLA is arachidonic acid
(AA). DGLA is the building block of many of the "good"
eicosanoids, whereas AA is the building block of "bad"
eicosanoids, and therefore excess amounts of AA will
accelerate the development of chronic disease. Ultimately,
it is the balance between DGLA and AA in every one of
your sixty trillion cells that determines which types of
eicosanoids you will produce. You need some AA to pro-

duce some "bad" eicosanoids, but in the case of excess production of AA, the balance of eicosanoids will shift toward accelerated aging and chronic disease.

Many of the eicosanoids derived from arachidonic acid can be considered "bad" because they promote inflammation (PGE_2 and LTB_4) and decrease blood flow (TXA_2). In addition, the inflammatory "bad" eicosanoids can also promote the release of other pro-inflammatory cytokines.

While eicosanoids from arachidonic acid are bewilderingly complex, only a very limited number of eicosanoids come from dihomo gamma linolenic acid, as shown below.

Some of the Eicosanoids Derived from Arachidonic Acid

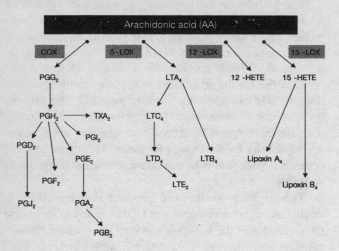

Eicosanoids Derived from DGLA

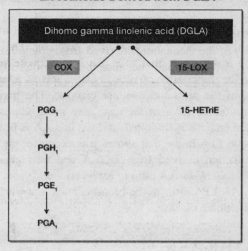

The primary eicosanoid derived from DGLA is PGE_1, one of the most highly studied "good" eicosanoids, as it is a very powerful vasodilator and inhibitor of platelet aggregation. It also reduces the secretion of insulin and increases the synthesis of a wide variety of hormones that normally decrease during the aging process. PGE_1 is able to carry out these diverse functions because it causes an increase in the production of cyclic AMP. Another eicosanoid derived from DGLA is PGA_1, which is the most powerful suppressor of viral replication, especially HIV transcription. PGA_1 also inhibits the nuclear transcription factor (NF kappa B), necessary for synthesis of a wide variety of pro-inflammatory cytokines, thus making it another anti-inflammatory eicosanoid. Finally, the 15-LOX enzyme can convert DGLA into a powerful inhibitor (15 = HETriE) of the 5-LOX enzyme that decreases leukotriene synthesis. You can see that having higher levels of DGLA relative to AA is an important factor in decreasing inflammation and increasing blood flow.

How do you help your body block excess AA formation and tilt the balance back toward a favorable DGLA/AA ratio? By making sure that your diet has adequate amounts of EPA. The importance of EPA is that it acts as a feedback inhibitor of the delta 5-desaturase enzyme. The higher the concentration of EPA in the diet, the more the delta 5-desaturase enzyme is inhibited, and the less AA is produced. As a result, EPA in the diet allows you to control the rate of AA production derived from DGLA and thus generate a favorable DGLA-to-AA ratio in each cell membrane. This is why the AA/EPA ratio in the blood is such a powerful predictor of chronic disease.

Omega-3 Fatty Acids

The synthesis of long-chain omega-3 fatty acids is much more complex, as shown on the next page.

The synthesis of EPA is seemingly relatively straightforward from the short-chain omega-3 fatty acid, alpha linolenic acid (ALA), just as the synthesis of arachidonic acid is from its short-chain precursor, linoleic acid. However, ALA is an inhibitor of the delta 6-desaturase enzyme. This inhibition makes the formation of EPA much more difficult than it should be. This is why human studies have indicated that the efficiency of making EPA from ALA is extremely limited. Therefore, if you want to get the greatest benefit of EPA, it will have to come from eating fish oil as opposed to vegetable sources rich in ALA (such as flaxseed).

Synthesis of Long-Chain Omega-3 Fatty Acids

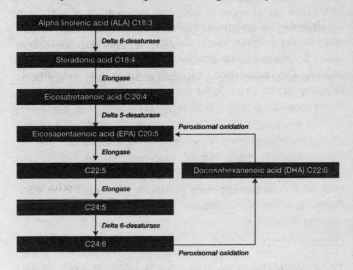

The situation is even more complex when EPA must further be metabolized to make DHA, which is critical for the brain. The EPA must be elongated twice more and then converted again by the delta 6-desaturase enzyme to the actual precursor of DHA, which then must be shortened by peroxisomal enzymes into DHA. The result is that the synthesis of DHA from ALA is even more difficult than the synthesis of EPA (which isn't very good to begin with). Furthermore, DHA acts as a feedback inhibitor of the delta 6-desaturase enzyme that further reduces the flow of ALA to EPA and DHA. You can begin to see why before modern humans started eating shellfish some 150,000 years ago, their ability to obtain adequate levels of long-chain omega-3 fatty acids for the brain was highly compromised.

DHA can also be retroconverted into EPA by the same

peroxisomal enzymes used to make DHA in the first place. Although the process is not very efficient, it at least is a mechanism by which vegetarian sources (genetically modified algae) of DHA can provide EPA. This retroconversion process appears to be a more efficient way of making EPA for someone following a vegetarian diet than is its synthesis from ALA.

This is why long-chain omega-3 fatty acids, like EPA, are so important in my dietary program. EPA inhibits the delta 5-desaturase enzyme, thereby restricting the flow of any omega-6 fatty acids into arachidonic acid and decreasing the production of "bad" eicosanoids. As long as you are consuming very moderate amounts of omega-6 fatty acids with adequate levels of EPA, the dietary omega-6 fatty acids tend to accumulate at the level of DGLA (because of the inhibition of delta 5-desaturase by the EPA), and this increases the production of "good" eicosanoids. However, the total amount of omega-3 and omega-6 fatty acid you need is relatively low. This means that you still have to add some fat to your diet to help slow the rate of entry of carbohydrate and thus control insulin secretion. And the fat should be primarily monounsaturated fat. Monounsaturated fats can't be made into eicosanoids ("good" or "bad"). Because they have no effect on eicosanoids or insulin, monounsaturated fats can provide the necessary amount of fat for controlling the entry rate of carbohydrates into the bloodstream without disturbing the hormonal balances that you are trying to achieve in the Omega Rx Zone.

THE SPILLOVER EFFECT

In the early days, I thought that simply providing low levels of EPA and adding the right amount of GLA would be all that I needed to control eicosanoids. Taking all the data into account, including the increasing overconsumption of omega-6 fatty acids in general, I believed that one ratio of EPA to GLA would work for everyone. In retrospect this thinking was obviously flawed, but since I had a background in pharmaceutical drug delivery, it seemed logical at the time. So I started out with one particular ratio, made some soft gelatin capsules containing both fish oil (the source of EPA) and borage oil (the source of GLA), and found some friends who were willing to be guinea pigs. I gave them my standard phrase, "Trust me."

Since I was working only on changing fatty acid levels during this early phase of my research, my initial observations on eicosanoids were not confounded by other potentially hormonal-modulating approaches, like controlling insulin. I had a very targeted approach, focusing solely on manipulating eicosanoid levels through dietary supplementation with defined amounts of activated essential fatty acids. And many of the physiological changes I observed occurred within weeks, if not days.

The time frame for these physiological actions was important because it was much shorter than the reported responses for treatments that focus on the restoration of endocrine hormones. With those treatments, it usually takes weeks, if not months, to see measurable effects.

After several months, however, I noticed that strange things seemed to be happening. Virtually all those who took the combination of EPA and GLA felt much better initially. After all, they were now making more "good" and fewer "bad" eicosanoids, since I was changing the DGLA/AA balance in the cells. With time, some people mentioned that they seemed to have stabilized or that they were even seeing a drop-off in the benefits they had experienced at first. Nonetheless, they still felt better than they had before they started. However, there was another, smaller group, who saw their initial benefits erode completely and actually began to feel worse than when they started. Some of my friends were no longer quite so friendly, until I figured out what was happening. I called it the "spillover" effect.

Initially, as the ratio of DGLA to AA improves, a person begins making more "good" eicosanoids and fewer "bad" ones. Everything just keeps getting better. But there will be some point in time, depending on your biochemistry, when the initial DGLA/AA ratio begins to degrade as more of the DGLA gets converted into AA. People still feel better than they did when they started, but not quite as good as at first. For some people, this degradation of the DGLA/AA ratio continues to a point when they begin to feel worse than they felt when they first started the program, because they are now making many more "bad" eicosanoids. This is shown in the figure below.

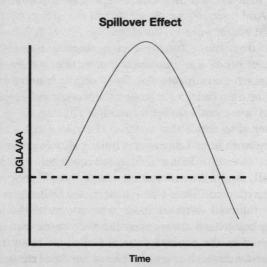

Spillover Effect

These people had developed a buildup of DGLA in their cells. The increased levels of DGLA were providing more substrate for the delta 5-desaturase enzyme to make more AA. The increase in DGLA was overwhelming the amount of EPA being supplied to inhibit the delta 5-desaturase enzyme. This spillover effect seemed to occur more often in females than in males. So much for the "one size fits all" ratio of GLA to EPA.

So I decided that if one size does not fit all, I had better start making a wide array of different EPA and GLA combinations and fine-tune them for each individual. But how could I do this? Fortunately, eicosanoids leave a biochemical audit trail that gives an insight into their actual balance in different organs in the body. That's what led me to develop my Eicosanoid Status Report to provide information on how to alter the amounts and ratios of activated essential fatty acids to fine-tune these exceptionally powerful hormones. (Now the AA/EPA test makes it even more precise.)

By 1989, I thought I had finally gotten this concept down to a science—although a more complex science than I had originally thought, but one still governed by some basic biochemical rules. However, what finally gave me the insight into the Omega Rx Zone was my work with elite athletes.

I began to notice that some of the elite athletes I was working with would have great training sessions but then not do as well during competition. Others would do extremely well. When I started to ask them if they were doing anything different with regard to diet before a competition, it turned out that those who were carbohydrate-loading beforehand always appeared to do worse than those who maintained a consistent diet. I racked my brain trying to understand what had gone wrong or what had changed to explain this sudden shift in their eicosanoid status. Then it struck me. It was carbohydrate-loading that was increasing their insulin levels.

A trip to the bowels of the MIT library confirmed my suspicion. There I found published research demonstrating that high levels of insulin activate the delta 5-desaturase enzyme. All the hormonal benefits I had carefully crafted for each athlete to manipulate the ratio of DGLA to AA were being undermined by the surge of insulin caused by elevated carbohydrate intake. This increase in insulin stimulated the delta 5-desaturase enzyme to increase the production of AA at the expense of DGLA. For these athletes, the result was that a highly favorable DGLA/AA ratio created during training quickly became a very undesirable ratio at the time of competition. It was the same spillover effect that I had observed in the early days of learning how to fine-tune eicosanoid levels. At this point I knew that I would never be able to control eicosanoid levels without controlling insulin first. It was back to the drawing board.

Is there any confirming evidence that high levels of insulin would affect the DGLA/AA ratio in humans? Fortunately, this information was published in 1991. In that research, a high level of insulin was maintained for six hours in both normal subjects and patients with type 2 diabetes (who characteristically have excessive insulin levels). After only six hours of exposure to elevated insulin levels, the ratio of DGLA to AA in the bloodstream in both healthy individuals and type 2 diabetics had dropped by nearly 50 percent. The elite athletes who were carbo-loading before competition were suffering the same decrease in the DGLA/AA ratio by eating more high-density carbohydrates (grains, pasta, and starches), thus increasing insulin, which caused a rapid deterioration of the DGLA/AA ratio and a decrease in their performance.

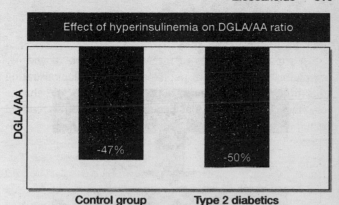

Effect of hyperinsulinemia on DGLA/AA ratio

DGLA/AA

-47%   -50%

Control group   Type 2 diabetics

Now the metabolism of activated essential fatty acids had to be modified to take into account the role of insulin on the delta 5-desaturase enzyme. This is shown above.

Insulin was an activator of the delta 5-desaturase enzyme. The role of excess insulin in negatively affecting the eicosanoid balance also explained why excess insulin was highly associated with heart disease. Insulin was not a direct cause, but it drove the metabolism of essential fatty acids to make more arachidonic acid and therefore more "bad" eicosanoids. The more "bad" eicosanoids you make, the more likely you are to promote platelet aggregation and increased vasoconstriction, the underlying factors for a heart attack.

I knew that the only way to control insulin was to control the protein-to-carbohydrate ratio at every meal. Again I was confronted by a question: What was the optimal ratio of protein to carbohydrate? A good beginning was to attempt to estimate the protein-to-carbohydrate ratio consumed by neo-Paleolithic humans some 10,000 to 40,000 years ago, since our genes haven't changed very much since then.

Fortunately, such an estimate did exist in research pub-

Effect of Elevated Insulin on the Synthesis of Activated

Omega-6 Essential Fatty Acids

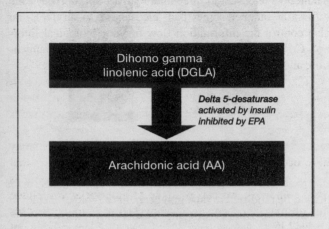

lished in 1985 in the *New England Journal of Medicine*. Using anthropological data and comparing a large number of existing hunter-gatherer tribes, the researchers estimated the average protein-to-carbohydrate ratio in the neo-Paleolithic diet as approximately 3 grams of protein for every 4 grams of carbohydrate, or 0.75. Using this research as a starting point, I began developing a diet that would maintain the protein-to-carbohydrate ratio in a range between 0.5 and 1.0 at every meal so that the balance of insulin and glucagon would be maintained from meal to meal. This is the foundation of the insulin-control component of my dietary recommendations.

Thus, my dietary program controls both the ratio of long-chain omega-3 fatty acids to omega-6 fatty acids and the balance of protein to carbohydrate at every meal. This dietary strategy maintains the dynamic balance of eicosanoids by controlling the levels of the actual precursors and the hormones responsible for activating the critical enzymes in essential fatty acid metabolism. By keeping the balance of eicosanoid precursors in an appropriate zone (after all, you need some "bad" eicosanoids to survive), you also control the information flow of your biological Internet. Control that flow to avoid hormonal miscommunication, and you have begun to reverse the aging process.

The development of chronic diseases associated with aging (heart disease, diabetes, cancer, and arthritis) does not occur overnight but is a result of constant hormonal insults to your body. But by the time these diseases do appear, significant (and potentially irreversible) organ damage may have occurred. If eicosanoids act as master hormones that control this complex hormonal communication system, is there some way we can continue to monitor and fine-tune this ultimate mechanism of aging before chronic diseases appear? If so, then you could tell when you are moving out of the appropriate eicosanoid zone and take immediate dietary steps to restore that balance. There are very few direct diagnostic tests for eicosanoids. However, the ratio of AA to EPA plasma phospholipids in blood will provide a remarkably good insight into your eicosanoid status. More important, this is a blood parameter that can be changed rapidly within thirty days by following the Omega Rx Zone diet.

Understanding Carbohydrates

Success in controlling insulin using my dietary program depends on restricting the amount of carbohydrates consumed while maximizing the vitamins and minerals derived from them. Your first step is to recognize what a carbohydrate is. Yes, carbohydrates include pasta and sweets, but they also include fruits and vegetables. An easy way to distinguish carbohydrates from protein is this mnemonic: "Carbohydrates grow in the ground and don't move around." Obviously pasta must be a carbohydrate, since it comes from wheat, which grows in the ground. Likewise, vegetables, such as broccoli, grow in the ground, so they, too, must be carbohydrates. Finally, fruits, such as apples, come from trees that grow in the ground, and this makes them carbohydrates as well. Protein (with the exception of soy) comes from animal sources that move around—like fish, chickens, and cows.

INSULIN-STIMULATING CARBOHYDRATE CONTENT

Since my dietary plan requires consistent insulin control, you need to realize that not all carbohydrates affect insulin secretion equally. Every complex carbohydrate must be broken down into simple sugars, which eventually enter the bloodstream as glucose. High levels of blood sugar trigger insulin secretion. Although fiber (both soluble and insoluble) is technically a carbohydrate, it cannot be broken down into simple sugars, and therefore will have no impact on insulin. On food labels, total carbohydrate content includes both fiber and carbohydrates. Taking this into account, I developed the concept of *insulin-stimulating carbohydrate content* for foods. This simply is the total amount of carbohydrate a food source contains minus its fiber content.

If a carbohydrate source (such as pasta) has very little fiber content, then virtually all of its listed carbohydrate content will be insulin-stimulating carbohydrate. On the other hand, if a carbohydrate source (such as broccoli) is rich in fiber, its insulin-stimulating carbohydrate content will be significantly reduced. This means that a much greater volume of a fiber-rich carbohydrate source must be consumed to have the same impact on insulin secretion as a much smaller volume of a low-fiber-content carbohydrate, as I show on the next page.

Amount of Insulin-Stimulating Carbohydrates in Various Food Volumes

Food	Volume	Total Carbohydrates (grams)	Fiber (grams)	Insulin-Stimulating Carbohydrates (grams)
Pasta	1 cup (cooked)	40	2	38
Apple	1 medium	20	4	16
Broccoli	1 cup	7	4	3

As you see, you would have to eat a tremendous volume of broccoli (approximately 12 cups) to have the same impact on insulin as eating a relatively small amount (1 cup) of cooked pasta. This is why starches and grains are considered high-density carbohydrates, fruits are medium-density carbohydrates, and vegetables are low-density carbohydrates. My dietary program relies heavily on low-density carbohydrates, so large volumes of food must be consumed in order to have an appreciable impact on insulin. This not only stabilizes your insulin response but also ensures that you are never deprived of an adequate volume of food. You should now see why high-density carbohydrates are used in moderation in my plan: even very small amounts can stimulate excess insulin production.

CARBOHYDRATE BLOCKS

Food Blocks are an integral part of my original dietary recommendations. They were designed to put various carbohydrates on an equal footing with regard to their insulin-stimulating effect. I define a Block of carbohydrate as a volume containing 9 grams of insulin-stimulating carbohydrate. Let's return to the example above and determine the approximate amount of Carbohydrate Food Blocks in each of the sources.

Food Block Calculations

Food	Volume	Insulin-stimulating Carbohydrates (grams)	Approximate Carbohydrate Blocks
Pasta	1 cup	38	38/9 = 4
Apple	1 medium	16	16/9 = 2
Broccoli	1 cup	3	3/9 = ⅓

These numbers aren't easy to remember, so I have simplified them by standardizing the volume of the carbohydrate source required to make one Carbohydrate Food Block. This is accomplished by dividing the volume of a carbohydrate, listed in the table above, by the number of Carbohydrate Food Blocks in that source. Then you round the number to an approximate volume that you can easily remember, as shown below.

Carbohydrate Block Calculations Simplified

Food	Blocks in a Volume	Volume for One Zone Block
Pasta	1 cup has 4 Zone Food Blocks	¼ cup
Apple	1 medium has 2 Zone Food Blocks	½ apple
Broccoli	1 cup has ⅓ Zone Food Block	3 cups

Now you have a way to compare carbohydrates directly with their ability to stimulate insulin secretion. A more complete listing of these Food Blocks, including carbohydrates, protein, and fat, is found in appendix F.

THE CONCEPTS OF GLYCEMIC INDEX AND GLYCEMIC LOAD

One nutritional breakthrough has been the concept of the glycemic index. It was always thought that there were only simple and complex carbohydrates. The simple ones would enter the bloodstream rapidly, whereas the complex carbohydrates would be slowly broken down, thus providing sustained release over time. From this seemingly reasonable concept came the nutritional "wisdom" that eventually led to the development of the USDA Food Pyramid.

Then, nutrition researchers began to ask whether or not this thinking was factual. Lo and behold, it wasn't. Some simple carbohydrates, such as fructose, entered the bloodstream as glucose very slowly. On the other hand, some complex carbohydrates, such as potatoes, entered the bloodstream at a faster rate than table sugar. The explanation of this apparent paradox led to the development of the glycemic index.

The glycemic index is a measure of the entry rates of various carbohydrate sources into the bloodstream. The faster the rate of entry, the greater the effect on insulin secretion. There are three factors that affect the glycemic index of a particular carbohydrate. The first is the amount of fiber (especially soluble fiber) it contains; the second is the amount of fat (the more fat consumed with the carbohydrate, the slower the rate of entry into the bloodstream); the third is the composition of the complex carbohydrate itself. The greater the amount of glucose it contains, the higher the glycemic index; the more fructose it contains, the lower the glycemic index. This is because fructose cannot enter the bloodstream without first being converted into glucose—a relatively slow process that takes place in the liver.

With time the glycemic index became the new fashionable guideline for which carbohydrates to eat. However, the glycemic index had significant experimental problems in dealing with low-density carbohydrates, such as vegetables.

The difficulties arose because in order to determine the glycemic index of a food, a person must consume a sufficient amount of carbohydrates (usually 50 grams) to see a rise in blood sugar. But for most vegetables, it is simply too difficult to consume this amount of carbohydrate at a sitting. For instance, it would require consuming about 16 cups of steamed broccoli. As a result, nearly all work with the glycemic index has been done with grains, starches, and some fruits, and virtually nothing is known about the glycemic index of the low-density vegetables that are the backbone of my dietary program.

These difficulties have given rise to a more sophisticated concept, the *glycemic load,* which is far more important than the glycemic index in determining the insulin output of a meal. The glycemic load is the actual amount of an insulin-stimulating carbohydrate consumed multiplied by the glycemic index for that carbohydrate. This reflects the reality that a small volume of high-glycemic carbohydrates has the same impact on insulin as a large volume of low-glycemic carbohydrates. Therefore, eating too many low-glycemic carbohydrates can still increase insulin production significantly. For example, black beans have a low glycemic index because of their high fiber content. However, they are also very dense in carbohydrate content. As a result, eating too many black beans at a meal can have a very great stimulating effect on insulin.

Ultimately, a healthy diet is obtained through insulin moderation, which can best be achieved by consuming primarily low-density carbohydrates that also have a low-glycemic index. That means eating a lot of vegetables. To illustrate this concept, the table below shows three distinct carbohydrate sources in the volumes in which they are typically consumed. The glycemic load is the product of the number of grams of insulin-stimulating carbohydrate times the glycemic index for that carbohydrate. The lower the glycemic load, the lower the insulin stimulation from that carbohydrate.

Comparison of Different Glycemic Loads

Source	Typical Volume (grams)	Glycemic Index	Glycemic Load
Pasta	1 cup	59	3068
Apple	1	54	972
Broccoli	1 cup	50*	150

*Estimated.

Even though the glycemic index of each of these carbohydrates is about the same, 1 cup of pasta generates twenty times as much insulin response as 1 cup of broccoli. And a single apple generates about six times as much insulin response as the 1 cup of broccoli. It is clear that a glycemic load based on the serving size of a carbohydrate is a much more valuable tool than the glycemic index. The chart on the following pages lists the glycemic loads of a wide variety of carbohydrates. For vegetables that have never been tested for their glycemic index, I have used an estimate of 50 (although it probably is considerably lower).

Glycemic Loads of Various Tested Carbohydrates

Source	Typical Volume	Grams	Glycemic Index	Glycemic Load
Fruits				
Apple	1	18	54	972
Apple juice	8 ounces	29	57	1,653
Apricot	1	4	81	324
Banana (medium)	1	32	79	2,528
Cantaloupe	1 cup	15	65	975
Cherries	10	10	31	310
Grapefruit	1	10	36	360
Grapefruit juice	8 ounces	22	69	1,518
Grapes	1 cup	15	66	990
Kiwi	1	8	74	592
Mango (medium)	1	33	80	2,640
Orange (medium)	1	10	63	630
Orange juice	8 ounces	26	66	1,716
Papaya (medium)	1	28	83	2,324
Peach	1	7	40	280
Pear	1	21	54	1,134
Plum	1	7	56	392
Raisins	1 cup	112	91	10,192
Watermelon	1 cup	11	103	1,133
Legumes				
Black beans (boiled)	1 cup	41	43	1,763
Black bean soup	1 cup	38	91	3,458
Chickpeas (boiled)	1 cup	46	47	2,162
Fava beans (boiled)	1 cup	34	113	3,978
Kidney beans (boiled)	1 cup	40	39	1,560
Kidney beans (canned)	1 cup	38	74	2,812
Lentils (boiled)	1 cup	32	43	1,376

Glycemic Loads of Various Tested Carbohydrates

Source	Typical Volume	Grams	Glycemic Index	Glycemic Load
Navy beans (boiled)	1 cup	38	54	2,052
Pinto beans (canned)	1 cup	36	64	2,304
Soy beans (boiled)	1 cup	20	26	520
Breads and pasta				
Bagel, small	1	38	103	3,914
Bread, dark rye	1 slice	18	109	1,962
Bread, sourdough	1 slice	20	74	1,480
Bread, white	1 slice	12	100	1,200
Bread, whole wheat	1 slice	13	99	1,287
Croissant (medium)	1	27	96	2,592
Hamburger bun	1	22	86	1,892
Kaiser roll	1	34	104	3,536
Linguine pasta (thin)	1 cup	56	79	4,424
Macaroni	1 cup	52	64	3,328
Pita bread	1	35	81	2,835
Pizza	1 slice	28	86	2,408
Spaghetti	1 cup	52	59	3,086
Starches, grains, and cereals				
Barley (boiled)	1 cup	44	36	1,584
Bulgur (cooked)	1 cup	31	69	2,139
Cheerios	1 cup	23	106	2,438
Couscous (cooked)	1 cup	42	93	3,906
Corn, sweet (canned)	1 cup	30	79	2,370
Corn Chex	1 cup	26	119	3,094
Corn Flakes	1 cup	24	120	2,880
Grapenuts	1 cup	108	96	10,368
Oatmeal (slow-cooking)	1 cup	24	70	1,680
Potato, red (boiled)	1	15	126	1,890

Glycemic Loads of Various Tested Carbohydrates

(continued)

Source	Typical Volume	Grams	Glycemic Index	Glycemic Load
Starches, grains, and cereals (continued)				
Potato, white (boiled)	1	24	90	2,160
Potato, white (mashed)	1 cup	40	100	4,000
Rice cakes	3	23	117	2,691
Rice Chex	1 cup	22	127	2,794
Rice Krispies	1 cup	21	117	2,457
Rice, white	1 cup	42	103	4,326
Rice, brown	1 cup	37	79	2,923
Dairy products				
Milk (low-fat)	1 cup	11	43	473
Soy milk	1 cup	14	44	616
Frozen tofu	1 cup	42	164	6,888
Yogurt (plain)	1 cup	17	20	340
Vegetables (cooked)				
Artichoke hearts	1 cup	7	50*	350
Bok choy	1 cup	2	50*	100
Broccoli	1 cup	2	50*	100
Cabbage	1 cup	2	50*	100
Collard greens	1 cup	3	50*	150
Eggplant	1 cup	5	50*	250
Kale	1 cup	3	50*	150
Mushrooms	1 cup	3	50*	150
Onions	1 cup	14	50*	700
String beans	1 cup	5	50*	250
Swiss chard	1 cup	4	50*	200
Spinach	1 cup	2	50*	150
Zucchini	1 cup	4	50*	200

*Estimated glycemic index of 50.

Glycemic Loads of Various Tested Carbohydrates

Source	Typical Volume	Grams	Glycemic Index	Glycemic Load
Others				
Coca-Cola (regular)	1	39	90	3,510
Fructose	1 packet	3	33	100
Gatorade	8 ounces	14	111	1,554
Granola bar	1	23	87	2,001
Honey	1 tablespoon	16	83	1,328
Power Bar	1	45	83	3,735
Snickers bar	1	36	59	2,124
Table sugar	1 teaspoon	4	93	372

A good rule of thumb is to keep your glycemic load below 3,000 in any one meal. As you can see from the data, if you are eating low-density carbohydrates, you'll have no trouble avoiding a high glycemic load. On the other hand, eating typical volumes of grain and other starch-based carbohydrates gives a very high glycemic load and results in a far greater insulin response.

Now you understand why many of the carbohydrates found in traditional grain-based diets are likely to increase insulin levels dramatically. For example, white rice generates a tremendous insulin response compared with the same volume of oatmeal or barley because rice has a greater glycemic load. Likewise, most breakfast cereals will have the same impact on insulin as a Snickers bar, since their glycemic loads are approximately the same. By contrast, cooked vegetables represent a very low glycemic load—that is why they are a critical component of my dietary recommendations.

Also remember that the more processed a food, the higher the glycemic load. This is why boiled beans have a much lower glycemic load than the same volume of canned beans. And when you make any bean (like black beans) into a soup, the glycemic load skyrockets because the prolonged cooking breaks down the cell walls of the bean, making it easier for the body to digest it into simple sugars for absorption.

Thus, the concept of the glycemic load makes it clear why consuming most of your carbohydrates from high-quality vegetables is the key to maintaining insulin levels within the appropriate zone.

Food Blocks

Any long-term dietary program is simply an accounting system to keep track of your balance of macronutrients (fat, carbohydrates, protein). Some of these systems are based on counting calories, fat grams, or carbohydrates during the course of a day. With such systems, beyond a certain limit, you won't be successful in achieving your weight loss goal. My dietary program is based on a different concept—balancing every meal. You are trying to maintain a balance of protein to carbohydrate at each meal and snack to generate the appropriate hormonal response. If you get the right balance, you will lose excess body fat. In addition, you'll also live longer with less chronic disease.

My dietary plan is like balancing your checkbook. You use your checkbook to track money coming in and money going out. You don't have to balance it to the penny, but you do want to make sure you have enough money to write a check that won't bounce. Your diet is no different. You don't have to be obsessive; you just need to have a general idea that you have a close enough balance of hormones to ensure that you don't bounce any hormonal checks in the next four to six hours. I believe the easiest way to balance your hormonal checkbook is my Food Block method.

Remember, when it comes to carbohydrates, you need to count only the amount of insulin-stimulating carbohydrate in a meal; this means that you have to subtract the fiber content. All these calculations are done for you when you use my Food Blocks.

Similarly, only about 70 percent of the protein in vegetarian sources is absorbed, because of the fiber content. The lower the fiber content in a protein source, the higher the percentage of protein absorbed. Many of the soybean proteins listed below are low in fiber, so that most of the protein will be absorbed.

Making Omega Rx Zone meals requires simply balancing the number of protein, carbohydrate, and fat block servings in equal proportions. The typical female will need 3 blocks of *each* macronutrient at every meal, whereas the typical male will need 4 blocks of *each* macronutrient at every meal. Omega Rx Zone snacks consist of 1 block of *each* macronutrient. But let me emphasize again, don't be obsessive about the exact amounts.

Thus for a typical female, each Omega Rx Zone meal would consist of 3 protein blocks, 3 carbohydrate blocks, and 3 fat blocks. For the typical male, each meal would consist of 4 protein blocks, 4 carbohydrate blocks, and 4 fat blocks. Feel free to mix and match the Food Blocks within each macronutrient group as long as they add up pretty closely to your required number of blocks at the end of the meal.

Be aware that many vegetarian protein sources also contain some carbohydrate blocks, so take this into account when constructing Omega Rx Zone meals.

Protein Blocks

*(Each portion contains approximately 7 grams
of absorbable protein per block.)*

Protein-Rich Source	Per Block
Mackerel	1½ ounces
Salmon	1½ ounces
Tuna	1½ ounces
Tuna (canned)	1 ounce
Lobster	1½ ounces
Scallops	1½ ounces
Trout	1½ ounces
Sea bass	1½ ounces
Beef tenderloin	1 ounce
Pork tenderloin	1 ounce
Chicken breast	1 ounce
Turkey breast	1 ounce
Protein powder	7 grams
Soybean hamburger crumbles	½ cup
Soybean Canadian bacon	3 slices
Soybean frozen sausage	1 link
Soybean hot dog	1 link
Tofu, extra-firm	2 ounces
Tofu, firm	3 ounces

Mixed Protein Sources*	Per Block	Associated Carbohydrate Blocks
Soybeans, boiled	¼ cup	⅔
Soy milk	8 ounces	1
Soybean hamburger	⅔ patty	⅓
Tempeh	1½ ounces	1
Tofu, soft	4 ounces	½
Milk, skim	6 ounces	1
Yogurt, skim	8 ounces	1

*These contain more carbohydrates. Read the labels carefully.

Carbohydrate Blocks

(Each portion contains approximately 9 grams of insulin-stimulating carbohydrates per block.)

Cooked Vegetables	Per Block
Artichoke	4 large
Artichoke hearts	1 cup
Asparagus	12 spears
Beans, green or wax	1½ cups
Beans, black	¼ cup
Bok choy	3 cups
Broccoli	3 cups
Brussels sprouts	1½ cups
Cabbage (red or green)	3 cups
Cauliflower	4 cups
Chickpeas	¼ cup
Collard greens, chopped	2 cups
Eggplant	1½ cups
Kale	2 cups
Kidney beans	¼ cup
Leeks	1 cup
Lentils	¼ cup
Mushrooms, whole, boiled	2 cups
Onions (all types), chopped, boiled	½ cup
Okra, sliced	1 cup
Squash, yellow, sliced and boiled	2 cups
Spinach	3½ cups
Swiss chard	2½ cups
Tomato, canned, chopped	1 cup
Tomato, puree	½ cup
Tomato sauce	½ cup
Turnip greens, chopped, boiled	4 cups
Zucchini	2 cups

Carbohydrate Blocks

*(Each portion contains approximately 9 grams of
insulin-stimulating carbohydrates per block.)*

Raw Vegetables	Per Block
Alfalfa sprouts	10 cups
Bamboo shoots	4 cups
Bean sprouts	3 cups
Beans, green	2 cups
Bell peppers (green or red)	2
Broccoli	4 cups
Brussels sprouts	1½ cups
Cabbage, shredded	4 cups
Cauliflower	4 cups
Celery, sliced	2 cups
Chickpeas	¼ cup
Cucumber (medium)	1½
Endive, chopped	10 cups
Escarole, chopped	10 cups
Jalapeno peppers	2 cups
Lettuce, iceberg	2 heads
Lettuce, romaine, shredded	10 cups
Mushrooms, chopped	4 cups
Onion, chopped	1½ cups
Radishes, sliced	4 cups
Scallions	3 cups
Shallots, diced	1½ cups
Snow peas	1½ cups
Spinach, chopped	20 cups
Tomato	2
Tomato, cherry	2 cups
Tomato, chopped	1½ cups

Carbohydrate Blocks (continued)

*(Each portion contains approximately 9 grams of
insulin-stimulating carbohydrates per block.)*

Fruits (Fresh, Frozen, or Canned Light)	Per Block
Apple	½
Applesauce (unsweetened)	⅓ cup
Apricots	3
Blackberries	¾ cup
Blueberries	½ cup
Boysenberries	½ cup
Cherries	8
Grapes	½ cup
Grapefruit	½
Kiwi	1
Nectarine	½
Orange	½
Orange, mandarin canned in water	⅓ cup
Peach	1
Pear	½
Plum	1
Raspberries	1 cup
Strawberries, diced fine	1 cup

Grains	Per Block
Barley, dry	½ tablespoon
Oatmeal, dry (slow cooking)	½ ounce
Oatmeal, cooked (slow cooking)	⅓ cup

Fat Sources
(Approximately 3 grams of fat per block.)

Best (Rich in Monounsaturated Fats)	Per Block
Almonds	3
Almond butter, natural	1 teaspoon
Almond oil	⅔ teaspoon
Avocado	1 tablespoon
Canola oil	⅔ teaspoon
Cashews	3
Guacamole	2 tablespoons
Macadamia nuts	2
Olives, black (medium)	5
Olive oil	⅔ teaspoon
Peanuts	6
Pistachios	3

Resources

SUPPLIERS OF PHARMACEUTICAL-GRADE FISH OILS

There are currently only two suppliers of pharmaceutical-grade fish oil in this country. I predict that in time there will be others.

Sears Labs
Tel: 1-800-404-8171
www.searslabs.com

Omega Rx

This product uses a 2:1 combination of EPA and DHA. This is the ratio of long-chain omega-3 fatty acids that has been used in most clinical studies conducted with pharmaceutical-grade fish oil. This oil is available in either soft gelatin capsules containing 0.6 gram of long-chain omega-3 fatty acids (400 mg EPA and 200 mg DHA) or in highly palatable lime-flavored liquid form containing 2.7 grams of long-chain omega-3 fatty acids (1.8 g EPA and 0.9 g DHA) per teaspoon.

Omega Natural Health
Tel: 1-888-57-OMEGA
www.omegabrite.com

OmegaBrite

This product contains primarily EPA and very little DHA. As a result, it may not be as useful for neurological conditions, as most studies have used the combination of EPA and DHA found in Omega Rx. This oil is only available in soft gelatin capsules that contain 0.4 gram of long-chain omega-3 fatty acids consisting primarily of EPA and very little DHA.

BLOOD TESTING

In order to follow my dietary recommendations correctly, especially with regard to supplementary high-dose fish oil, you should periodically monitor your blood to make sure you are getting the optimal results from the Omega Rx Zone diet. I believe the most important blood test you can ever take to determine your state of wellness is the one that measures your AA/EPA ratio. This is a specialized test that relatively few laboratories offer.

The laboratory with which I have had the greatest success is Your Future Health (YFH):

Your Future Health
Tel: 1-877-468-6934

This is the only service that an individual can access without going first to a physician. This is because YFH has physicians on staff who can authorize your blood to be taken at more than 2,000 specified drawing centers around the country. In addition, YFH can send a qualified health care professional to your home or work to take the necessary blood sample. Furthermore, YFH measures the ratio of AA/EPA in the plasma phospholipids, which yields very different results than a blood sample that uses the red blood cell as a source of the fatty acids. The plasma phospholipids provide a more consistent standard that is necessary for reproducibility. All of the AA/EPA ratios that I discuss in this book are based upon the plasma phospholipids as opposed to the red blood cell membranes.

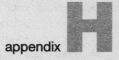

Calculation of Percent Body Fat

A rapid way to determine your percent body fat is simply to use a tape measure. You should make all measurements on bare skin (not through clothing), and make sure that the tape fits snugly but does not compress the skin and underlying tissue. Take all measurements three times and calculate the average. All measurements should be in inches.

CALCULATING BODY-FAT PERCENTAGES FOR FEMALES

There are five steps you must take to calculate your percentage of body fat:

1. While keeping the tape level, measure your hips at their widest point, and your waist at the umbilicus (i.e., belly button). It is critical that you measure at the belly button and not at the narrowest point of your waist. Take each of these measurements three times and compute the average.

2. Measure your height in inches without shoes.
3. Record your height, waist, and hip measurements on the accompanying worksheet.
4. Find each of these measurements in the appropriate column in the accompanying tables and record the constants on the worksheet.
5. Add constants A and B, then subtract constant C for this sum and round to the nearest whole number. That figure is your percentage of body fat.

Conversion Constants for Calculation of Percentage of Body Fat in Females

Hips		Abdomen		Height	
Inches	Constant A	Inches	Constant B	Inches	Constant C
30	33.48	20	14.22	55	33.52
30.5	33.83	20.5	14.40	55.5	33.67
31	34.87	21.0	14.93	56	34.13
31.5	35.22	21.5	15.11	56.5	34.28
32	36.27	22	15.64	57	34.74
32.5	36.62	22.5	15.82	57.5	34.89
33	37.67	23	16.35	58	35.35
33.5	38.02	23.5	16.53	58.5	35.50
34	39.06	24	17.06	59	35.96
34.5	39.41	24.5	17.24	59.5	36.11
35	40.46	25	17.78	60	36.57
35.5	40.81	25.5	17.96	60.5	36.72
36	41.86	26	18.49	61	37.18
36.5	42.21	26.5	18.67	61.5	37.33
37	43.25	27	19.20	62	37.79
37.5	43.60	27.5	19.38	62.5	37.94
38	44.65	28	19.91	63	38.40
38.5	45.32	28.5	20.27	63.5	38.70
39	46.05	29	20.62	64	39.01

Hips		Abdomen		Height	
Inches	Constant A	Inches	Constant B	Inches	Constant C
39.5	46.40	29.5	20.80	64.5	39.16
40	47.44	30	21.33	65	39.62
40.5	47.79	30.5	21.51	65.5	39.77
41	48.84	31	22.04	66	40.23
41.5	49.19	31.5	22.22	66.5	40.38
42	50.24	32	22.75	67	40.84
42.5	50.59	32.5	22.93	67.5	40.99
43	51.64	33	23.46	68	41.45
43.5	51.99	33.5	23.64	68.5	41.60
44	53.03	34	24.18	69	42.06
44.5	53.41	34.5	24.36	69.5	42.21
45	54.53	35	24.89	70	42.67
45.5	54.86	35.5	25.07	70.5	42.82
46	55.83	36	25.60	71	43.28
46.5	56.18	36.5	25.78	71.5	43.43
47	57.22	37	26.31	72	43.89
47.5	57.57	37.5	26.49	72.5	44.04
48	58.62	38	27.02	73	44.50
48.5	58.97	38.5	27.20	73.5	44.65
49	60.02	39	27.73	74	45.11
49.5	60.37	39.5	27.91	74.5	45.26
50	61.42	40	28.44	75	45.72
50.5	61.77	40.5	28.62	75.5	45.87
51	62.81	41	29.15	76	46.32
51.5	63.16	41.5	29.33		
52	64.21	42	29.87		
52.5	64.56	42.5	30.05		
53	65.61	43	30.58		
53.5	65.96	43.5	30.76		
54	67.00	44	31.29		
54.5	67.35	44.5	31.47		

Hips		Abdomen		Height	
Inches	Constant A	Inches	Constant B	Inches	Constant C
55	68.40	45	32.00		
55.5	68.75	45.5	32.18		
56	69.80	46	32.71		
56.5	70.15	46.5	32.89		
57	71.19	47	33.42		
57.5	71.54	47.5	33.60		
58	72.59	48	34.13		
58.5	72.94	48.5	34.31		
59	73.99	49	34.84		
59.5	74.34	49.5	35.02		
60	75.39	50	35.56		

Worksheet for Women to Calculate Their Percentage of Body Fat

Average hip measurement _____ (used for constant A)

Average abdomen measurement _____ (used for constant B)

Height _____ (used for constant C)

Using the table on pages 348—350, look up each of the average measurements and your height in the appropriate column.

Constant A = _____

Constant B = _____

Constant C = _____

To determine your approximate percentage of body fat, add constants A and B. From that total, subtract constant C. The result is your percentage of body fat, as shown below.

(Constant A + Constant B) − Constant C = % Body Fat

CALCULATING BODY-FAT PERCENTAGES FOR MEN

There are four steps you must take to determine your body-fat percentage:

1. While keeping the tape level, measure the circumference of your waist at the umbilicus (i.e., belly button). Measure three times and compute the average.
2. Measure your wrist at the space between your dominant hand and your wrist bone, at the location where your wrist bends.
3. Record these measurements on the worksheet for men.
4. Subtract your wrist measurement from your waist measurement and find the resulting value listed in the table. On the left-hand side of this table, find your weight. Proceed to the right from your weight and down from your waist-minus-wrist measurement. Where these two points intersect, read your body fat percentage.

Worksheet for Men to Calculate Their Percentage of Body Fat

Average waist measurement _____ (inches)

Average wrist measurement _____ (inches)

Subtract the wrist measurement from the waist measurement. Use the table starting on page 352 to find your weight. Then find your "waist minus wrist" number. Where the two columns intersect is your approximate percentage of body fat.

Male Percentage Body Fat Calculations

Waist-Wrist (in inches)	22	22.5	23	23.5	24
Weight (in pounds)					
120	4	6	8	10	12
125	4	6	7	9	11
130	3	5	7	9	11
135	3	5	7	8	10
140	3	5	6	8	10
145		4	6	7	9
150		4	6	7	9
155		4	5	6	8
160		4	5	6	8
165		3	5	6	8
170		3	4	6	7
175			4	6	7
180			4	5	7
185			4	5	6
190			4	5	6
195			3	5	6
200			3	4	6
205				4	5
210				4	5
215				4	5
220				4	5
225				3	4
230				3	4
235				3	4
240					4
245					4
250					4
255					3
260					3
265					
270					
275					
280					
285					
290					
295					
300					

24.5	25	25.5	26	26.5	27	27.5
14	16	18	20	21	23	25
13	15	17	19	20	22	24
12	14	16	18	20	21	23
12	13	15	17	19	20	22
11	13	15	16	18	19	21
11	12	14	15	17	19	20
10	12	13	15	16	18	19
10	11	13	14	16	17	19
9	11	12	14	15	17	18
9	10	12	13	15	16	17
9	10	11	13	14	15	17
8	10	11	12	12	15	16
8	9	10	12	13	14	16
8	9	10	11	13	14	15
7	8	10	11	12	13	15
7	8	9	11	12	13	14
7	8	9	10	11	12	14
6	8	9	10	11	12	13
6	7	8	9	11	12	13
6	7	8	9	10	11	12
6	7	8	9	10	11	12
6	7	8	9	10	11	12
5	6	7	8	9	10	11
5	6	7	8	9	10	11
5	6	7	8	9	10	11
5	6	7	8	9	9	10
5	6	6	7	8	9	10
4	5	6	7	8	9	10
4	5	6	7	8	9	10
4	5	6	7	8	8	9
4	5	6	7	7	8	9
4	5	5	6	7	8	9
4	4	5	6	7	8	9
4	4	5	6	7	8	8
3	4	5	6	7	7	8
3	4	5	6	6	7	8
3	4	5	5	6	7	8

Waist-Wrist (in inches)	28	28.5	29	29.5	30	30.5	31
Weight (in pounds)							
120	27	29	31	33	35	37	39
125	26	28	30	32	33	35	37
130	25	27	28	30	32	34	36
135	24	26	27	29	31	32	34
140	23	24	26	28	29	31	33
145	22	23	25	27	28	30	31
150	21	23	24	26	27	29	30
155	20	22	23	25	26	28	29
160	19	21	22	24	25	27	28
165	19	20	22	23	24	26	27
170	18	19	21	22	24	25	26
175	17	19	20	21	23	24	25
180	17	18	19	21	22	23	25
185	16	18	19	20	21	23	24
190	16	17	18	19	21	22	23
195	15	16	18	19	20	21	22
200	15	16	17	18	19	21	22
205	14	15	17	18	19	20	21
210	14	15	16	17	18	19	21
215	13	15	16	17	18	19	20
220	13	14	15	16	17	18	19
225	13	14	15	16	17	18	19
230	12	13	14	15	16	17	18
235	12	13	14	15	16	17	18
240	12	13	14	15	16	17	17
245	11	12	13	14	15	16	17
250	11	12	13	14	15	16	17
255	11	12	13	14	14	15	16
260	10	11	12	13	14	15	16
265	10	11	12	13	14	15	15
270	10	11	12	13	13	14	15
275	10	11	11	12	13	14	15
280	9	10	11	12	13	14	14
285	9	10	11	12	12	13	14
290	9	10	11	11	12	13	14
295	9	10	10	11	12	13	14
300	9	9	10	11	12	12	13

31.5	32	32.5	33	33.5	34	34.5
41	43	45	47	49	50	52
39	41	43	45	46	48	50
37	39	41	43	44	46	48
36	38	39	41	43	44	46
34	36	38	39	41	43	44
33	35	36	38	39	41	43
32	33	35	36	38	40	41
31	32	34	35	37	38	40
30	31	33	34	35	37	38
29	30	31	33	34	36	37
28	29	30	32	33	34	36
27	28	29	31	32	33	35
26	27	28	30	31	32	34
25	26	28	29	30	31	33
24	26	27	28	29	30	32
24	25	26	27	28	30	31
23	24	25	26	28	29	30
22	23	25	26	27	28	29
22	23	24	25	26	27	28
21	22	23	24	25	26	28
20	22	23	24	25	26	27
20	21	22	23	24	25	26
19	20	21	22	23	24	25
19	20	21	22	23	24	25
18	19	20	21	22	23	24
18	19	20	21	22	23	24
18	18	19	20	21	22	23
17	18	19	20	21	22	23
17	18	19	19	20	21	22
16	17	18	19	20	21	22
16	17	18	19	19	20	21
16	16	17	18	19	20	21
15	16	17	18	19	19	20
15	16	17	17	18	19	20
15	15	16	17	18	19	19
14	15	16	17	17	18	19
14	15	16	16	17	18	19

Waist-Wrist (in inches)	35	35.5	36	36.5	37
Weight (in pounds)					
120	54				
125	52	54			
130	50	52	53	55	
135	48	50	51	53	55
140	46	48	49	51	53
145	44	46	47	49	51
150	43	44	46	47	49
155	41	43	44	46	47
160	40	41	43	44	46
165	38	40	41	43	44
170	37	39	40	41	43
175	36	37	39	40	41
180	35	36	37	39	40
185	34	35	36	38	39
190	33	34	35	37	38
195	32	33	34	35	37
200	31	32	33	35	36
205	30	31	32	34	35
210	29	30	32	33	34
215	29	30	31	32	33
220	28	29	30	31	32
225	27	28	29	30	31
230	26	27	28	30	31
235	26	27	28	29	30
240	25	26	27	28	29
245	25	26	27	27	28
250	24	25	26	27	28
255	24	24	25	26	27
260	23	24	25	26	27
265	22	23	24	25	26
270	22	23	24	25	25
275	22	22	23	24	25
280	21	22	23	24	24
285	21	21	22	23	24
290	20	21	22	23	23
295	20	21	21	22	23
300	19	20	21	22	22

37.5	38	38.5	39	39.5	40	40.5
54						
52	54	55				
50	52	53	55			
49	50	52	53	55		
47	48	50	51	53	54	
45	47	48	50	51	52	54
44	45	47	48	49	51	52
43	44	45	47	48	49	51
41	43	44	45	47	48	49
40	41	43	44	45	46	48
39	40	41	43	44	45	46
38	39	40	41	43	44	45
37	38	39	40	41	43	44
36	37	38	39	40	41	43
35	36	37	38	39	40	42
34	35	36	37	38	39	40
33	34	35	36	37	38	39
32	33	34	35	36	37	38
32	33	34	35	36	37	38
31	32	33	34	35	36	37
30	31	32	33	34	35	36
29	30	31	32	33	34	35
29	30	31	31	32	33	34
28	29	30	31	32	33	34
27	28	29	30	31	32	33
27	28	29	29	30	31	32
26	27	28	29	30	31	31
26	27	27	28	29	30	31
25	26	27	28	29	29	30
25	26	26	27	28	29	30
24	25	26	27	27	28	29
24	25	25	26	27	28	28
23	24	25	26	26	27	28

Waist-Wrist (in inches)	41	41.5	42	42.5	43	43.5
Weight (in pounds)						
120						
125						
130						
135						
140						
145						
150						
155						
160						
165	55					
170	54	55				
175	52	53	55			
180	50	52	53	54		
185	49	50	51	53	54	55
190	48	49	50	51	52	54
195	46	47	49	50	51	52
200	45	46	47	48	50	51
205	44	45	46	47	48	49
210	43	44	45	46	47	48
215	42	43	44	45	46	47
220	41	42	43	44	45	46
225	40	41	42	43	44	45
230	39	40	41	42	44	44
235	38	39	40	41	42	43
240	37	38	39	40	41	42
245	36	37	38	39	40	41
250	35	36	37	38	39	40
255	34	35	36	37	38	39
260	34	35	35	36	37	38
265	33	34	35	36	36	37
270	32	33	34	35	36	37
275	32	32	33	34	35	36
280	31	32	33	33	34	35
285	30	31	32	33	34	34
290	30	31	31	32	33	34
295	29	30	31	32	32	33
300	29	29	30	31	32	33

44	44.5	45	45.5	46	46.5	47
55						
53	55					
52	53	54	55			
51	52	53	54	55		
49	50	51	53	54	55	
48	49	50	51	52	53	54
47	48	49	50	51	52	53
46	47	48	49	50	51	52
45	46	47	48	49	50	51
44	45	46	47	48	49	50
43	44	45	46	46	47	48
42	43	44	44	45	46	47
41	42	43	44	44	45	46
40	41	42	43	44	44	45
39	40	41	42	43	43	44
38	39	40	41	42	43	43
37	38	39	40	41	42	43
37	38	38	39	40	41	42
36	37	38	38	39	40	41
35	36	37	38	39	39	40
35	35	36	37	38	39	39
34	35	36	36	37	38	39
33	34	35	36	36	37	38

Waist-Wrist (in inches)	47.5	48	48.5	49	49.5	50
Weight (in pounds)						
120						
125						
130						
135						
140						
145						
150						
155						
160						
165						
170						
175						
180						
185						
190						
195						
200						
205						
210						
215	55					
220	54	55				
225	53	54	55			
230	52	53	54	55		
235	51	51	52	53	54	55
240	49	50	51	52	53	54
245	48	49	50	51	52	53
250	47	48	49	50	51	52
255	46	47	48	49	50	51
260	45	46	47	48	49	50
265	44	45	46	47	48	49
270	43	44	45	46	47	48
275	43	43	44	45	46	47
280	42	43	43	44	45	46
285	41	42	43	43	44	45
290	40	41	42	43	43	44
295	39	40	41	42	43	43
300	39	39	40	41	42	43

References

Journal Abbreviation	Journal Name
Acta Derm Venerol	*Acta Dermato-Venerologica*
Acta Endocrinol	*Acta Endocrinologica*
Acta Med Scand	*Acta Medica Scandinavica*
Acta Neurol Scand	*Acta Neurologica Scandinavica*
Acta Neuropathol	*Acta Neuropathologica*
Acta Obstet Gynecol Scand	*Acta Obstetrica and Gynecologica Scandinavica*
Acta Paediactr	*Acta Paediactrica*
Acta Physiol Hungarica	*Acta Physiologica Hungarica*
Acta Physiol Scan	*Acta Physiologica Scandinavica*
Adv Exp Med Bio	*Advances in Experimental Medicine and Biology*
Adv Lipid Res	*Advances in Lipid Research*
Adv Neuroimmunol	*Advances in Neuroimmunology*
Adv Pros Throm Leuko Res	*Advances in Prostaglandin, Thromboxane, Leukotriene Research*
Alcohol Clin Exp Res	*Alcoholism-Clinical Experimental Research*
Altern Med Rev	*Alternative Medicine Review*
Altern Ther Health Med	*Alternative Therapeutic Health and Medicine*

Am Heart J	*American Heart Journal*
Am J Cardiol	*American Journal of Cardiology*
Am J Clin Nutr	*American Journal of Clinical Nutrition*
Am J Epidemiol	*American Journal of Epidemiology*
Am J Med	*American Journal of Medicine*
Am J Med Sci	*American Journal of Medical Science*
Am J Obstet Gynecol	*American Journal of Obstetrics and Gynecology*
Am J Physiol	*American Journal of Physiology*
Am J Physiol Endocrinol Metab	*American Journal of Physiology— Endocrinology and Metabolism*
Am J Psychiatry	*American Journal of Psychiatry*
Am J Pub Health	*American Journal of Public Health*
Am J Respir Critical Care Med	*American Journal of Respiratory and Critical Care Medicine*
Am J Sports Med	*American Journal of Sports Medicine*
Ann Intern Med	*Annals of Internal Medicine*
Ann Med	*Annals of Medicine*
Ann Neurology	*Annals of Neurology*
Ann Nutr Metab	*Annals of Nutrition and Metabolism*
Ann NY Acad Sci	*Annals of the New York Academy of Science*
Ann Rev Anthropol	*Annual Review of Anthropology*
Ann Rev Immunol	*Annual Review of Immunology*
Ann Rev Med	*Annual Review of Medicine*
Ann Rev Neurosci	*Annual Review of Neuroscience*
Ann Rev Nutr	*Annual Review of Nutrition*
Ann Rev Public Health	*Annual Review of Public Health*
Ann Rheum Dis	*Annals of Rheumatic Disease*
Ann Surg	*Annals of Surgery*
Anticancer Res	*Anticancer Research*
Arch Biochem Biophys	*Archives of Biochemistry and Biophysics*
Arch Dermatol Res	*Archives of Dermatological Research*
Arch Dis Child	*Archives of Disease in Childhood*

Arch Gen Psychiatry	*Archives of General Psychiatry*
Arch Intern Med	*Archives of Internal Medicine*
Arch Med Res	*Archives of Medical Research*
Arch Pediatri Adolesc	*Archives of Pediatric and Adolescent Medicine*
Arterioscler	*Arteriosclerosis*
Arterioscler Thromb Vasc Biol	*Arteriosclerosis, Thrombosis, and Vascular Biology*
Arthritis Rheum	*Arthritis and Rheumatism*
Athero	*Atherosclerosis*
Biochem Biophys Res Comm	*Biochemical and Biophysical Research Communications*
Biochem Pharmacol	*Biochemical Pharmacology*
Biochem Int	*Biochemistry International*
Biochim Biophys Acta	*Biochimica et Biophysica Acta*
Blood Coagul Fibrinolysis	*Blood Coagulation and Fibrinolysis*
Bio Psychiatry	*Biological Psychiatry*
Brain Res	*Brain Research*
Brain Res Mol Brain Res	*Brain Research and Molecular Brain Research*
Br Heart J	*British Heart Journal*
Br J Cancer	*British Journal of Cancer*
Br J Haematology	*British Journal of Haematology*
Br J Med	*British Journal of Medicine*
Br J Nutr	*British Journal of Nutrition*
Br J Obstet Gynecol	*British Journal of Obstetrics and Gynecology*
Br J Sports Med	*British Journal of Sports Medicine*
Br J Surgery	*British Journal of Surgery*
Br Med J	*British Medical Journal*
Bull Environ Contam Toxicol	*Bulletin of Environmental Contamination and Toxicology*
Calcif Tissue Int	*Calcified Tissue International*
Cancer Biol	*Cancer Biology*

Cancer Chemother Pharmacol	*Cancer Chemotherapy and Pharmacology*
Cancer Epidemiol Biomarkers Prev	*Cancer Epidemiology Biomarkers and Prevention*
Cancer Lett	*Cancer Letters*
Cancer Metastasis Rev	*Cancer Metastasis Review*
Cancer Res	*Cancer Research*
Cardiovasc Drugs Ther	*Cardiovascular Drugs and Therapy*
Cardiovasc Res	*Cardiovascular Research*
Cell Biol Toxicol	*Cell Biology and Toxicology*
Cell Regul	*Cellular Regulation*
Circ Res	*Circulation Research*
Clin Cancer Res	*Clinical Cancer Research*
Clin Chem	*Clinical Chemistry*
Clin Chim Acta	*Clinical and Chimica Acta*
Clin Endocrinol	*Clinical Endocrinology*
Clin Endocrinol Metab	*Clinical Endocrinology and Metabolism*
Clin Exp Metastasis	*Clinical and Experimental Metastasis*
Clin Invest Med	*Clinical and Investigative Medicine*
Clin Neuropharmacol	*Clinical Neuropharmacology*
Clin Neurophysiology	*Clinical Neurophysiology*
Clin Rheumatol	*Clinical Rheumatology*
Clin Sci	*Clinical Science*
Coronary Artery Dis	*Coronary Artery Disease*
Curr Atheroscler Rep	*Current Atherosclerosis Reports*
Curr Biol	*Current Biology*
Curr Med Chem	*Current Medical Chemistry*
Curr Opin Clin Nutr Metab Care	*Current Opinion in Clinical Nutrition and Metabolic Care*
Curr Opinion Lipidol	*Current Opinion in Lipidology*
Curr Pharma Design	*Current Pharmaceutical Design*
Curr Ther Res Clin Exp	*Current Therapeutic Research—Clinical Experimental*

Curr Top Microbiol Immunol	*Current Topics in Microbiology and Immunology*
Cytokine Growth Factor Rev	*Cytokine and Growth Factor Review*
Dev Neurosci	*Developmental Neuroscience*
Diabetes Metab	*Diabetes and Metabolism*
Diabetes Metab Res Rev	*Diabetes-Metabolism Research and Reviews*
Diabetes Res Clin Prac	*Diabetes Research and Clinical Practice*
Dis Colon Rectum	*Diseases of the Colon and Rectum*
Drug Development Res	*Drug Development Research*
EMBO J	*European Molecular Biology Organization Journal*
Endocrine Rev	*Endocrine Reviews*
Environ Health Perspect	*Environmental Health Perspectives*
Ernst Schering Res Foundation Workshop	*Ernst Schering Research Foundation Workshop*
Eur Cytokine Netw	*European Cytokine Network*
Eur Heart J	*European Heart Journal*
Eur J Appl Physiol Occup Physiol	*European Journal of Applied Physiology and Occupational Physiology*
Eur J Cancer	*European Journal of Cancer*
Eur J Cancer Prev	*European Journal of Cancer Prevention*
Eur J Clin Nutr	*European Journal of Clinical Nutrition*
Eur J Pharmacol	*European Journal of Pharmacology*
Eur Respir J	*European Respiratory Journal*
Exp Bio Med	*Experimental Biology and Medicine*
Exp Cell Res	*Experimental Cell Research*
Exp Clin Endocrinol Diabetes	*Experimental and Clinical Endocrinology and Diabetes*
Exp Gerontology	*Experimental Gerontology*
FASEB J	*Federation of American Society of Experimental Biology Journal*
Fert Steril	*Fertility and Sterility*
Free Radical Biol Med	*Free Radicals in Biology and Medicine*

Front Biosci	*Frontiers in Bioscience*
Gastroenterol Clin North Am	*Gastroenterology Clinics of North America*
Gen Pharmacol	*General Pharmacology*
Glycoconjugate J	*Glycoconjugate Journal*
Harvard Rev of Psychiatry	*Harvard Review of Psychiatry*
Horm Metab Res	*Hormone and Metabolism Research*
Hormones Behav	*Hormones and Behavior*
Immunol Rev	*Immunological Reviews*
Inflamm Res	*Inflammation Research*
Int J Biochem	*International Journal of Biochemistry*
Int J Cancer	*International Journal of Cancer*
Int J Clin Pharmacol Ther	*International Journal of Clinical Pharmacology and Therapeutics*
Int J Environ Anal Chem	*International Journal of Environmental and Analytical Chemistry*
Int J Mol Med	*International Journal of Molecular Medicine*
Int J Neurosci	*International Journal of Neuroscience*
Int J Obesity	*International Journal of Obesity*
Int J Obes Relat Metab Disorders	*International Journal of Obesity-Related Metabolic Disorders*
Int J Oncol	*International Journal of Oncology*
Int J Sports Med	*International Journal of Sports Medicine*
Int J Sports Nutr	*International Journal of Sports Nutrition*
Int J Vitam Nutr Res	*International Journal for Vitamin and Nutrition Research*
Invest Ophthalmol Vis Sci	*Investigative Ophthalmology and Visual Science*
Isr J Med	*Israeli Journal of Medicine*
J Affect Dis	*Journal of Affective Disorders*
J Agric Food Chem	*Journal of Agriculture and Food Chemistry*

JAMA	*Journal of the American Medical Association*
J Am Chem Soc	*Journal of the American Chemistry Society*
J Am Coll Cardiology	*Journal of the American College of Cardiology*
J Am Coll Nutr	*Journal of the American College of Nutrition*
J Am Dietetic Assoc	*Journal of the American Dietetic Association*
J Am Geriatrics Soc	*Journal of the American Geriatrics Society*
J Am Oil Chem Soc	*Journal of the American Oil Chemists Society*
J Am Soc Nephrol	*Journal of the American Society of Nephrology*
J Appl Physiol	*Journal of Applied Physiology*
J Biol Chem	*Journal of Biological Chemistry*
J Biol Regul Homeost Agents	*Journal of Biological Regulators and Homeostatic Agents*
J Bio Response Mod	*Journal of Biological Response Modifiers*
J Cardiovasc Pharmacol	*Journal of Cardiovascular Pharmacology*
J Cardiovasc Risk	*Journal of Cardiovascular Risk*
J Clin Endocrinol	*Journal of Clinical Endocrinology*
J Clin Endocrinol Metab	*Journal of Clinical Endocrinology and Metabolism*
J Clin Epidemiol	*Journal of Clinical Epidemiology*
J Clin Invest	*Journal of Clinical Investigation*
J Clin Lab Med	*Journal of Clinical Laboratory Medicine*
J Clin Ligand Assay	*Journal of Clinical Ligand Assay*
J Clin Oncol	*Journal of Clinical Oncology*
J Clin Pharmacol	*Journal of Clinical Pharmacology*
J Clin Ther Med	*Journal of Clinical Therapy in Medicine*
J Endocrinol	*Journal of Endocrinology*

J Exp Med	*Journal of Experimental Medicine*
J Gen Virol	*Journal of General Virology*
J Gerontol A Biol Sci Med Sci	*Journal of Gerontology Series A—Biological Sciences and Medical Sciences*
J Human Hypertension	*Journal of Human Hypertension*
J Immunol	*Journal of Immunology*
J Intern Med	*Journal of Internal Medicine*
J Invest Med	*Journal of Investigative Medicine*
J Lab Clin Med	*Journal of Laboratory and Clinical Medicine*
J Lipid Res	*Journal of Lipid Research*
J Mol Neurosci	*Journal of Molecular Neuroscience*
J Natl Cancer Inst	*Journal of the National Cancer Institute*
J Neural Transm	*Journal of Neural Transmission*
J Neurochem	*Journal of Neurochemistry*
J Neurochem Res	*Journal of Neurochemical Research*
J Neuroimmunol	*Journal of Neuroimmunology*
J Neuro Sci	*Journal of Neuroscience*
J Neurosci Res	*Journal of Neuroscience Research*
J Nutr	*Journal of Nutrition*
J Nutr Biochem	*Journal of Nutritional Biochemistry*
J Nutr Sci Vitaminol	*Journal of Nutritional Science and Vitaminology*
J Pain Symptom	*Journal of Pain and Symptom Management*
J Pediatr	*Journal of Pediatrics*
J Physiol (London)	*Journal of Physiology (London)*
J Physiol Pharmacol	*Journal of Physiology and Pharmacology*
J Recept Signal Transduc Res	*Journal of Receptor and Signal Transduction Research*
J Reprod Fertil	*Journal of Reproduction and Fertility*
J Reprod Med	*Journal of Reproductive Medicine*
J Rheumatol	*Journal of Rheumatology*

J Surg Res	*Journal of Surgical Research*
J Vas Res	*Journal of Vascular Research*
Kidney Int	*Kidney International*
Lab Invest	*Laboratory Investigation*
Life Sci	*Life Sciences*
Mech Ageing Dev	*Mechanisms of Ageing and Development*
Med Hypotheses	*Medical Hypotheses*
Med J Austr	*Medical Journal of Australia*
Med Sci Sports Exerc	*Medicine and Science in Sports and Exercise*
Metab	*Metabolism*
Mol Cell Biochem	*Molecular and Cellular Biochemistry*
Mol Cell Endocrinol	*Molecular and Cellular Endocrinology*
Mol Med	*Molecular Medicine*
Mol Psychiatry	*Molecular Psychiatry*
Mutation Res	*Mutation Research*
Nature Cell Bio	*Nature Cell Biology*
Nature Neurosci	*Nature Neuroscience*
Nature New Biol (England)	*Nature New Biology* (England)
N Engl J Med	*New England Journal of Medicine*
Neurobio	*Neurobiology*
Neurobiol Aging	*Neurobiology and Aging*
Neurochem Res	*Neurochemistry Research*
Neurosci	*Neuroscience*
Neurosci Biobehav Rev	*Neuroscience and Biobehavioral Reviews*
Neurosci Lett	*Neuroscience Letters*
Nutr	*Nutrition*
Nutr Cancer	*Nutrition and Cancer*
Nutr Res	*Nutrition Research*
Nutr Rev	*Nutrition Reviews*
Obesity Res	*Obesity Research*
Obstet Gynecol	*Obstetrics and Gynecology*
Obstet Gynecol Surv	*Obstetrics and Gynecology Surveys*
Pediatr Res	*Pediatric Research*

Percept Mot Skills	*Perceptive Motor Skills*
Perspect Bio Med	*Perspectives in Biology and Medicine*
Pharmacol Biochem Behav	*Pharmacology and Biochemistry of Behavior*
Pharmacol Res	*Pharmacology Research*
Pharmacol Therap	*Pharmacology and Therapeutics*
Pharm World Sci	*Pharmacy World and Science*
Philos Trans R Soc Lond B Biol Sci	*Philosophical Transactions of the Royal Society of London Series B—Biological Sciences*
Physiol Behav	*Physiology and Behavior*
Physiol Rev	*Physiological Reviews*
Prev Med	*Preventive Medicine*
Proc Nat Acad Sci USA	*Proceedings of the National Academy of Sciences of the USA*
Proc Nutr Soc	*Proceedings of the Nutrition Society*
Proc Soc Exp Biol Med	*Proceedings of the Society of Experimental Biology and Medicine*
Prog Cardio Dis	*Progress in Cardiovascular Diseases*
Prog Clin Biol Res	*Progress in Clinical and Biological Research*
Prog Histochem Cytochem	*Progress in Histochemistry and Cytochemistry*
Prog Lipid Res	*Progress in Lipid Research*
Prostaglandins Leuko Essen Fatty Acids	*Prostaglandins, Leukotrienes, and Essential Fatty Acids*
Prostaglandins Leukot Med	*Prostaglandins and Leukotrienes in Medicine*
Prostaglandins Other Lipid Mediat	*Prostaglandins and Other Lipid Mediators*
Psychiat Clin North Am	*Psychiatry Clinics of North America*
Psychiatry Res	*Psychiatry Research*
Psychol Bull	*Psychological Bulletin*
Psychol Med	*Psychological Medicine*

Psychol Reports	*Psychological Reports*
Psychol Rev	*Psychological Reviews*
Psychopharmacology Bull	*Psychopharmacology Bulletin*
Reprod Nutr Dev	*Reproductive Nutrition and Development*
Res Exp Med (Berlin)	*Research in Experimental Medicine* (Berlin)
Rheum Dis Clin North Am	*Rheumatological Disease Clinics of North America*
Scand J Nutr	*Scandinavian Journal of Nutrition*
Schizophr Res	*Schizophrenia Research*
Sci Am	*Scientific American*
Sem Arthr Rheum	*Seminars in Arthritis and Rheumatism*
Sem Gastrointest Dis	*Seminars in Gastrointestinal Disease*
Sports Med	*Sports Medicine*
Surg Today	*Surgery Today*
TEM	*Trends in Endocrinology and Metabolism*
TIPS	*Trends in Pharmacological Sciences*
Toxicological Sci	*Toxicological Sciences*
Trends in Pharm Sci	*Trends in Pharmacological Sciences*
Tumor Diol	*Tumor Biology*
World Rev Nutr Diet	*World Review of Nutrition and Diet*

Introduction

Kromann, N., and A. Green. "Epidemiological studies in the Upernavik district, Greenland. Incidence of some chronic diseases 1950–1974." *Acta Med Scand* 208:401–406 (1980).

Lands, W. E. M. *Fish and Human Health.* New York: Academic Press, 1986.

Oates, J. A. "The 1982 Nobel Prize in physiology or medicine." *Science* 218:765–768 (1982).

Sears, Barry. *The Zone.* New York: Regan Books, 1995.

———. *Mastering the Zone.* New York: Regan Books, 1997.

———. *Zone-Perfect Meals in Minutes.* New York: Regan Books, 1997.

———. *Zone Food Blocks.* New York: Regan Books, 1998.

———. *The Anti-Aging Zone.* New York: Regan Books, 1999.

———. *The Soy Zone.* New York: Regan Books, 2000.

———. *A Week in the Zone*. New York: Regan Books, 2000.

———. *100 Top Zone Foods*. New York: Regan Books, 2001.

Chapter 1 The Continuing Evolution of the Zone

Cao G., E. Sofic, and R. L. Prior. "Antioxidant capacity of tea and common vegetables." *J Agric Food Chem* 44:3426–3431 (1996).

De Groot, L. J., M. Besser, H. G. Burger, J. L. Jameson, D. L. Loriaux, J. C. Marshall, W. D. Odell, J. T. Potts, and A. H. Rubenstein, eds. *Endocrinology,* 3rd edition. Philadelphia, Pa.: W. B. Saunders Company, 1995.

Felig, P., J. D. Baxter, and L. A. Frohman. *Endocrinology and Metabolism.* 3rd edition. New York: McGraw-Hill, 1995.

Lands, W. E. M. *Fish and Human Health.* New York: Academic Press, 1986.

Norman, A. W., and G. Litwack. *Hormones.* 2d edition. New York: Academic Press, 1997.

Oates, J. A. "The 1982 Nobel Prize in physiology or medicine." *Science* 218:765–768 (1982).

Sears, Barry. *The Zone*. New York: Regan Books, 1995.

———. *Mastering the Zone*. New York: Regan Books, 1997.

———. *Zone-Perfect Meals in Minutes*. New York: Regan Books, 1997.

———. *Zone Food Blocks*. New York: Regan Books, 1998.

———. *The Anti-Aging Zone*. New York: Regan Books, 1999.

———. *The Soy Zone*. New York: Regan Books, 2000.

———. *A Week in the Zone*. New York: Regan Books, 2000.

———. *100 Top Zone Foods*. New York: Regan Books, 2001.

Timiras, P. S., W. B. Quay, and A. Vernakdakis, eds. *Hormones and Aging.* Boca Raton, Fla.: CRC Press, 1995.

Wang, H., G. Cao, and R. L. Prior. "Total antioxidant capacity of fruits." *J Agric Food Chem* 44:701–705 (1996).

Wilson, J. D., and D. W. Foster, eds. *Williams Textbook of Endocrinology.* 8th edition. Philadelphia, Pa.: W. B. Saunders Company, 1992.

Chapter 2 The Beginnings of Modern Man

Aiello, L. C., and P. Wheeler. "The expensive-tissue hypothesis." *Current Anthropology* 36:199–221 (1995).

Berger, L. R. *In the Footsteps of Eve: The Mystery of Human Origins.* Washington, D.C.: National Geographic, 2000.

Broadhurst, C. L., S. C. Cunnane, and M. A. Crawford. "Rift valley lake fish and shellfish provided brain-specific nutrition for early *Homo*." *Br J Nutr* 79:3–21 (1998).

Chamberlain, J. G. "The possible role of long-chain omega-3 fatty acids in human brain phylogeny." *Perspect Bio Med* 39:436–445 (1996).

Cordain, L., J. B. Miller, S. B. Eaton, N. Mann, S. H. A. Holt, and J. D. Speth. "Plant-animal subsistence ratios and macronutrient energy estimations in worldwide hunter-gatherer diets." *Am J Clin Nutr* 71:682–692 (2000).

Crawford, M. A. "Fatty acid ratios in free-living and domestic animals." *Lancet* i:1329–1333 (1968).

Crawford, M. A., M. M. Gale, and M. H. Woodford. "Comparative studies on fatty acid composition of wild and domestic animals." *Int J Biochem* 1:295–305 (1970).

Crawford, M. A., and D. Marsh. *The Driving Force: Food, Evolution, and the Future.* New York: Harper and Row, 1989.

Crawford, M. A., M. Bloom, C. L. Broadhurst, W. F. Schmidt, S. C. Cunnane, C. Galli, K. Gehremeskel, F. Linseisen, J. Lloyd-Smith, and J. Parkington. "Evidence for the unique function of docosahexaenoic acid during the evolution of the modern hominid brain." *Lipids* 34:S39–S47 (1999).

Crawford, M. A., M. Bloom, S. Cunnane, H. Holmsen, K. Ghebremeskel, J. Parkington, W. Schmidt, A. J. Sinclair, and C. L. Broadhurst. "Docosahexaenoic acid and cerebral evolution." *Fatty Acids and Lipids—New Findings,* H. Hamazaki and H. Okuyama, pp. 6–17. Basel, Switzerland: S. Krager, 2001.

Diamond, J. *The Third Chimpanzee: The Evolution and Future of the Human Animal.* New York: HarperCollins, 1992.

Eaton, S. B., and M. J. Konner. "Paleolithic nutrition." *N Engl J Med* 312:283–289 (1985).

Eaton, S. B., M. Shostak, and M. Konner. *The Paleolithic Prescription.* New York: Harper and Row, 1988.

Eaton, S. B. "Humans, lipids, and evolution." *Lipids* 27:814–820 (1992).

Eaton, S. B. "An evolutionary perspective enhances understanding of human nutritional requirements." *J Nutr* 126:1732–1740 (1996).

———. "Paleolithic nutrition revisited: A twelve-year retrospective on its nature and implications." *Eur J Clin Nutr* 51:207–216 (1997).

Eaton, S. B., M. Konner, and M. Shostak. "Stone agers in the fast lane: Chronic degenerative diseases in evolutionary perspective." *Am J Med* 84: 739–749 (1998).

Eaton, S. B., A. J. Sinclair, L. Cordain, and N. J. Mann. "Dietary intake of long-chain polyunsaturated fatty acids during the Paleolithic." *World Rev Nutr Diet* 83:12–23 (1998).

Foley, R. A., and P. C. Lee. "Ecology and energetics of encephalization in hominid evolution." *Philos Trans R Soc Lond B Bio Sci* 334:223–231 (1991).

Relenthford, J. H. "Genetics of modern human origins and diversity." *Ann Rev Anthropol* 27:1–23 (1998).

Relenthford, J. H. "Genetic history of the human species." In *Handbook of Statistical Genetics,* ed. D. J. Balding et al., pp. 813–845. New York: John Wiley and Sons, 2001.

Ruff, C. B, E. Trinkaus, and T. W. Holliday. "Body mass and encephalization in Pleistocene *Homo.*" *Nature* 387:173–176 (1997).

Stringer, C., and R. McKie. *African Exodus: The Origins of Modern Humanity.* New York: Henry Holt and Company, 1996.

Sykes, B. *The Seven Daughters of Eve.* New York: W. W. Norton, 2001.

Viglant, L., M. Stonemaking, H. Harpending, K. Hawkes, and A. C. Wilson. "African populations and evolution of human mitochrondrial DNA." *Science* 253: 1503–1507 (1991).

Chapter 3 The Fats That Made Us Human

Anderson, G. J. "Developmental sensitivity of the brain to dietary n-3 fatty acids." *J Lipid Res* 35:105–111 (1994).

Anderson, J. W., B. M. Johnstone, and D. T. Remley. "Breast-feeding and cognitive development: A meta analysis." *Am J Clin Nutr* 70:535–535 (1999).

Brozoski, T. J., R. M. Brown, H. E. Rosvold, and P. S. Goldman. "Cognitive deficit caused by regional depletion of dopamine in prefrontal cortex of rhesus monkey." *Science* 205:929–932 (1979).

Carlson, S. E., S. H. Werkman, P. G. Rhodes, and E. A. Tolley. "Visual acuity development in healthy preterm infants: Effect of marine-oil supplements." *Am J Clin Nutr* 58:35–42 (1993).

Carlson, S. E., S. H. Werkman, J. M. Peeples, and W. M. Wilson. "Long-chain fatty acids and early visual and cognitive development of preterm infants." *Eur J Clin Nutr* 48:S27–S30 (1994).

Cunnane, S. C., V. Francescutti, J. T. Brenna, and M. A. Crawford. "Breast-fed infants achieve a higher rate of brain and whole body docosahexaenoate accumulation than formula-fed infants not consuming dietary docosahexaenoate." *Lipids* 35:105–111 (2000).

Delion, S., S. Chalon, J. Herault, D. Guilloteau, J. C. Besnard, and G. Durand. "Chronic dietary alpha-linolenic acid deficiency alters dopaminergic and serotoninergic neurotransmitters in rats." *J Nutr* 124:2466–2476 (1994).

Delion, S., S. Chalon, D. Guilloteau, J. C. Besnard, and G. Durand.

"Alpha-linolenic acid deficiency alters age-related changes of dopaminergic and serotoninergic neurotransmitters in the rat frontal cortex." *J Neurochem* 66:1582–1591 (1996).

Dyerberg, J., H. O. Bang, and N. Hjorne. "Fatty acid composition of the plasma lipids in Greenland Eskimos." *Am J Clin Nutr* 28:958–966 (1975).

Farquharson, J., F. Cockburn, W. A. Patrick, E. C. Jamieson, and R. W. Logan. "Infant cerebral cortex phospholipid fatty acid composition and diet." *Lancet* 340:810–814 (1992).

Farquharson, J., E. C. Jamieson, K. A. Abbasi, W. J. A. Patrick, R. W. Logan, and F. Cockburn. "Effect of diet on fatty acid composition of major phospholipids of intact cerebral cortex." *Arch Dis Child* 72:198–203 (1995).

Francois, C. A., S. L. Connor, R. C. Wander, and W. E. Connor. "Acute effects of dietary fatty acids on the fatty acids of human milk." *Am J Clin Nutr* 67:301–308 (1998).

Gibson, R. A., and G. M. Kneebone. "Fatty acid composition of human colostrums and mature breast milk." *Am J Clin Nutr* 34:252–257 (1981).

Gibson, R. A., M. A. Neumann, and M. Makrides. "Effect of dietary docosahexaenoic acid on brain composition and neural function in term infants." *Lipids* 31:S177–S181 (1996).

Ikemoto, A., T. Kobayashi, S. Watanabe, and H. Okuyama. "Membrane fatty acid modifications of PC12 cells by arachidonate or docosahexaenoic acid affect neurite outgrowth but not norepinephrine release." *Neurochem Res* 22:671–678 (1997).

Horrocks, L. A., and Y. K. Yeo. "Health benefits of docosahexaenoic acid (DHA)." *Pharmacol Res* 40:211–225 (1999).

Innis, S. M. "The role of dietary n-6 and n-3 fatty acids in the developing brain." *Dev Neurosci* 22:474–480 (2000).

Lim, S-Y., and H. Suzuki. "Intakes of dietary docosahexaenoic acid ethyl ester and egg phosphatidylcholine improve maze-learning ability in young and old mice." *J Nutr* 130:1629–1632 (2000).

———. "Changes in maze behavior of mice occur after sufficient accumulation of docosahexaenoic acid in brain." *J Nutr* 131:319–324 (2001).

Lucas, A., R. Morley, T. J. Cole, G. Lister, and C. Leeson-Payne. "Breast milk and subsequent intelligence quotient in children born preterm." *Lancet* 339:261–264 (1992).

Makrides, M., M. A. Neumann, R. W. Byard, K. Simmer, and R. A. Gibson. "Fatty acid composition of the brain, retina, and erythrocytes in breast-fed and formula-fed infants." *Am J Clin Nutr* 60:189–194 (1994).

Neuringer, M. "Cerebral cortex docosahexaenoic acid is lower in formula-fed than in breast-fed infants." *Nutr Rev* 51:238–241 (1993).

Schmidt, M. A. *Smart Fats*. Berkeley, Calif.: Frog, Ltd., 1997.

Suzuki, H., S. Park, M. Tamura, and S. Ando. "Effect of the long-term feeding of dietary lipids on the learning ability, fatty acid composition of brain stem phospholipids and synaptic membrane fluidity in adult mice: A comparison of sardine oil diet with palm oil diet." *Mech Ageing Dev* 101:119–128 (1998).

Willatts, P., and J. S. Forsyth. "The role of long-chain polyunsaturated fatty acids in infant cognitive development." *Prostaglandins Leuko Essen Fatty Acids* 63:95–100 (2000).

Yonekubo, A., S. Honda, T. Kanno, K. Takahashi, and Y. Yamamoto. "Physiological role of docosahexaenoic acid in mother's milk and infant formulas." In *Essential Fatty Acids and Eicosanoids,* ed. A. Sinclair and R. Gibson, pp. 214–217. Champaign, Ill.: American Oil Chemists Press, 1992.

Zimmer, L., S. Hembert, G. Durand, P. Breton, D. Guilloteau, J. C. Besnard, and S. Chalon. "Chronic n-3 polyunsaturated fatty acid diet deficiency acts on dopamine metabolism in the rat frontal cortex." *Neurosci Lett* 240:177–181 (1998).

Zimmer, L., P. Breton, G. Durand, D. Guilloteau, J. C. Besnard, and S. Chalon. "Prominent role of n-3 polyunsaturated fatty acids in cortical dopamine metabolism." *Nutr Neurosci* 2:257–265 (1999).

Zimmer, L., S. Delpal, D. Guilloteau, J. Aioun, G. Durand, and S. Chalon. "Chronic n-3 polyunsaturated fatty acid deficiency alters dopamine vesicle density in the rat frontal cortex." *Neurosci Lett* 284:25–28 (2000).

Chapter 4   Eicosanoids: Hormones That Harm, Hormones That Heal

Brenner, R. R. "Nutrition and hormonal factors influencing desaturation of essential fatty acids." *Prog Lipid Res* 20:41–48 (1982).

Chakrin, L. W., and D. M. Bailey, eds. *The Leukotrienes*. New York: Academic Press, 1984.

Connor, W. E. "Importance of n-3 fatty acids in health and disease." *Am J Clin Nutr* 71:S171–S175 (2000).

Dek, S. B., and Walsh, M. F. "Leukotrienes stimulate insulin release from rat pancreas." *Proc Nat Acad Sci USA* 81:2199–2202 (1985).

Despres, J-P., B. Lamarche, P. Mauriege, B. Cantin, G. R. Dagenais, S. Moorjani, and P-J Lupien. "Hyperinsulinemia as an independent risk factor for ischemic heart disease." *N Engl J Med* 334:952–957 (1996).

El Boustani, S., J. E. Gausse, B. Descomps, L. Monnier, F. Mendy, and A. Crastes de Paulet. "Direct in vivo characterization of delta 5-desaturase activity in humans by deuterium labeling: Effect of insulin." *Metabolism* 38:315–321 (1989).

Ferreria, S. H., S. Moncada, and J. R. Vane. "Indomethacin and aspirin abolish prostaglandin release from the spleen." *Nature New Biol* (England) 231:237–239 (1971).

Gaziano, J. M., P. J. Skerrett, and J. E. Buring. "Aspirin in the treatment and prevention of cardiovascular disease." *Haemostasis* 30:1–13 (2000).

Herman, A. G., P. M. Vanhoutle, H. Denolin, and A. Goossons, eds. *Cardiovascular Pharmacology of Prostaglandins*. New York: Raven Press, 1982.

Lakshmanan, M. R., C. M. Nepokroeff, G. C. Ness, R. E. Dugan, and J. W. Porter. "Stimulation by insulin of rat liver beta hydroxy methyl HMG-CoA and cholesterol synthesizing activities." *Biochem Biophys Res Comm* 50:704–710 (1973).

Lands, W. E. M. *Fish and Human Health*. New York: Academic Press, 1986.

Metz, S., W. Fujimoto, and R. O. Robertson. "Modulation of insulin secretion by cyclic AMP and prostaglandin E." *Metabolism* 31:1014–1033 (1982).

Metz, S., M. van Rollins, R. Strife, W. Fujimoto, and R. P. Robertson. "Lipoxygenase pathway in islet endocrine cells: Oxidative metabolism of arachidonic acid promotes insulin release." *J Clin Invest* 71:1191–1205 (1983).

Oates, J. A. "The 1982 Nobel Prize in physiology or medicine." *Science* 218:765–768 (1982).

Pek, S. B., and M. F. Walsh. "Leukotrienes stimulate insulin released from rat pancreas." *Proc Nat Acad Sci USA* 82:2199–2202 (1984).

Pelikonova, T., M. Kohout, J. Base, Z. Stefka, J. Kovar, L. Kerdova, and J. Valek. "Effect of acute hyperinsulinemia on fatty acid composition of serum lipids in non-insulin dependent diabetics and healthy men." *Clin Chim Acta* 203:329–337 (1991).

Robertson, R. P., D. J. Gavarenski, D. Porte, and E. L. Bierman. "Inhibition of in vivo insulin secretion by prostaglandin E₁." *J Clin Invest* 54:310–315 (1974).

Robertson, R. P. "Prostaglandins, glucose homeostasis, and diabetes mellitus." *Ann Rev Med* 34:1–12 (1983).

Sacca, L., G. Perez, F. Pengo, I. Pascucci, and M. Conorelli. "Reduction of circulating insulin levels during the infusion of different prostaglandins in the rat." *Acta Endocrinol* 79:266–274 (1975).

Schror, K., and H. Sinziner, eds. *Prostaglandins in Clinical Research*. New York: Liss, 1989.

Sears, Barry. *The Zone*. New York: Regan Books, 1995.

———. *The Anti-Aging Zone*. New York: Regan Books, 1999.

Vane, J. R., and J. O'Grady, eds. *Therapeutic Applications of Prostaglandins*. London: Edward Arnold, 1993.

Watkins, W. D., M. B. Petersen, and J. R. Fletcher, eds. *Prostaglandins in Clinical Practice*. New York: Raven Press, 1989.

Willis, A. L. *Handbook of Eicosanoids, Prostaglandins, and Related Lipids*. Boca Raton, Fla.: CRC Press, 1987.

Chapter 5 What Is Wellness?

Brod, S. A. "Unregulated inflammation shortens human functional longevity." *Inflamm Res* 49:561–570 (2000).

Dalen, J. E. "Health care in America: The good, the bad, and the ugly." *Arch Intern Med* 160:2573–2576 (2000).

Despres, J-P., B. Lamarche, P. Mauriege, B. Cantin, G. R. Dagenais, S. Moorjani, and P-J. Lupien. "Hyperinsulinemia as an independent risk factor for ischemic heart disease." *N Engl J Med* 334:952–957 (1996).

Eaton, S. B., M. Konner, and M. Shostak. "Stone agers in the fast lane: Chronic degenerative diseases in evolutionary perspective." *Am J Med* 84:739–749 (1998).

Jeppesen, J., H. O. Hein, P. Suadicani, and F. Gyntelberg. "Relation of high TG low HDL cholesterol and LDL cholesterol to the incidence of ischemic heart disease—An 8-year follow-up in the Copenhagen Male Study." *Arterioscler Thromb Vasc Biol* 17:1114–1120 (1997).

Lamarche, B., I. Lemieux, and J-P. Despres. "The small, dense LDL phenotype and the risk of coronary heart disease: Epidemiology, pathphysiology, and therapeutic aspects." *Diabetes Metab* 25:199–211 (1999).

Lane, M. A., D. K. Ingram, and G. S. Roth. "Calorie restriction in nonhuman primates: effects on diabetes and cardiovascular disease risk." *Toxicological Sci* 52:41–48 (1999).

Sears, Barry. *The Zone*. New York: Regan Books, 1995.

———. *The Anti-Aging Zone*. New York: Regan Books, 1999.

Chapter 6 Brain Wellness

Aisen, P. S. "Anti-inflammatory therapy for Alzheimer's disease." *Neurobiol Aging* 21:447–448 (2000).

Endres, S., R. Ghorbani, V. E. Kelley, K. Georgilis, G. Lonnemann, J. W. van der Meer, J. G. Cannon, T. S. Rogers, M. S. Klempner, and P. C.

Weber. "The effect of dietary supplementation with n-3 polyunsaturated fatty acids on the synthesis of interleukin-1 and tumor necrosis factor by mononuclear cells." *N Engl J Med* 320:265–271 (1989).

Jones, C. R., T. Aria, and S. I. Rapaport. "Evidence for the involvement of docohexaenoic acid in cholinergic simulated signal transduction at the synapse." *J Neurochem Res* 22:663–670 (1997).

Khalsa, D. S. Brain Longevity. New York: Warner Books, 1997.

Lands, W. E. M. *Fish and Human Health*. New York: Academic Press, 1986.

Sapolsky, R. M. S*tress, the Aging Brain, and the Mechanisms of Neuron Death*. Cambridge, Mass.: MIT Press, 1992.

Schmidt, M. A. *Smart Fats*. Berkeley, Calif.; Frog, Ltd., 1997.

Sears, Barry. *The Zone*. New York: Regan Books, 1995.

———. *The Anti-Aging Zone*. New York: Regan Books, 1999.

Simopoulos, A. P., and J. Robinson. *The Omega Plan*. New York: Harper-Collins, 1998.

Stoll, A. L. *The Omega-3 Connection*. New York: Simon and Schuster, 2001.

Unger, R. H., and P. J. Lefebvre. *Glucagon: Molecular Physiology, Clinical and Therapeutic Implications*. Oxford: Pergamon Press, 1972.

Yehuda, S., S. Rabinovitz, R. L. Carasso, and D. I. Mostofsky. "Essential fatty acid preparation improves Alzheimer's patients' quality of life." *Int J Neurosci* 87:141–149 (1996).

Chapter 7 The Basic Plan

Agus, M. S. D., J. F. Swain, C. L. Larson, E. A. Eckert, and D. S. Ludwig. "Dietary composition and physiologic adaptations to energy restriction." *Am J Clin Nutr* 71:901–907 (2000).

Ascherio, A., and W. C. Willett. "Health effects of trans fatty acids." *Am J Clin Nutr* 66:1006S–10010S (1997).

Ballschmiter, K., and M. Zell. "Baseline studies of the global pollution. I. Occurrence of organohalogens in pristine European and antarctic aquatic environments." *Int J Environ Anal Chem* 8:15–35 (1980).

Bertoni-Freddari, C. L., P. Fattoretti, U. Caselli, T. Casoi, G. Di Stefano, and S. Algeri. "Dietary restriction modulates synaptic structural dynamics in the aging hippocampus." *Age* 22:107–113 (1999).

Bodkin, N. L., H. K. Ortmeyer, and B. C. Hansen. "Long-term dietary restriction in older-aged rhesus monkeys: Effects on insulin resistance." *J Gerontol A Biol Sci Med Sci* 50:B142–B147 (1995).

Cao, G., E. Sofic, and R. L. Prior. "Antioxidant capacity of tea and common vegetables." *J Agric Food Chem* 44:3426–3431 (1996).

Cao, G., S. L. Booth, J. A. Sadowski, and R. L. Prior. "Increases in human plasma antioxidant capacity after consumption of controlled diets high in fruits and vegetables." *Am J Clin Nutr* 68:1081–1087 (1998).

Campbell, L. A., and F. J. Smith. "Transient declines in blood glucose signal meal initiation." *Int J Obesity* 14:15–23 (1990).

Cefalu, W. T., J. D. Wagner, Z. Q. Wang, A. D. Bell-Farrow, J. Collins, D. Haskell, R. Bechtold, and T. Morgan. "A study of caloric restriction and cardiovascular aging in cynomolgus monkeys: A potential model for aging research." *J Gerontol A Biol Sci Med Sci* 52:B98–B102 (1997).

Cefalu, W. T., Z. Q. Wang, A. D. Bell-Farrow, J. G. Terry, W. Sonntag, M. Waite, and J. Parks. "Chronic caloric restriction alters muscle membrane fatty acid content." *Exp Gerontology* 35:331–341 (2000).

Coulston, A. M., G. C. Liu, and G. M. Reaven. "Plasma glucose, insulin, and lipid responses to high-carbohydrate, low-fat diets in normal humans." *Metab* 32:52–56 (1983).

DeLongeril, M., P. Salen, J. L. Martin, I. Monjaud, J. Delaye, and N. Mamelle. "Mediterranean diet, traditional risk factors, and the rate of cardiovascular complications after myocardial infarction: Final report of the Lyon Diet Heart Study." *Circulation* 99:79–785 (1999).

Farquhar, J. W., A. Frank, R. C. Gross, and G. M. Reaven. "Glucose, insulin, and triglyceride responses to high and low carbohydrate diets in man." *J Clin Invest* 45:1648–1656 (1966).

Hansen, B. C., N. L. Bodkin, and H. K. Ortmeyer. "Calorie restriction in nonhuman primates: Mechanisms of reduced morbidity and mortality." *Toxicological Sci* 52:56–60 (1999).

———. "Calorie restriction: Effects on body composition, insulin signaling and aging." *J Nutr* 131:900S–902S (2001).

Hill, E. G., S. B. Johnson, L. D. Lawson, M. M. Mahfouz, and R. T. Holman. "Perturbation of the metabolism of essential fatty acids by dietary partially hydrogenated vegetable oil." *Proc Natl Acad Sci USA* 79:953–957 (1982).

Himaya, A., M. Fantino, J. M. Antoine, L. Brondel, and J. Louis-Sylvestre. "Satiety power of dietary fat: A new appraisal." *Am J Clin Nutr* 65:1410 (1997).

Holt, S., J. Brand, C. Soveny, and J. Hansky. "Relationship to satiety of postprandial glycaemic, insulin, and cholecystokinin responses." *Appetite* 8:129–141 (1992).

Jenkins, D. J. A., T. M. S. Wolever, and R. H. Taylor. "Glycemic index of foods: A physiological basis for carbohydrate exchange." *Am J Clin Nutr* 34:362–366 (1981).

Jenkins, D. J. A., T. M. S. Wolever, S. Vukson, F. Brighenti, S. C. Cunnane,

A. V. Rao, A. L. Jenkins, G. Buckley, and W. Singer. "Nibbling versus gorging: Metabolic advantages of increased meal frequency." *N Engl J Med* 321:929–934 (1989).

Katan, M. B., S. M. Grundy, and W. C. Willett. "Should a low-fat, high-carbohydrate diet be recommended for everyone? Beyond low-fat diets." *N Engl J Med* 337:563–567 (1997).

Kemnitz, J. W., R. Weindruch, E. B. Roecker, K. Crawford, P. L. Kaufman, and W. B. Ershler. "Dietary restriction of adult male rhesus monkey: Design, methodology, and preliminary findings from the first year of study." *J Gerontol A—Biol Sci Med Sci* 48:B17–B26 (1993).

Kemnitz, J. W., E. B. Roecker, R. Weindruch, D. F. Elson, S. T. Baum, and R. N. Bergman. "Dietary restriction increases insulin sensitivity and lowers blood glucose in rhesus monkeys." *Am J Physiol* 266:E540–E547 (1994).

Kim, M. J., E. B. Roecher, and R. Weindruch. "Influences of aging and dietary restriction on red blood cell density profiles and antioxidant enzyme activities in rhesus monkeys." *Exp Gerontology* 28:515–527 (1993).

Laganiere, S., and B. P. Yu. "Anti-lipoperoxidation action of food restriction." *Biochem Biophys Res Comm* 45:1185–1189 (1987).

———. "Effect of chronic food restriction in aging rats: Liver cytosolic antioxidants and related enzymes." *Mech Ageing Dev* 48:221–226 (1989).

Lampe, J. W. "Health effects of vegetables and fruit: Assessing mechanisms of action in human experimental studies." *Am J Clin Nutr* 70:475S–490S (1999).

Lane, M. A., S. S. Ball, D. K. Ingram, R. G. Cutler, J. Engel, V. Read, and G. S. Roth. "Diet restriction in rhesus monkeys lowers fasting and glucose-stimulated glucoregulatory end points." *Am J Physiol* 268:E941–E948 (1993).

Lane, M. A., A. Z. Reznick, E. M. Tilmont, A. Lanir, S. S. Ball, V. Read, D. K. Ingram, R. G. Cutler, and G. S. Roth. "Aging and food restriction alter some indices of bone metabolism in male rhesus monkeys." *J Nutr* 125:1600–1610 (1995).

Lane, M. A., D. J. Baer, W. V. Rumpler, R. Weindruch, D. K. Ingram, E. M. Tilmont, R. G. Cutler, and G. S. Roth. "Calorie restriction lowers body temperature in rhesus monkeys, consistent with a postulated anti-aging mechanism in rodents." *Proc Natl Acad Sci USA* 93:4159–4164 (1996).

Lane, M. A., D. K. Ingram, S. S. Ball, and G. S. Roth. "Dehydroepiandrosterone sulfate: A biomarker of primate aging slowed by calorie restriction." *J Clin Endocrinol Metab* 82:2093–2096 (1997).

Lane, M. A., D. K. Ingram, and G. S. Roth. "Calorie restriction in nonhuman primates: Effects on diabetes and cardiovascular disease risk." *Toxicological Sci* 52:41–48 (1999).

Lane, M. A., E. M. Tilmont, H. De Angelis, A. Handy, D. K. Ingram, J. W. Kemnitz, and G. S. Roth. "Short-term calorie restriction improves disease-related markers in older male rhesus monkeys." *Mech Ageing Devel* 112:185–196 (1999).

Lee, C-K., R. G. Kloop, R. Weindruch, and T. A. Prolia. "Gene expression profile of aging and its retardation by caloric restriction." *Science* 285:1390–1393 (1999).

Lee, D. W., and B. P. Yu. "Modulation of free radicals and superoxide dimutase by age and dietary restriction." *Aging* 2:357–362 (1991).

Li, D., A. Ng, N. J. Mann, and A. J. Sinclair. "Contribution of meat fat to dietary arachidonic acid." *Lipids* 33:437–440 (1998).

Liu, D., E. Moberg, M. Kollind, P. E. Lins, and U. Adamson. "A high concentration of circulating insulin suppresses the glucagon response to hypoglycemia in normal men." *J Clin Endocrinol Metab* 73:1123–1128 (1991).

Louis-Sylvestre, J. "Glucose utilization dynamics and food intake." *Br J Nutr* 82:427–429 (1999).

Ludwig, D. S., J. A. Majzoub, A. Al-Zahrani, G. E. Dallal, I. Blanco, and S. B. Roberts. "High glycemic index foods, overeating, and obesity." *Pediatrics* 103:E26 (1999).

Masoro, E. J. "Antiaging action of caloric restriction: Endocrine and metabolic aspects." *Obesity Res* 3:241S–247S (1995).

———. "Assessment of nutritional components in prolongation of life and health by diet." *Proc Soc Exp Biol Med* 193:31–34 (1990).

———. "Retardation of aging process by food restriction: An experimental tool." *Am J Clin Nutr* 55:1250S–1252S (1992).

———. "Caloric restriction and aging." *Exp Gerontology* 35:299–305 (2000)

Masoro, E. J., B. P. Yu, and H. A. Bertrand. "Action of food restriction in delaying the aging process." *Proc Natl Acad Sci USA* 79:4239–4241 (1982).

Masoro, E. J., R. J. M. McCarter, M. S. Katz, and McMahan. "Dietary restriction alters characteristics of glucose fuel use." *J Gerontol A— Biol Sci Med Sci* 47:B202–B208 (1992).

McCarty, M. F. "Vegan proteins may reduce risk of cancer, obesity, and cardiovascular disease by promoting increased glucagon activity." *Med Hypothesis* 53:459–485 (1999).

McCay, C. M., M. F. Crowell, and L. A. Maynard. "The effect of retarded growth upon the length of life span and the ultimate body size." *J Nutr* 10:63–79 (1935).

McCullough, M. L., D. Feskanich, E. B. Rimm, E. L. Giovannucci, A. Ascherio, J. N. Variyam, D. Spegelman, M. J. Stampfer, and W. C. Willett. "Adherence to the Dietary Guidelines for Americans and the risk of major chronic disease in men." *Am J Clin Nutr* 72:1223–1231 (2000).

McCullough, M. L., D. Feskanich, M. J. Stampfer, B. A. Rosner, F. B. Hu, D. J. Hunter, J. N. Variyam, G. A. Colditz, and W. C. Willett. "Adherence to Dietary Guidelines for Americans and risk of major chronic disease in women." *Am J Clin Nutr* 72:1214–1222 (2000).

McManus, K., L. Antinoro, and F. Sachs. "A randomized controlled trial of a moderate-fat, low-energy diet compared with a low-fat, low-energy diet for weight loss in overweight adults." *Int J Obesity* 25:1503–1511 (2001).

Means, L. W., J. L. Higgins, and T. J. Fernandez. "Mid-life onset of dietary restriction extends life and prolongs cognitive functioning." *Physiol Behav* 54:503–508 (1993).

Melanson, K. J., M. S. Weserterp, F. J. Smith, L. A. Campfield, and W. H. M. Saris. "Blood glucose patterns and appetite in time-blinded humans: Carbohydrate versus fat." *Am J Physiol* 46:337–345 (1999).

Mensiak, R. P., and M. B. Katan. "Effect of monounsaturated fatty acids versus complex carbohydrates on high-density lipoproteins in healthy men and women." *Lancet* i:122–125 (1897).

Metges, C. C., K. J. Petzke, and V. R. Young. "Dietary requirements for indispensable amino acids in adult humans: New concepts, methods of estimation, uncertainties, and challenges." *Ann Nutr Metab* 43:267–276 (1999).

Parr, T. "Insulin exposure and aging theory." *Gerontology* 43:182–200 (1997).

Rissanen, T., S. Voutilainen, K. Myyssonen, T. A. Lakka, and J. T. Salonen. "Fish oil–derived fatty acids, docosahexaenoic acid, and docosapentaenoic acid, and the risk of acute coronary events." *Circulation* 102:2677–2679 (2000).

Salonen, J. T., K. Seppanen, T. A. Lakka, R. Salonen, and G. A. Kaplan. "Mercury accumulation and accelerated progression of carotid atherosclerosis." *Atherosclerosis* 148:265–273 (1999).

Sadur, C. N., and R. H. Eckel. "Insulin stimulation of adipose tissue lipoprotein lipase." *J Clin Invest* 69:1119–1123 (1982).

Schwartz, M. W., D. P. Figlewicz, D. G. Baskin, S. C. Woods, and D. Porte.

384   References

"Insulin in the brain: A hormonal regulation of energy balance." *Endocrine Rev* 43:387–414 (1992).

Sears, Barry. *The Zone.* New York: Regan Books, 1995.

———. *Mastering the Zone.* New York: Regan Books, 1997.

———. *Zone-Perfect Meals in Minutes.* New York: Regan Books, 1997.

———. *Zone Food Blocks.* New York: Regan Books, 1998.

———. *The Anti-Aging Zone.* New York: Regan Books, 1999.

———. *The Soy Zone.* New York: Regan Books, 2000.

———. *A Week in the Zone.* New York: Regan Books, 2000.

Skov, A. R., S. Toubro, B. Renn, L. Holm, and A. Astrup. "Randomized trial on protein vs. carbohydrate in ad libitum fat reduced diet for the treatment of obesity." *Int J Obes Relat Metab Disord* 23:528–536 (1999).

Sohal, R. S., and R. Weindruch. "Oxidative stress, caloric restriction, and aging." *Science* 273:59–63 (1996).

Soucy, J., and J. LeBlanc. "The effects of a beef and fish meal on plasma amino acids, insulin, and glucagon levels." *Nutr Res* 19:17–24 (1999).

Walford, R. L., S. B. Harris, and M. W. Gunion. "The calorically restricted low-fat nutrient dense diet in Biosphere 2 significantly lowers blood glucose, total leukocyte count, cholesterol, and blood pressure in humans." *Proc Natl Acad Sci USA* 89:11533–11537 (1992).

Wang, H., G. Cao, and R. L. Prior. "Total antioxidant capacity of fruits." *J Agric Food Chem* 44:701–705 (1996).

Weed, J. L., M. A. Lane, G. S. Roth, D. L. Speer, and D. K. Ingram. "Activity measures in rhesus monkeys on long-term calorie restriction." *Physiol Behav* 62:97–103 (1997).

Weindruch, R. "Caloric restriction and aging." *Sci Am* 274:46–52 (1996).

Weindruch, R., T. Kayo, C-K. Lee, and T. A. Prolla. "Microarry profiling of gene expression in aging and its alteration by caloric restriction in mice." *J Nutr* 131:918S–923S (2001).

Westphal, S. A., M. C. Gannon, and F. Q. Nutrall. "Metabolic response to glucose ingested with various amounts of protein." *Am J Clin Nutr* 62:267–272 (1990).

Willett, W. C. *Eat, Drink, and Be Healthy.* New York: Simon and Schuster, 2001.

Wolever, T. M. S., D. J. A. Jenkins, G. R. Collier, R. Lee, G. S. Wong, and R. G. Josse. "Metabolic response to test meals containing different carbohydrate foods: Relationship between rate of digestion and plasma insulin response." *Nutr Res* 8:573–581 (1988).

Wolever, T. M. S. "Relationship between dietary fiber content and composition in foods and the glycemic index." *Am J Clin Nutr* 51:72–75 (1990).

Wolever, T. M. S., D. J. A. Jenkins, A. A. Jenkins, and R. G. Josse. "The glycemic index: methodology and chemical implications." *Am J Clin Nutr* 54:846–854 (1991).

Wolfe, B. M., and L. A. Piche. "Replacement of carbohydrate by protein in a conventional-fat diet reduces cholesterol and triglyceride concentrations in healthy normolipidemic subjects." *Clin Invest Med* 22:140–148 (1999).

Unger, R. H. "Glucagon and the insulin glucagon ratio in diabetes and other catabolic illnesses." *Diabetes* 20:834–838 (1971).

Unger, R. H., and P. J. Lefebvre. *Glucagon: Molecular Physiology, Clinical and Therapeutic Implications.* Oxford: Pergamon Press, 1972.

Van Vliet, T., and M. B. Katan. "Lower ratio of n-3 to n-6 fatty acids in cultured than in wild fish." *Am J Clin Nutr* 51:1–2 (1990).

Young, V. R., D. M. Bier, and P. L. Pellert. "A theoretical basis for increasing current estimates of the amino acid requirements in adult men with experimental support." *Am J Clin Nutr* 50:80–92 (1989).

Young, V. R. "Protein and amino acid requirements in humans." *Scand J Nutr* 36:47–56 (1992).

Chapter 8 Fish Oil Supplements: Knowledge Is Power

Addison, R. F., M. E. Zinck, R. G. Ackman, and J. C. Sipos. "Behavior of DDT, polychlorinated biphenyls (PCBs), and dieldrin at various stages of refining of marine oils for edible use." *J Am Oil Chem Soc* 55:391–394 (1978).

Axelrod, L., J. Carnuso, E. Williams, K. Kleiman, E. Briones, and D. Schoenfeld. "Effects of a small quantity of n-3 fatty acids on cardiovascular risk factors in NIDDM: A randomized, prospective, double-blind, controlled study." *Diabetes Care* 17:37–44 (1994).

Ballschmiter, K., and M. Zell. "Baseline studies of the global pollution. I. Occurrence of organohalogens in pristine European and antarctic aquatic environments." *Int J Environ Anal Chem* 8:15–35 (1980).

Bang, H. O., and J. Dyerberg. "Fish consumption and mortality for coronary heart disease." *N Engl J Med* 313:822–823 (1985).

Barber, M. D., and K. C. H. Fearon. "Tolerance and incorporation of a high-dose eicosapentaenoic acid diester emulsion by patients with pancreatic cancer cachexia." *Lipids* 36:347–351 (2001).

Blanck, H. M., M. Marcus, P. E. Tolbert, C. Rubin, A. K. Henderson, V. S. Hertzberg, R. H. Zhang, and L. Cameron. "Age at menarch and Tanner stage in girls exposed in utero and postnatally to polybrominated biphenyl." *Epidemiology* 11:641–647 (2000).

Bowles, M. H., D. Klonis, T. G. Plavac, B. Gonzales, D. A. Francisco,

R. W. Roberts, G. R. Boxberger, L. R. Poliner, and J. P. Galichia. "EPA in the prevention of restenois post PTCA." *Angiology* 42:187–194 (1991).

Cao, G., E. Sofic, and R. L. Prior. "Antioxidant capacity of tea and common vegetables." *J Agric Food Chem* 44:3426–3431 (1996).

Donnelly, S. M., M. A. Ali, and D. N. Churchill. "Effect of n-3 fatty acids from fish oil on hemostasis, blood pressure, and lipid profile of dialysis patients." *J Am Soc Nephrol* 2:1634–1639 (1992).

Dyerberg, J., and H. O. Bang. "Homeostatic function and platelet polyunsaturated fatty acids in Eskimos." *Lancet* ii:433–435 (1979).

Eaton, S. B. "An evolutionary view of dietary recommendations." *National Institutes of Health Workshop on the Essentiality of and Dietary Reference Intakes for Omega-6 and Omega-3 Fatty Acids* (1999).

Eaton, S. B., A. J. Sinclair, L. Cordain, and N. J. Mann. "Dietary intake of long-chain polyunsaturated fatty acids during the Paleolithic." *World Rev Nutr Diet* 83:12–23 (1998).

Eritsland, J., H. Arnesen, I. Seljeflot, and P. Kierulf. "Long-term effects of n-3 polyunsaturated fatty acids on haemostatic variables and bleeding episodes in patients with coronary artery disease." *Blood Coagul Fibrinolysis* 6:17–22 (1995).

Eritsland, J., H. Arnesen, K. Gronseth, N. B. Fjeld, and M. Abdelnoor. "Effect of dietary supplementation with n-3 fatty acid on coronary artery bypass graft patency." *Am J Cardiol* 77:31–36 (1996).

Eritsland, J. "Safety considerations of polyunsaturated fatty acids." *Am J Clin Nutr* 71:197S–201S (2000).

Fairchild, W. L., E. O. Swansburg, J. T. Arsenault, and S. B. Brown. "Does an association between pesticide use and subsequent declines in catch of Atlantic salmon represent a case of endocrine disruption?" *Environ Health Perspect* 107:349–358 (1999).

Freidberg, C. E., M. J. Janssen, R. J. Heine, and D. E. Grobbee. "Fish oil and glycemic control in diabetes: A meta analysis." *Diabetes Care* 19:21:494–500 (1998).

GISSI-Prevenzione Investigators. "Dietary supplementation with n-3 polyunsaturated fatty acids and vitamin E after myocardial infarction: Results of the GISSI-Prevenzione trial." *Lancet* 354:447–455 (1999).

Glauber, H., P. Wallace, K. Griver, and G. Brechtel. "Adverse metabolic effects of omega-3 fatty acids in non-insulin diabetes mellitus." *Ann Intern Med* 108:663–668 (1988).

Goodnight, S. H., W. S. Harris, and W. E. Connor. "The effects of dietary omega-3 fatty acids on platelet composition and function in man: A prospective, controlled study." *Blood* 58:880–885 (1981).

Harris, W. S., S. L. Windsor, and C. A. Dujovne. "Effects of four doses of n-3 fatty acids given to hyperlipidemic patients for six months." *J Am Coll Nutr* 10:220–227 (1991).

Haglund, O., R. Wallin, R. Luostarinen, and T. Saldeen. "Effects of a new fluid fish oil concentration on triglycerides, cholesterol, fibrinogen, and blood pressure." *J Intern Med* 227:347–353 (1990).

Haumann, B. F. "Alternative sources for n-3 fatty acids." *Inform* 9:1108–1119 (1998).

Hilbert, G., L. Lillemark, S. Balchen, and C. S. Hojskov. "Reduction of organochlorine contaminants from fish oil during refining." *Chemosphere* 37:1241–1252 (1998).

Horrocks, L. A., and Y. K. Yeo. "Health benefits of docosahexaenoic acid (DHA)." *Pharmacol Res* 40:211–225 (1999).

Jacobs, M. N., D. Santillo, P. A. Johnston, C. L. Wyatt, and M. C. French. "Organochlorine residues in fish oil dietary supplements: Comparison with industrial grade oils." *Chemosphere* 37:1709–1721 (1998).

Jeppesen, J., H. O. Hein, P. Suadicani, and F. Gyntelber. "Low triglycerides–high high-density lipoprotein cholesterol and the risk of ischemic heart disease." *Arch Intern Med* 161:361–366 (2001).

Jorgensen, K-A., A. H. Nielsen, and J. Dyerberg. "Hemostatic factors and rennin in Greenland Eskimos on a high eicosapentaenoic acid intake." *Acta Med Scand* 219:473–479 (1986).

Knapp, H. R., I. A. G. Reilly, P. Alessandrini, and G. A. FitzGerald. "In vivo indexes of platelet and vascular function during fish-oil administration in patients with atherosclerosis." *N Engl J Med* 314:937–942 (1986).

Knapp, H. R. "Dietary fatty acids in human thrombosis and hemostasis." *Am J Clin Nutr* 65:1687S–1698S, (1997).

Krauss, R. M., R. H. Eckel, B. Howard, L. J. Appel, S. R. Daniels, R. J. Deckelbaum, J. W. Erdman, P. Kris-Etherton, I. J. Goldberg, T. A. Kotchen, A. H. Lichtenstein, W. E. Mitch, R. Mullis, K. Robinson, J. Wylie-Rosett, S. St. Jeor, J. Suttie, D. L. Tribble, and T. L. Bazzarre. "American Heart Association Guidelines." *Circulation* 102:2284–2299 (2000).

Leaf, A., M. B. Jorgenson, A. K. Jacobs, et al. "Do fish oils prevent restenosis after coronary angioplasty?" *Circulation* 90:2248–2257 (1994).

Li, D., N. J. Mann, and A. J. Sinclair. "Comparison of n-3 polyunsaturated fatty acids from vegetable oils, meat, and fish in raising platelet eicosapentaenoic acid levels in humans." *Lipids* 34:S309 (1999).

Mueller, B. A., R. L. Talker, C. H. Tegeler, and T. J. Prihoda. "The bleeding time effects of a single dose of aspirin in subjects receiving omega-3 fatty acid dietary supplementation." *J Clin Pharmacol* 31:185–190 (1991).

Nelson, G. J., P. S. Schmidt, G. L. Bartolini, D. S. Kelley, and D. Kyle. "The effect of dietary docosahexaenoic acid on platelet function, platelet fatty acid composition, and blood coagulation in humans." *Lipids* 32:1129–1136 (1997).

Parkinson, A. J., A. L. Cruz, W. L. Heyward, L. R. Bulkow, D. Hall, L. Barstae, and W. E. Connor. "Elevated concentrations of plasma omega-3 polyunsaturated fatty acids among Alaskan Eskimos." *Am J Clin Nutr* 59:383–388 (1994).

Pedersen, H. S., G. Muvad, K. N. Sedelin, G. T. Malcom, and D. A. Boudreau. "N-3 fatty acids as a risk factor for haemorrhagic stroke." *Lancet* 353:812–813 (1999).

Phinney, S. "Potential risk of prolonged gamma-linolenic acid use." *Ann Intern Med* 120:692 (1994).

Raz, A., N. Kamin-Belsky, F. Przedecki, and M. Obukowicz. "Dietary fish oil inhibits delta-6 desaturase activity in vivo." *J Am Oil Chem Soc* 75:241–245 (1998).

Rissanen, T., S. Voutilainen, K. Nyyssonen, T. A. Lakka, and J. T. Salonen. "Fish oil–derived fatty acids, docosahexaenoic acid and docosapentaenoic acid, and the risk of acute coronary events: The Kuopio ischaemic heart disease risk factor study." *Circulation* 102:2677–2679 (2000).

Rivellese, A. A., A. Maffettone, C. Iovine, L. Di Marino, G. Annuzzi, M. Mancini, and G. Riccardi. "Long-term effects of fish oil on insulin resistance and plasma lipoproteins in NIDDM patients with hypertriglyceridemia." *Diabetes Care* 19:1207–1213 (1996).

Rogan, W. J. "Persistent pesticides and polychlorinated biphenyls." *Ann Rev Public Health* 4:381–390 (1983).

Salonen, J. T., K. Seppanen, T. A. Lakka, R. Salonen, and G. A. Kaplan. "Mercury accumulation and accelerated progression of carotid atherosclerosis." *Atherosclerosis* 148:265–273 (1999).

Sargent, J. R. "Fish oil and human diet." *Br J Nutr* 78:S5–S13 (1997).

Sims, G. G., C. E. Cosham, J. R. Campbell, and M. C. Murray. "DDT residues in cod livers from the Maritime Provinces of Canada." *Bull Environ Contam Toxicol* 14:505–512 (1975).

Simopoulos, A. P., A. Leaf, and N. Salem. "Workshop on the essentiality of recommended dietary intakes of omega-6 and omega-3 fatty acids." *J Am Coll Nutr* 18:487–489 (1999).

Sirtori, C. R., R. Paoletti, M. Mancini, G. Crepaldi, E. Manzato, A. Rivellese, F. Pamparana, and E. Stragliotto. "N-3 fatty acids do not lead to an increased diabetic risk in patients with hyperlipidemia and abnormal glucose tolerance: Italian fish oil multicenter trial." *Am J Clin Nutr* 65:1874–1881 (1997).

Stoll, A. L., E. Sverus, M. P. Freeman, S. Rueter, H. A. Zhoyan, E. Diamond, K. K. Cress, and L. B. Marangell. "Omega-3 fatty acids in bipolar depression: A preliminary double-blind, placebo-controlled trial." *Arch Gen Psychiatry* 56:407–412 (1999).

"Substances affirmed as generally recognized as safe: Menhaden oil." *Federal Register* 62:30751–30757 (1997).

Thies, F., G. Nebe-von-Caron, J. R. Powell, P. Yaqoob, E. A. Newsholme, and P. C. Calder. "Dietary supplementation with eicosapentaenoic acid, but not with other long-chain n-3 or n-6 polyunsaturated fatty acids, decreases natural killer cell activity in healthy subjects aged >55 y." *Am J Clin Nutr* 73:539–548 (2001).

Tsigouri, A. D., and A. E. Tyrpenou. "Determination of organochlorine compounds (OCPs and PCBs) in fish oil and fish liver oil by capillary gas chromatography and electron capture detection." *Bull Environ Contam Toxicol* 65:244–252 (2000).

Van Vliet, T., and M. B. Katan. "Lower ratio of n-3 to n-6 fatty acids in cultured than in wild fish." *Am J Clin Nutr* 51:1–2 (1990).

Yamada, T., J. P. Strong, T. Ishii, T. Ueno, M. Koyama, H. Wagayama, A. Shimizu, T. Sakai, G. T. Malcom, and M. A. Guzman. "Atherosclerosis and omega-3 fatty acids in the populations of fishing village and a farming village in Japan." *Athero* 153:469–481 (2000).

Zuijdgeest-van Leeuwen, S. D., P. C. Dagnelie, T. Rietveld, J. W. van den Berg, and J. H. Wilson. "Incorporation and washout of orally administered n-3 fatty acid ethyl esters in different plasma lipid fractions." *Br J Nutr* 82:481–488 (1999).

Chapter 9 Your Blood Will Tell Your Future

Allred, J. B. "Too much of a good thing? An over-emphasis on eating low-fat food may be contributing to the alarming increase in overweight amounts of US adults." *J Am Dietetic Assoc* 95:417–418 (1995).

Boizel, R., P. Y. Benhhamou, B. Lardy, F. Laporte, T. Foulon, and S. Halmi. "Ratio of triglycerides to HDL cholesterol is an indicator of LDL particle size in patients with type 2 diabetes and normal HDL cholesterol levels." *Diabetes Care* 23:1679–1683 (2000).

Colditz, G. A. "Economic costs of obesity." *Am J Clin Nutr* 55:503S–507S (1992).

Corti, M-C., J. M. Guraink, M. E. Saliva, T. Harris, T. S. Field, R. B. Wallace, L. F. Berkman, T. E. Seeman, R. J. Glynn, C. H. Hennekens, and R. J. Havlik. "HDL cholesterol predicts coronary heart disease mortality in older persons." *JAMA* 274:539–544 (1995).

Despres, J-P., B. Lamarche, P. Mauriege, B. Cantin, G. R. Dagenais, S. Moorjani, and P-J. Lupien. "Hyperinsulinemia as an independent risk factor for ischemic heart disease." *N Engl J Med* 334:952–957 (1996).

Drexel, H., F. W. Amann, J. Beran, K. Rentsch, R. Candinas, J. Muntwyler, A. Leuthy, T. Gasser, and F. Follath. "Plasma triglycerides and three lipoprotein cholesterol fractions are independent predictors of the extent of coronary atherosclerosis." *Circulation* 90:2230–2235 (1992).

Gould, K. L., D. Ornish, L. Scherwitz, S. Brown, R. P. Edens, M. J. Hess, Z. Mullani, L. Bolomey, F. Dobbs, W. T. Armstrong, T. Merritt, T. Potts, S. Sparler, and J. Billings. "Changes in myocardial perfusion abnormalities by positron emission tomography after long-term, intense risk factor modification." *JAMA* 274:894–901 (1995).

Gould, K. L. "Very low-fat diets for coronary heart disease: Perhaps, but which one?" *JAMA* 275:1402–1403 (1996).

Hamm, P., R. B. Shekelle, and J. Stamler. "Large fluctuations in body weight during young adulthood and 25-year risk of coronary death in men." *Am J Epidemiol* 129:312–318 (1989).

Heini, A. F., and R. L. Weinsier. "Divergent trends in obesity and fat intake patterns: An American paradox." *Am J Med* 102: 259–264 (1997).

Holman, R. T., L. Smythe, and S. Johnson. "Effect of sex and age on fatty acid composition of human serum lipids." *Am J Clin Nutr* 32:2390–2399 (1979).

Jeppesen, J., H. O. Hein, P. Suadicani, and F. Gyntelberg. "Low triglycerides–high high-density lipoprotein cholesterol and the risk of ischemic heart disease." *Arch Intern Med* 161:361–366 (2001).

Kagawa, Y., M. Nishizawa, M. Suzuki, T. Miyatake, T. Hamamoto, K. Goto, E. Montaonga, H. Izumikawa, H. Hirata, and A. Eibhara. "Eicosapolyenoic acids of serum lipids of Japanese islanders with incidence of cardiovascular diseases." *J Nutr Sci Vitaminol* 28:441–453 (1982).

Knopp, R. H., C. E. Walden, B. M. Retzlaff, B. S. McCann, A. A. Dowdy, J. J. Albers, G. O. Gey, and M. N. Copper. "Long-term cholesterol-lowering effects of 4 fat-restricted diets in hypercholesterolemic and combined hyperlipidemic men." *JAMA* 278:1509–1515 (1997).

Knopp, R. H. "Serum lipids after a low-fat diet." *JAMA* 279:1345–1346 (1998).

Kris-Etherton, P. M., T. A. Pearson, Y. War, R. L. Hargrove, K. Moriarty, V. Fishell, and T. D. Etherton. "High-monounsaturated fatty acid diets lower both plasma cholesterol and triacylglycerol concentrations." *Am J Clin Nutr* 70:1009–1015 (1999).

Kuczmarshi, R. J., K. M. Flegal, S. M. Campbell, and C. L. Johnson. "Increasing prevalence of overweight among U.S. adults." *JAMA* 272:205–211 (1994).

Lamarche, B., A. Tchernof, P. Mauriege, B. Cantin, G. R. Dagenais, P. J. Lupien, and J-P. Despres. "Fasting insulin and apolipoprotein levels as a predictor as risk factors for ischemic heart disease." *JAMA* 279:1955–1961 (1998).

Lamarche, B., J. Lemieux, and J-P. Despres. "The small dense phenotype and the risk of coronary heart disease: Epidemiology, pathophysiology, and therapeutic aspects." *Diabetes Metab* 25:199–211 (1999).

Laakso, M. "How good a marker is insulin level for insulin resistance?" *Am J Epidemiol* 137:959–965 (1993).

Laws, A., A. C. King, W. I. Haskell, and G. M. Reaven. "Relation of fasting plasma insulin concentrations to high density lipoprotein cholesterol and triglyceride concentrations in man." *Arteriosclerosis and Thrombosis* 11:1636–1642 (1991).

Lee, I. M., and R. S. Paffenbarger. "Change in body weight and longevity." *JAMA* 268:2045–2049 (1992).

Lee, H. Y., J. Woo, Z. Y. Chen, S. P. Leung, and X. H. Peng. "Serum fatty acid, lipid profiles, and dietary intake of Hong Kong Chinese omnivores and vegetarians." *Eur J Clin Nutr* 54:768–773 (2000).

Lemieux, I., A. Pascot, C. Couillard, B. Lamarche, A. Tchernof, N. Almeras, J. Bergeron, D. Gaudet, G. Tremblay, D. Prudhomme, A Nadeau, and J-P. Despres. "Hypertriglyceridemic waist: A marker of the atherogenic metabolic triad (hyperinsulinemia; hyperlipoprotein B; small, dense LDL) in men?" *Circulation* 102:179–184 (2000).

Lichtenstein, A. H., and L. van Horn. "Very low fat diets." *Circulation* 98:935–939 (1998).

Markovic, T. P., A. C. Fleury, L. V. Campbell, L. A. Simons, S. Balasubramanian, D. J. Chisholm, and A. B. Jenkins. "Benefical effect on average lipid levels from energy restriction and fat loss in obese individuals with or without type 2 diabetes." *Diabetes Care* 21:695–700 (1998).

Markovic, T. P., S. M. Furler, A. B. Jenkins, E. W. Kraegen, L. V. Campbell, and D. J. Chisholm. "The determinants of glycemic responses to diet restriction and weight loss in obesity and NIDDM." *Diabetes Care* 21:687–694 (1988).

Mathers, C. D., R. Sadana, J. A. Salomon, C. J. L. Murray, and A. D. Lopez. "Healthy life expectancy in 191 countries, 1999." *Lancet* 357:1685–1691 (2001).

Nakamura, T., K. Takebe, Y. Tando, Y. Arai, N. Yamada, M. Ishii, H. Kituchi, K. Machida, K. Imamura, and A. Terada. "Serum fatty acid composition in normal Japanese and its relationship with dietary fish and vegetable oil contents and blood lipid levels." *Ann Nutr Metab* 39:261–270 (1995).

Ornish, D., S. E. Brown, L. W. Scherwitz, J. H. Billings, W. T. Armstrong, T. A. Ports, S. M. McLanahan, R. L. Kirkeeide, R. J. Brand, and K. L. Gould. "Can lifestyle changes reverse coronary heart disease?" *Lancet* 336:129–133 (1990).

Parkinson, A. J., A. L. Cruz, W. L. Heyward, L. R. Bukow, D. Hall, L. Barstaed, and W. E. Connor. "Elevated concentrations of plasma omega-3 polyunsaturated fatty acids amoung Alaskan Eskimos." *Am J Clin Nutr* 59:384–388 (1994).

Patch, J. R., G. Miesenbock, F. Hopferwieser, V. Muhlberger, E. Knapp, J. K. Dunn, A. M. Gotto, and W. Patsch. "Relation of triglyceride metabolism and coronary artery disease." *Arteriosclerosis and Thrombosis* 12:1336–1345 (1992).

Pouliot, M. C., J-P. Despres, A. Nadeau, S. Moorjani, D. Prud'Homme, P. J. Lupien, A. Tremblay, and C. Bouchard. "Visceral obesity in men: Associations with glucose tolerance, plasma insulin, and lipoprotein levels." *Diabetes* 41:826–834 (1992).

Reaven, G. M., Y. D. Chen, J. Jeppesen, P. Maheux, and R. M. Krauss. "Insulin resistance and hyperinsulinemia in individuals with small, dense low density lipoproteins." *J Clin Invest* 92:141–146 (1993).

Sears, B. *The Zone*. New York: Regan Books, 1995.

———. *The Anti-Aging Zone*. New York: Regan Books, 1999.

Tchernof, A., B. Lamarche, D. Prud'Homme, A. Nadeau, S. Moorjani, F. Labrie, P. J. Lupien, and J-P. Despres. "The dense LDL phenotype: Associations with plasma lipoprotein levels, visceral obesity, and hyperinsulinemia." *Diabetes Care* 19:629–637 (1996).

Thompson, P. D. "More on low-fat diets." *N Engl J Med* 338:1623–1624 (1998).

Wang, H., G. Cao, and R. L. Prior. "Total antioxidant capacity of fruits." *J Agric Food Chem* 44:701–705 (1996).

Willett, W. C., J. E. Manson, M. I. Stampfer, G. A. Colditz, B. Rosner, F. E. Speizer, and C. H. Hennekens. "Weight, weight change, and coronary heart disease in women." *JAMA* 273:461–465 (1995).

Yamada, T., J. P. Strong, T. Ishii, T. Ueno, M. Koyama, H. Wagayama, A. Shimizu, T. Sakai, G. T. Malcom, and M. A. Guzman. "Atherosclerosis and omega-3 fatty acids in the populations of fishing village and a farming village in Japan." *Athero* 153:469–481 (2000).

Yeni-Komshian, H., M. Carntoni, F. Abbasi, and G. M. Reaven. "Relationship between several surrogate estimates of insulin resistance and quantification of insulin-mediated glucose disposal in 490 healthy nondiabetic volunteers." *Diabetes Care* 23:171–175 (2000).

Zeleniuch-Jacquotte, A., V. Chajes, A. L. van Kappel, E. Riboi, and P. Tonilo. "Reliability of fatty acid composition in human serum phospholipids." *Eur J Clin Nutr* 54:367–372 (2000).

Chapter 10 When the Brain Goes Wrong

Adams, P., S. Lawson, A. Sanigorski, and A. J. Sinclair. "Arachidonic acid to eicosapentaenoic acid ratio in blood correlates positively with clinical symptoms of depression." *Lipids* 31:S157–S161 (1996).

Agren, J. J., M. L. Tormala, M. J. Nenonem, and O. O. Haainea. "Fatty acid composition of erythrocyte, platelet, and serum lipids in strict vegetarians." *Lipids* 30:365–369 (1995).

Agostoni, C., S. Trojan, R. Bellu, E. Riva, M. G. Bruzzese, and M. Giovannini. "Development quotient at 24 months and fatty acid composition of the diet in early infancy." *Arch Dis Child* 76:421–424 (1997).

Ahmann, P. A., S. J. Waltonen, K. A. Olson, F. W. Theye, A. J. van Erem, and R. J. LePlant. "Placebo-controlled evaluation of Ritalin side effects." *Pediatrics* 91:1101–1106 (1993).

Aisen, P. S. "Anti-inflammatory therapy for Alzheimer's disease." *Neurobiol Aging* 21:447–448 (2000).

———. "Anti-inflammatory therapy for Alzheimer's disease: Implication of the prednisone trial." *Acta Neurol Scand* 176:85–89 (2000).

Akiyama, H., T. Arai, H. Kondo, E. Tanno, C. Haga, and K. Ikeda. "Cell mediators of inflammation in the Alzheimer disease brain." *Alzheimer Disease and Associated Disorders* 14:S47–S53 (2000).

Alvarez, J. C., D. Cremniter, P. Lesieur, A. Gregoire, A. Gilton, T. Macquin-Mavier, C. Jarreu, and C. Spreux-Varoquaux. "Low blood cholesterol and low platelet serotonin levels in violent suicide attempters." *Bio Psychiatry* 45:1066–1069 (1999).

Amen, D. G. *Change Your Brain, Change Your Life*. New York: Random House, 1998.

———. *Healing ADD*. New York: Putnam, 2001.

Attvall, S., J. Fowelin, I. Lager, H. Von Schenck, and U. Smith. "Smoking induces insulin resistance—A potential link with the insulin resistance syndrome." *J Intern Med* 233:327–332 (1993).

Blaylock, R. L. *Excitotoxins*. Santa Fe, N.M.: Health Press, 1995.

Bourre, J. M. "Function of polyunsaturated fatty acids in the nervous system." *Prostaglandins Leuko Essen Fatty Acids* 48:5–15 (1993).

Brozoski, T. J., R. M. Brown, H. E. Rosvold, and P. S. Goldman. "Cognitive deficit caused by regional depletion of dopamine in prefrontal cortex of rhesus monkey." *Science* 205:929–932 (1979).

Burdge, G. C., S. M. Wright, J. O. Warner, and A. D. Postle. "Fetal brain and liver phospholipid fatty acid composition in a guinea pig model of fetal alcohol syndrome: Effect of maternal supplementation with tuna oil." *J Nutr Biochem* 8:438–444 (1997).

Burgress, J. R., L. Stevens, and L. Peck. "Long-chain polyunsaturated fatty acids in children with attention-deficit hyperactivity disorder." *Am J Clin Nutr* 71:327S–330S (2000).

Bush, G., J. A. Frazier, S. L. Rauch, L. J. Seidman, P. J. Whalen, M. A. Jenike, B. R. Rosen, and J. Biederman. "Anterior cingulated cortex dysfunction in attention deficit/hyperactivity disorder revealed by fMRI and the counting stroop." *Bio Psychiatry* 45:1542–1552 (1999).

Carlson, S., and A. Werkman. "A randomized trial of visual attention of preterm infants fed docosahexaenoic acid until two months." *Lipids* 31:85–90 (1996).

Carrie, I., M. Clement, D. De Javel, H. Frances, and J. M. Bourre. "Learning deficits in the first generation OF1 mice deficient in (n-3) polyunsaturated fatty acids do not result from visual alteration." *Neurosci Lett* 266:69–72 (1999).

Centonze, D., P. Calabresi, P. Giacomini, and G. Berardi. "Neurophysiology of Parkinson's disease: From basic research to clinical correlates." *Clin Neurophysiology* 110:2006–2013 (1999).

Connor, W. E., M. Neuringer, and D. S. Lin. "Dietary effects on brain fatty acid composition: The reversibility of n-3 fatty acids deficiency and turnover of docosahexaenoic acid in the brain erythrocytes and plasma of rhesus monkeys." *J Lipid Res* 31:237–247 (1990).

Connor, W. E., M. Neuringer, and S. Reisbick. "Essential fatty acids: Importance of n-3 fatty acids in the retina and brain." *Nutr Rev* 50:21–29 (1992).

Cooper, N. R., R. N. Kalaria, P. L. McGeer, and J. Rogers. "Key issues in Alzheimer's disease inflammation." *Neurobiol Aging* 21:451–453 (2000).

Conquer, J. A., M. C. Tierney, J. Zecevic, W. J. Bettger, and R. H. Fisher. "Fatty acid analysis of blood plasma of patients with Alzheimer's disease, other types of dementia, and cognitive impairment." *Lipids* 35:1305–1312 (2000).

Delion, S., S. Chalon, J. Herault, D. Guilloteau, J. C. Besnard, and G. Durand. "Chronic dietary alpha-linolenic acid deficiency alters dopaminergic and serotoninergic neurotransmitters in rats." *J Nutr* 124:2466–2476 (1994).

Delion, S., S. Chalon, D. Guilloteau, J. C. Besnard, and G. Durand. "-Alpha-linolenic acid deficiency alters age-related changes of dopaminergic and serotoninergic neurotransmitters in the rat frontal cortex." *J Neurochem* 66:1582–1591 (1996).

Eliasson, B., and U. Smith. "Insulin resistance in smokers and other long-term users of nicotine." In *Contempory Endocrinology: Insulin Resistance*, ed. G. Reaven and A. Laws, pp. 121–136. Humana Press, 1999.

Ensel, M., H. Milon, and A. Malnoe. "Effect of low intake of n-3 fatty acids during development of brain phospholipid, fatty acid composition and exploratory behavior in rats." *Lipids* 26:203–208 (1991).

Fenton, W. S., J. Hibbeln, and M. Knable. "Essential fatty acids, lipid membrane abnormalities, and the diagnosis and treatment of schizophrenia." *Bio Psychiatry* 47:8–21 (2000).

Fernstrom, J. D. "Effects of dietary polyunsaturated fatty acids on neuronal function." *Lipids* 34:161–169 (1999).

Freychet, P. "Insulin receptors and insulin actions in the nervous system." *Diabetes Metab Res Rev* 16:390–392 (2000).

Gallai, V., P. Sarchielli, A. Trequattrini, M. Franceschini, A. Floridi, C. Firenze, A. Alberti, D. Di Benedetto, and E. Stragliotto. "Cytokine secretion and eicosanoid production in the peripheral blood mononuclear cells of MS patients undergoing dietary supplementation with n-3 polyunsaturated fatty acids." *J Neuroimmunol* 56:143–153 (1995).

Gayo, A., L. Mozo, A. Suarez, A. Tunon, C. Lahoz, and C. Gutierrez. "Interferon beta treatment modulates TNF and interferon gamma spontaneous gene expression in MS." *Neurology* 52:1764–1770 (1999).

Gibson, R. A., M. A. Neuman, and M. Makrides. "Effect of dietary docosahexaenoic acid on brain composition and neural function in term infants." *J Lipid Res* 34:S177–S181 (1996).

Gillman, M. W., A. Cupples, B. E. Millen, C. Ellison, and P. A. Wolf. "Inverse association of dietary fat with development of ischemic stroke in men." *JAMA* 278:2145–2150 (1997).

Glueck, C. J., M. Tieger, R. Kunkel, T. Tracy, J. Speirs, P. Streicher, and E. Illig. "Improvement in symptoms of depression and in an index of life stressors accompany treatment of severe hypertriglyceridemia." *Bio Psychiatry* 34:240–252 (1993).

Hamazaki, T., S. Sawazaki, M. Itomura, E. Asaoka, Y. Nagao, N. Nishimura, K. Yazawa, T. Kuwamori, and M. Kobayashi. "The effect of docosahexaenoic acid on aggression in young adults." *J Clin Invest* 97:1129–1134 (1996).

Hamazaki, T., S. Sawazaki, M. Itomura, Y. Nagao, A. Thienprasert,

T. Nagasawa, and S. Watanabe. "Effect of docosahexaenoic acid on hostility." *World Rev Nutr Diet* 88:47–52 (2001).

Harvey, B. H., and C. D. Bouwer. "Neuropharmacology of paradoxic weight gain with selective serotonin reuptake inhibitors." *Clin Neuropharmacol* 23:90–97 (2000).

Hibbeln, J. R., and N. Salem. "Dietary polyunsaturated fatty acids and depression: When cholesterol does not satisfy." *Am J Clin Nutr* 62:1–9 (1995).

Hibbeln, J. R. "Fish consumption and major depression." *Lancet* 351:1213 (1998).

———. "Seafood consumption and homicide mortality." *World Rev Nutr Diet* 88:41–46 (2001).

Hohlfeld, R., and H. Wiendl. "The ups and downs of multiple sclerosis therapeutics." *Ann Neurology* 49:281–284 (2001).

Holman, R. T., S. B. Johnson, and P. L. Ogburn. "Deficiency of essential fatty acids and membrane fluidity during pregnancy and lactation." *Proc Natl Acad Sci USA* 88:4835–4839 (1991).

Horrobin, D. F. "Essential fatty acids, prostaglandins, and alcoholism: An overview." *Alcohol Clin Exp Res* 11:2–9 (1987).

Horrocks, L. A., and Y. K. Yeo. "Health benefits of docosahexaenoic acid (DHA)." *Pharmacol Res* 40:211–225 (1999).

Hoozemans, J. J. M., A. J. M. Rozemuller, I. Janssen, C. J. A. De Groot, R. Veerhuls, and P. Eikelenboon. "Cyclooxygenase expression in microglia and neurons in Alzheimer's disease and control brain." *Acta Neuropathol* 101:2–8 (2001).

Hoozemans, J. J. M., R. Veerhuis, I. Janssen, A. J. M. Rozemuller, and P. Eikelenboon. "Interleukin-1 beta induced cyclooxygenase 2 expression and prostaglandin E2 secretion by human neuroblastoma cells: Implications for Alzheimer's disease." *Exp Gerontology* 36:559–570 (2001).

Holden, R. J., I. S. Pakula, and P. A. Mooney. "The role of brain insulin in the neurophysiology of serious mental disorders: Review." *Med Hypotheses* 52:193–200 (1999).

Ichiyama, T., K. Okada, J. M. Lipton, T. Matsubara, T. Hayashi, and S. Furukawa. "Sodium valproate inhibits production of TNF and IL-6 and activation of NF-kappa B." *Brain Res* 857:246–251 (2000).

Ikemoto, A., A. Nitta, S. Furukawa, M. Ohishi, A. Nakamure, Y. Fujii, and H. Okuyama. "Dietary n-3 fatty acid deficiency decreases nerve growth factor content in rat hippocampus." *Neurosci Lett* 285:99–102 (2000).

Iso, H., M. J. Stampfer, J. E. Manson, K. Rexrode, F. Hu, C. H. Hennekens,

G. A. Colditz, F. E. Speizer, and W. C. Willett. "Prospective study of fat and protein intake and risk of intraparenchymal hemorrhage in women." *Circulation* 103:856–863 (2001).

Kademi, M., E. Wallstrom, M. Andersson, F. Piehl, R. Di Marco, and T. Olsson "Reduction of both pro- and anti-inflammatory cytokines after 6 months of interferon beta-1a treatment of multiple sclerosis." *J Neurochem* 103:202–210 (2000).

Kalmijn, S., D. Foley, L. White, C. M. Burchfiel, J. D. Curb, H. Petrovitch, G. W. Ross, R. J. Havlik, and L. J. Launer. "Metabolic cardiovascular syndrome and risk of dementia in Japanese-American elderly men." *Arterioscler Thromb* 20:2255–2260 (2000).

Kawas, C. H., and R. Brookmeyer. "Aging and the public health: Effects of dementia." *N Engl J Med* 344:1160–1161 (2001).

Khalsa, D. S. *Brain Longevity*. New York: Warner Books, 1997.

Knapp, H. R., I. A. G. Reilly, P. Alessandrini, and G. A. FitzGerald. "In vivo indexes of platelet and vascular function during fish-oil administration in patients with atherosclerosis." *N Engl J Med* 314:937–942 (1986).

Kyle, D. J., E. Schaefer, G. Patton, and A. Beiser. "Low serum docosahexaenoic acid is a significant risk factor for Alzheimer's dementia." *Lipids* 34:S245 (1999).

Lauritzen, I., N. Blondeau, C. Heurteaux, C. Widmann, G. Romey, and M. Lazdunski. "Polyunsaturated fatty acids are potent neuroprotectors." *EMBO J* 19:1784–1793 (2000).

Lauritzen, L., H. S. Hansen, M. H. Jorgensen, and K. F. Michaelsen. "The essentiality of long-chain n-3 fatty acids in relation to development and function of the brain and retina." *Prog Lipid Res* 40:1–94 (2001).

Maes, M. "Fatty acid composition in major depression: Decreased n-3 fractions in cholesterol esters and increased C20:46/C20:5n3 ratio in cholesterol ester and phospholipids." *J Affect Dis* 38:35–46 (1996).

Maes, M., A. Christophe, J. Delanghe, C. Altamura, H. Neels, and H. Y. Meltzer. "Lowered omega-3 polyunsaturated fatty acids in serum phospholipids and cholesterol esters of depressed patients." *Psychiatry Res* 85:275–291 (1999).

Manev, H., U. Tolga, K. Sugaya, and T. Qu. "Putative role of neuronal 5-lipoxygenase in an aging brain." *FASEB J* 14:1464–1469 (2000).

Mayeux, R., R. Costa, K. Bell, C. Merchant, M. X. Tung, and D. Jacobs. "Reduced risk of Alzheimer's disease among individuals with low caloric intake." *Neurology* 59:S296–S297 (1999).

McGeer, P. L., M. Shulzer, and E. G. McGeer. "Arthritis and anti-inflammatory agents as possible protective factors for Alzheimer's disease: A review of 17 epidemiological studies." *Neurology* 47:425–432 (1996).

McGeer, P. L., E. G. McGeer, and K. Yasojima. "Alzheimer disease and neuroinflammation." *J Neural Transm* 59:53–57 (2000).

Mills, D. E., K. M. Prkochin, K. A. Harvey, and R. P. Ward. "Dietary fatty acid supplementation alters stress reactivity and performance in man." *J Human Hypertension* 3:111–116 (1989).

Minami, M., S. Kimura, T. Endo, N. Hamaue, M. Hirafuji, H. Togashi, M. Matsujoto, M. Yoshika, H. Saito, S. Watanabe, T. Kobayashi, and H. Okuyama. "Dietary docosahexaenoic acid increases cerebral acetylcholine levels and improves passive avoidance performance in stroke-prone spontaneously hypertensive rats." *Pharmacol Biochem Behav* 58:1123–1129 (1997).

Mischoulon, D., and M. Fava. "Docosahexaenoic acid and omega-3 fatty acids in depression." *Psychiat Clin North Am* 23:785–794 (2000).

Miyanga, K., K. Yonemura, T. Takagi, R. Kifune, Y. Kishi, F. Miyakawa, K. Yazawa, and Y. Shirota. "Clinical effects of DHA in demented patients." *J Clin Ther Med* 11:881–901 (1995).

Montine, T. J., K. R. Sidell, B. C. Crews, W. R. Markesbery, L. J. Marnett, L. J. Roberts, and J. D. Morrow. "Elevated CSF prostaglandin E2 levels in patients with probable AD." *Neurology* 53:1495–1498 (1999).

Moriguchi, T., R. S. Greiner, and N. Salem, Jr. "Behavioral deficits associated with dietary induction of decreased brain docosahexaenoic acid concentration." *J Neurochem* 75:2563–2573 (2000).

Moses, H., and S. Sriram. "Interferon beta and the cytokine trial: Where are we going?" *Neurology* 52:1729–1730 (1999).

Nagatsu, T., M. Mogi, H. Ichinose, and A. Togari. "Cytokines in Parkinson's disease." *J Neural Transm* 58:143–151 (2000).

Nelson, G. J., P. S. Schmidt, G. L. Bartolini, D. S. Kelley, and D. Kyle. "The effect of dietary docosahexaenoic acid on platelet function, platelet fatty acid composition, and blood coagulation in humans." *Lipids* 32:1129–1136 (1997).

Neuroinflammation Working Group. "Inflammation and Alzheimer's disease." *Neurobiol Aging* 21:383–421 (2000).

Nightingale, S., E. Woo, A. D. Smith, J. M. French, M. M. Gale, H. M. Sinclair, D. Bates, and D. A. Shaw. "Red blood cell and adipose tissue fatty acids in active and inactive multiple sclerosis patients." *Acta Neurol Scand* 82:43–50 (1990).

Nishino, S., R. Ueno, K. Ohishi, T. Sakai, and O. Tayaishi. "Salivary prostaglandin concentrations: Possible state indicators for major depression." *Am J Psychiatry* 146:365–368 (1989).

Norden, M. Beyond Prozac. New York: Regan Books, 1996.

Nordvik, I., K-M. Myhr, H. Nyland, and K. S. Bjerve. "Effects of dietary advice and n-3 supplementation in newly diagnosed MS patients." *Acta Neurol Scand* 102:143–149 (2000).

Ohishi, K., R. Uneo, S. Nishino, T. Sakai, and O. Hayaishi. "Increased level of salivary prostaglandins in patients with major depression." *Bio Psychiatry* 15:326–334 (1988).

Pasinetti, G. M., and P. S. Aisen. "Cyclooxygenase-2 expression is increased in frontal cortex of Alzheimer's disease brain." *Neuroscience* 87:319–324 (1997).

Pawlosky, R. J., and N. Salem. "Ethanol exposure causes a decrease in docosahexaenoic acid and an increase in docosapentaenoic acid in feline brain and retina." *Am J Clin Nutr* 61:1284–1289 (1995).

Peet, M. "Essential fatty acid deficiency in erythrocyte membranes from chronic schizophrenic patients and clinical effects of dietary supplementation." *Prostaglandins Leuko Essen Fatty Acids* 55:71–75 (1996).

Peet, M., J. Brind, C. N. Ramchand, S. Shah, and G. K. Vankar. "Two double-blind placebo-controlled pilot studies of eicosapentaenoic acid in the treatment of schizophrenia." *Schizophr Res* 49:243–251 (2001).

Pratico, D., and J. Q. Rojanowski. "Inflammatory hypothesis: Novel mechanisms of Alzheimer's neurodegradation and new therapeutic targets?" *Neurobiol Aging* 21:441–445 (2000).

Rasmuson, S., R. Andrew, B. Nasman, J. R. Seckl, B. R. Walker, and T. Olsson. "Increased glucocorticoid production and altered cortisol metabolism in women with mild to moderate Alzheimer's disease." *Bio Psychiatry* 49:547–552 (2001).

Remarque, E. J., E. L. E. M. Bollen, A. W. E. Weverling-Rijnsburger, J. C. Laterveer, G. J. Blauw, and R. G. J. Westendorp. "Patients with Alzheimer's disease display a pro-inflammatory phenotype." *Exp Gerontology* 36:171–176 (2001).

Reisbick, S., M. Neuringer, R. Hasnain, and W. E. Connor. "Home cage behavior of rhesus monkey with long term deficiency of omega-3 fatty acids." *Physiol Behav* 55:231–239 (1994).

Riviere, S., I. Biroluez-Aragon, and B. Vellas. "Plasma protein glycation in Alzheimer's disease." *Glycoconjugate* J 15:1039–1042 (1998).

Roses, A. D., W. J. Strittmatter, M. A. Pericak-Vance, E. H. Corden, A. M. Saunders, and D. E. Schmechel. "Clinical application of apoplipoprotein E genotyping to Alzheimer's disease." *Lancet* 343:1564–1565 (1994).

Sachdev, P. "Attention deficit hyperactivity disorder in adults." *Psychol Med* 29:507–514 (1999).

Seung Kim, H. F., E. J. Weeber, J. D. Sweatt, A. L. Stoll, and L. B. Marangell. "Inhibitory effects of omega-3 fatty acids on protein kinase C activity in vitro." *Mol Psychiatry* 6:246–248 (2001).

Shoulson, I. "DATATOP: A decade of neuroprotective inquiry. Parkinson Study Group. Deprenyl and tocopherol antioxidative therapy of Parkinsonism." *Ann Neurology* 44:S160–S166 (1998).

Simopoulos, A. P., and J. Robinson. *The Omega Plan.* New York: Harper-Collins, 1998.

Sinclair, A. J., and M. A. Crawford. "The effect of a low fat maternal diet on neonatal rats." Br *J Nutr* 29:127–137 (1973).

Sonderberg, M., C. Edlund, K. Kristensson, and G. Dallner. "Fatty acid composition of brain phospholipids in aging and Alzheimer's disease." *Lipids* 26:421–423 (1991).

Stein, J. "The neurobiology of reading difficulties." *Prostaglandins Leuko Essen Fatty Acids* 63:109–116 (2000).

Stevens, L. J., and J. Burgess. "Omega-3 fatty acids in boys with behavior, learning, and health problems." *Physiol Behav* 59:915–920 (1996).

Stevens, L. J., S. S. Zentall, J. L. Deck, M. L. Abate, B. A. Watkins, S. A. Lipp, and J. R. Burgess. "Essential fatty acid metabolism in boys with attention-deficit hyperactivity disorder." *Am J Clin Nutr* 62:761–768 (1995).

Stewart, W. F., C. Kawas, M. Corrada, and E. J. Metter. "Risk of Alzheimer's disease and duration of NSAID use." *Neurology* 48:626–632 (1997).

Stoll, A. L., and E. Severus. "Mood stabilizers: Shared mechanisms of action at postsynaptic signal transduction and kindling process." *Harvard Rev Psychiatry* 59:915–920 (1999).

Stoll, A. L., E. Severus, M. P. Freeman, S. Reuter, H. A. Zhoyan, E. Diamond, K. K. Cress, and L. B. Marangell. "Omega-3 fatty acids in bipolar depression: A preliminary double-blind, placebo-controlled trial." *Arch Gen Psychiatry* 56:407–412 (1999).

Stoll, A. L. *The Omega-3* Connection. New York: Simon and Shuster, 2001.

Stordy, B. J. "Benefit of docosahexaenoic acid supplements to dark adaption in dyslexics." *Lancet* 346:385 (1995).

Tanner, C. M. "Dopamine agonists in early therapy: Promise and problems." *JAMA* 284:1971–1973 (2000).

Tanskanen, A. "Fish consumption, depression, and suicidality in a general population." *Arch Gen Psychiatry* 58:512–513 (2001).

Tatton, W. G., J. S. Wadia, W. Y. Ju, R. M. Chalmers-Redman, and N. A. Tatton. "Deprenyl reduces neuronal apoptosis and facilitates neuronal outgrowth by altering protein synthesis without inhibiting monoamine oxidase." *J Neural Transm* 48:45–59 (1996).

Taylor, K. E., and A. J. Richardson. "Visual function, fatty acids, and dyslexia." *Prostaglandins Leuko Essen Fatty Acids* 63:89–93 (2000).

Terano, T., S. Fujishiro, T. Ban, K. Yamamoto, T. Tanaka, Y. Noguchi, Y. Tamura, K. Yazawa, and T. Hirayama. "Docosahexaenoic acid supplementation improves moderately severe dementia from thrombotic cerebrovascular diseases." *Lipids* 34:S345–S346 (1999).

Uauy, R., P. Peirano, D. Hoffman, P. Mena, D. Birch, and E. Birch. "Role of essential fatty acids in the function of the developing nervous system." *Lipids* 31:S167–S176 (1996)

Venters, H. D., R. Dantzer, and K. W. Kelly. "A new concept in neurodegeneration: TNF is a silencer of survival signals." *Trends in Neuroscience* 23:175–180 (2000).

Virkkunen, M. E., D. F. Horrobin, K. Douglas, K. Jenkins, and M. S. Manku. "Plasma phospholipid essential fatty acids and prostaglandin in alcholic, habitually violent, and impulsive offenders." *Bio Psychiatry* 22:1087–1096 (1987).

Vitkovic, L., J. Bockaer, and C. Jacque. "Inflammatory cytokines: Neuromodulators in normal brain?" *J Neurochem* 74:457–471 (2000).

Voigt, R. G., A. M. Llorente, C. L. Jensen, J. K. Fraley, M. C. Berretta, and W. C. Heird. "A randomized, double-blind, placebo-controlled trial of docosahexaenoic acid supplementation in children with attention-deficit/hyperactivity disorder." *J Pediatr* 139:189–196 (2001).

Willatts, P., J. S. Forsyth, M. K. DiModugno, S. Varma, and M. Colvin. "Effect of long-chain polyunsaturated fatty acids in infant formula on problem solving at 10 months of age." *Lancet* 352:688–691 (1998).

Yamada, T., J. P. Strong, T. Ishii, T. Ueno, M. Koyama, H. Wagayama, A. Shimizu, T. Sakai, G. T. Malcom, and M. A. Guzman. "*Athero*sclerosis and omega-3 fatty acids in the populations of a fishing village and a farming village in Japan." *Athero*sclerosis 153:469–481 (2000).

Yehuda, S., S. Rabinovitz, R. L. Carasso, and D. I. Mostofsky. "Essential fatty acid preparation improves Alzheimer's patients' quality of life." *J Neurosci* 87:141–149 (1996).

Yehuda, S., S. Rabinovitz, and D. I. Mostofsky. "Essential fatty acids are mediators of brain biochemistry and cognitive functions." *J Neurosci Res* 56:565–570 (1999).

Zametkin, A. J., T. E. Nordahl, et al. "Cerebral glucose metabolism in adults with hyperactivity of childhood onset." *N Engl J Med* 323:1361–1366 (1990).

Zametkin, A. J., and M. Ernst. "Problems in the management of attention-deficit-hyperactivity disorder." *N Engl J Med* 340:40–46 (1999).

Zimmer, L., S. Hembert, G. Durand, P. Breton, D. Guilloteau, J. C. Besnard, and S. Chalon. "Chronic n-3 polyunsaturated fatty acid diet deficiency acts on dopamine metabolism in the rat frontal cortex." *Neurosci Letter* 240:177–181 (1998).

Zuijdgeest-van Leeuwen, S. D., P. C. Dagnelie, T. Rietveld, J. W. van den Berg, and J. H. Wilson. "Incorporation and washout of orally administered n-3 fatty acid ethyl esters in different plasma lipid fractions." Br *J Nutr* 82:481–488 (1999).

Chapter 11 Who Wants to Die of a Heart Attack?

Albert, C. M., C. H. Hennekens, C. I. O'Donnel, U. A. Ajani, V. J. Carey, and W. C. Willett. "Fish consumption and risk of sudden cardiac death." *JAMA* 279:23–28 (1998).

Albert, M. A., E. Danielson, N. Rifai, and P. M. Ridker. "Effect of statin therapy on C-reactive protein levels: The Pravastatin inflammation/CRP evaluation (PRICE)." *JAMA* 286:64–70 (2001).

Angerer, P., and C. von Schacky. "N-3 polyunsaturated fatty acids and cardiovascular system." *Curr Opinion Lipidol* 11:57–63 (2000).

Ascherio, A., C. H. Hennekens, J. E. Buring, C. Master, M. J. Stampfer, and W. C. Willett. "Trans fatty acid intake and risk of myocardial infarction." *Circulation* 89:94–101 (1994).

Ascherio, A., E. B. Rimm, M. J. Stampfer, E. L. Giovannucci, and W. C. Willett. "Dietary intake of marine n-3 fatty acids, fish intake, and risk of coronary heart disease among men." *N Engl J Med* 332:977–982 (1995).

Ascherio, A., and W. C. Willett. "Health effects of trans fatty acids." *Am J Clin Nutr* 66:1006S–1010S (1997).

Austin, M. A., J. L. Breslow, C. H. Hennekens, J. E. Buring, W. C. Willett, and R. M. Krauss. "Low density lipoprotein subclass patterns and risk of myocardial infarction." *JAMA* 260:1917–1920 (1988).

Austin, M. A. "Plasma triglyceride and coronary heart disease." *Arterioscler Thromb* 11:2–14 (1991).

Baba, T., and S. Neugebauer. "The link between insulin resistance and hypertension: Effects of antihypertensive and antihyperlipidaemic drugs on insulin sensitivity." *Drugs* 47:383–404 (1994).

Bang, H. O., J. Dyerberg, and A. B. Nielsen. "Plasma lipid and lipoprotein pattern in Greenlandic west-coast Eskimos." *Lancet* i:1143–1145 (1971).

Bao, W., S. R. Srinivasan, and G. S. Berenson. "Persistent elevation of plasma insulin levels is associated with increased cardiovascular risk in children and young adults." *Circulation* 93:54–59 (1996).

Bataile, R., and B. Klein. "C-reactive protein levels as a direct indicator of interleukin-6 levels in humans in vivo." *Arthritis Rheum* 35:982–983 (1992).

Baum, C. L., and M. Brown. "Low-fat, high-carbohydrate diets and atherogenic risk." *Nutr Rev* 58:148–151 (2000).

Bellamy, C. M., P. M. Schofield, E. B. Faragher, and D. R. Ramsdale. "Can supplementation of diet with omega-3 polyunsaturated fatty acids reduce coronary angioplasty restenosis rate?" *Eur Heart J* 13:1626–1631 (1992).

Bellosta, S., N. Ferri, F. Bernini, R. Paoletti, and A. Corsini. "Non-lipid related effects of statins." *Ann Med* 32:164–176 (2000).

Biderman, A., and J. Herman. "Risk markers are not without risk." *J Clin Epidemiol* 53:635–636 (2000).

Bigger, J. T., and T. El-Sherif. "Polyunsaturated fatty acids and cardiovascular events." *Circulation* 623–625 (2001).

Billman, G. E., J. X. Kang, and A. Leaf. "Prevention of ischemia-induced cardiac death by n-3 polyunsaturated fatty acids in dogs." *Lipids* 32:1161–1168 (1997).

———. "Prevention of sudden cardiac death by dietary pure omega-3 polyunsaturated fatty acids in dogs." *Circulation* 99:2452–2457 (1999).

Black, H. R. "The coronary artery disease paradox: The role of hyperinsulinemia and insulin resistance and implications for therapy." *J Cardiovasc Pharmacol* 15:26S–38S (1990).

Bonora, E., J. Willeit, S. Kiechl, F. Oberhollenzer, G. Egger, R. Bonadonna, and M. Meggeo. "U-shaped and J-shaped relationships between serum insulin and coronary heart disease in the general population." *Diabetes Care* 21:221–230 (1998).

Bowles, M. H., D. Klonis, T. G. Plavac, B. Gonzales, D. A. Francisco, R. W. Roberts, G. R. Boxberger, L. R. Poliner, and J. P. Galichia. "EPA in the prevention of restenois post PTCA." *Angiology* 42:187–194 (1991).

Braunwald, E. "Cardiovascular medicine at the turn of the millennium: Triumphs, concerns, and applications." *N Engl J Med* 337:1360–1369 (1997).

Brenner, R. R. "Nutrition and hormonal factors influencing desaturation of essential fatty acids." *Prog Lipid Res* 20:41–48 (1982).

Burr, M. L., A. M. Fehily, J. F. Gilbert, S. Rogers, R. M. Holliday, P. M. Sweetnam, P. C. Elwood, and N. M. Deadman. "Effects of changes in fat, fish, and fibre intakes on death and myocardial reinfarction: Diet and reinfarction trial (DART)." *Lancet* ii:757–761 (1989).

Burr, M. L. "Lessons from the story of n-3 fatty acids." *Am J Clin Nutr* 71:397S–398S (2000).

Busse, R., and I. Flemining. "Endothelial dysfunction in atherosclerosis." *J Vas Res* 33:181–194 (1996).

Carantoni, M., F. Abbasi, F. Warmerdan, M. Klebanov, P. W. Wang, Y. D. Chen, S. Azhar, and G. M. Reaven. "Relationship between insulin resistance and partially oxidized LDL particles in healthy, nondiabetic volunteers." *Arterioscler Thromb* 18:762–767 (1998).

Christensen, J. H., M. S. Christensen, J. Dyerberg, and E. B. Schmidt. "Heart rate variability and fatty acid content of blood cell membranes: A dose-response study with n-3 fatty acids." *Am J Clin Nutr* 70:331–337 (1999).

Cleland, S. J., N. Sattar, J. R. Petrie, N. G. Forouhi, H. L. Elliott, and J. M. C. Connell. "Endothelial dysfunction as a possible link between C-reactive protein and cardiovascular disease." *Clin Sci* 98:531–535 (2000).

Coresh, J., P. O. Kwiterovich, and H. H. Smith. "Association of plasma triglyceride concentration and LDL particle diameter, density, and chemico-composition with premature coronary artery disease." *J Lipid Res* 34:1687–1697 (1993).

Corti, M-C., J. M. Guraink, M. E. Saliva, T. Harris, T. S. Field, R. B. Wallace, L. F. Berkman, T. E. Seeman, R. J. Glynn, C. H. Hennekens, and R. J. Havlik. "HDL cholesterol predicts coronary heart disease mortality in older persons." *JAMA* 274:539–544 (1995).

Coulston, A. M., G. C. Liu, and G. M. Reaven. "Plasma glucose, insulin, and lipid responses to high-carbohydrate, low-fat diets in normal humans." *Metab* 32:52–56 (1983).

Cushman, M., C. Legault, E. Barrett-Connor, M. L. Stefanick, C. Kessler, H. L. Judd, P. A. Sakkienen, and R. P. Tracy. "Effect of postmenopausal hormones on inflammation-sensitive proteins." *Circulation* 100:717–722 (1999).

Davi, G., M. Avenra, I. Catalano, C. Barbugallo, A. Ganci, A. Notarbartolo, G. Ciabattoni, and C. Patrono. "Increased thromboxane biosynthesis in type IIa hypercholesterolemia." *Circulation* 85:1792–1798 (1992).

Daviglus, M. L., M. Stamler, A. J. Orencia, A. R. Dyer, K. Liu, P. Greenland, M. K. Walsh, D. Morris, and R. B. Shekelle. "Fish consumption and the 30-year risk of myocardial infarction." *N Engl J Med* 336:1046–1053 (1997).

Davignon, J., and J. S. Cohn. "Triglycerides: A risk factor for coronary heart disease." *Athero*sclerosis 124:S57–S64 (1996).

De Caterina, R., M. I. Cybulsk, S. K. Clinton, M. A. Gimbrone, and

P. Libby. "The omega-3 fatty acid docosahexaenoate reduces cytokine-induced expression of proatherogenic and proinflammatory protein in human endothelial cells." *Arterioscler Thromb* 14:1829–1836 (1994).

Dehmer, G. J., J. J. Popma, E. K. van den Berg, E. J. Eichorn, J. B. Prewitt, W. B. Campbell, L. Jennings, J. T. Willerson, and J. M. Schmitz. "Reduction in the rate of early restenosis after coronary angioplasty by a diet supplemented with n-3 fatty acids." *N Engl J Med* 319:733–740 (1988).

DeLongeril, M., S. Renaud, N. Mamelle, P. Salen, J. L. Martin, I. Monjaud, J. Guidollet, P. Touboul, and J. Delaye. "Mediterranean alpha-linolenic acid rich diet in secondary prevention of coronary heart disease." *Lancet* 343:1454–1459 (1994).

DeLongeril M., P. Salen, and J. Delaye. "Effect of a Mediterranean type of diet on the rate of cardiovascular complications in patients with coronary artery disease." *J Am Coll Cardiology* 28:1103–1108 (1996).

DeLongeril, M., P. Salen, J. L. Martin, I. Monjaud, J. Delaye, and N. Mamelle. "Mediterranean diet, traditional risk factors, and the rate of cardiovascular complications after myocardial infarction: Final report of the Lyon Diet Heart Study." *Circulation* 99:779–785 (1999).

DeMartin, R., M. Hoeth, R. Hofer-Warbinek, and J. A. Schmid. "The transcription factor NF kappa B and the regulation of vascular cell function." *Arterioscler Thromb* Vasc Biol 20: e83–e88 (2000).

Despres, J-P., B. Lamarche, P. Mauriege, B. Cantin, G. R. Dagenais, S. Moorjani, and P-J. Lupien. "Hyperinsulinemia as an independent risk factor for ischemic heart disease." *N Engl J Med* 334:952–957 (1996).

Despres, J. P., B. Lamarche, P. Mauriege, B. Cantin, P-J. Lupien, and G. R. Dagenais. "Risk factors for ischaemic heart disease: Is it time to measure insulin?" *Eur Heart J* 17:1453–1454 (1996).

Dolecek, T. A., and G. Grandits. "Dietary polyunsaturated fatty acids and mortality in the multiple risk factor intervention trial (MRFIT)." *World Rev Nutr Diet* 66:205–216 (1991).

Draznin, B., P. Miles, Y. Kruszynska, J. Olefsky, J. Friedman, J. Golovchenko, R. Stjernholm, K. Wall, M. Reitman, D. Accili, R. Cooksey, D. McClain, and M. Goalstone. "Effects of insulin on the prenylation as a mechanism of potentially detrimental influence of hyperinsulinemia." *Endocrinology* 141:1310–1316 (2000).

Dreon, D., H. A. Fernstrom, B. Miller, and R. M. Krauss. "Low-density lipoprotein subclass patterns and lipoprotein response to a reduced-fat diet in men." *FASEB J* 8:121–126 (1994).

Dreon, D. M., H. A. Fernstrom, P. T. Williams, and R. M. Krauss. "A very-low fat diet is not associated with improved lipoprotein profiles in men with a predominance of large, low-density lipoproteins." *Am J Clin Nutr* 69:411–418 (1999).

Drexel, H., F. W. Amann, J. Beran, K. Rentsch, R. Candinas, J. Muntwyler, A. Leuthy, T. Gasser, and F. Follath. "Plasma triglycerides and three lipoprotein cholesterol fractions are independent predictors of the extent of coronary atherosclerosis." *Circulation* 90:2230–2235 (1992).

Ducimetiere, P., E. Eschwege, G. Papoz, J. L. Richard, J. R. Claude, and G. Rosselin. "Relationship of plasma insulin to the incidence of myocardial infarction and coronary heart disease mortality in a middle-aged population." *Diabetologia* 19:205–210 (1980).

Durrington, P. N. "Triglycerides are more important in atherosclerosis than epidemiology has suggested." *Atherosclerosis* 141:S57–S62 (1998).

Dyerberg, J., H. O. Bang, E. Stofferson, S. Moncada, and J. R. Vane. "Eicosapentaenoic acid and prevention of thrombosis and atherosclerosis." *Lancet* ii:117–119 (1978).

Dyerberg, J., and H. O. Bang. "Haemostatic function and platelet polyunsaturated fatty acids in Eskimos." *Lancet* ii:433–435 (1979)

Eliasson, B., and U. Smith. "Insulin resistance in smokers and other long-term users of nicotine." In *Contemporary Endocrinology: Insulin Resistance*, ed. G. Reaven and A. Laws, pp. 121–136. Totowa, N.J.: Humana Press, 1999.

Eritsland, J., H. Arnesen, K. Bronseth, N. B. Fjeld, and M. Abdelnoor. "Effect of dietary supplementation with n-3 fatty acids on coronary artery bypass graft patency." *Am J Cardiol* 77:31–36 (1996).

Eschwege, E., J. L. Richard, N. Thibult, P. Ducimetiere, J. M. Warnet, J. R. Claude, and G. E. Rosselin. "Coronary heart disease mortality in relation with diabetes, blood glucose, and plasma insulin levels." *Horm Metab Res* 15:41–46 (1985).

Fanaian, M., J. Szilasi, L. Storlien, and G. D. Calvert. "The effect of modified fat diet on insulin resistance and metabolic parameters in type II diabetes." *Diabetologia* 39:A7 (1996).

Farquhar, J. W., A. Frank, R. C. Gross, and G. M. Reaven. "Glucose, insulin, and triglyceride responses to high and low carbohydrate diets in man." *J Clin Invest* 45:1648–1656 (1966).

Fischer, S., P. C. Weber, and J. Dyerberg. "The prostacyclin/thromboxane balance is favourably shifted in Greenland Eskimos." *Prostaglandins* 32:235–241 (1986).

Fontbonne, A., E. Eschwege, F. Cambien, P. Ducimetiere, N. Thibult, J. M. Warnet, J. R. Claude, and G. E. Rosselin. "Hypertriglyceridemia as a risk factor of coronary heart disease in subjects with impaired glucose tolerance or diabetes: Results from the 11-year follow-up of the Paris Prospective Study." *Diabetologia* 32:300–304 (1989).

Fontbonne, A., M. A. Charles, N. Thibult, J. L. Richard, J. R. Claude, J. M. Warnet, G. E. Rosselin, and E. Eschwege. "Hyperinsulinemia as a predictor of coronary heart disease mortality in a healthy population: The Paris Prospective Study, 15-year follow-up." *Diabetologia* 34:356–361 (1991).

Fontbonne, A. "Why can high insulin levels indicate a risk for coronary heart disease?" *Diabetologia* 37:953–955 (1994).

Ford, E. S., and S. Liu. "Glycemic index and serum high-density lipoprotein cholesterol concentration among U.S. adults." *Arch Intern Med* 161:572–576 (2001).

Foster, D. "Insulin resistance—A secret killer?" *N Engl J Med* 320:733–734 (1989).

Garcia-Closas, R., L. Serra-Majem, and L. Segura. "Fish consumption, omega-3 fatty acids, and the Mediterranean diet." *Eur J Clin Nutr* 47:585–590 (1993).

Gaziano, J. M., C. H. Hennekens, C. J. O'Donnell, J. L. Breslow, and J. E. Buring. "Fasting triglycerides, high-density lipoproteins, and risk of myocardial infarction." *Circulation* 96:2520–2525 (1997).

Gaziano, J. M., P. J. Skerrett, and J. E. Buring. "Aspirin in the treatment and prevention of cardiovascular disease." *Haemostasis* 30:1–13 (2000).

Gertler, M., H. E. Leetma, E. Saluste, J. L. Rosenberger, and R. G. Guthrie. "Ischemic heart disease, insulin, carbohydrate, and lipid interrelationship." *Circulation* 46:103–111 (1972).

Gillman, M. W., A. Cupples, B. E. Millen, C. Ellison, and P. A. Wolf. "Inverse association of dietary fat with development of ischemic stroke in men." *JAMA* 278:2145–2150 (1997).

Ginsberg, H. N. "Insulin resistance and cardiovascular disease." *J Clin Invest* 106:453–458 (2000).

Ginsburg, G. S., C. Safran, and R. C. Pasternak. "Frequency of low serum high-density lipoprotein cholesterol levels in hospitalized patients with 'desirable' total cholesterol levels." *Am J Cardiol* 1:187–192 (1991).

GISSI-Prevenzione Investigators. "Dietary supplementation with n-3 polyunsaturated fatty acids and vitamin E after myocardial infarction: Results of the GISSI-Prevenzione trial." *Lancet* 354:447–455 (1999).

Glueck, C. J., J. E. Lang, T. Tracy, L. Sieve-Smith, and P. Wang. "Contribution of fasting hyperinsulinemia to prediction of atherosclerotic cardiovascular disease status in 293 hyperlipidemic patients." *Metab* 48:1437–1444 (1999).

Golovchenko, I., M. L. Goalstone, P. Watson, M. Brownlee, and B. Draznin. "Hyperinsulinemia enhances transcriptional activity of nuclear factor kappa B induced by angiotensin II, hyperglycemia, and advanced glycosylation end products in vascular smooth muscle cells." *Circ Res* 87:746–752 (2000).

Gould, K. L. "Very low-fat diets for coronary heart disease: Perhaps, but which one." *JAMA* 275:1402–1403 (1996).

Gould, K. L., D. Ornish, L. Scherwitz, R. P. Edens, M. J. Hess, L. Bolomey, F. Dobbs, W. T. Armstrong, T. Merrit, T. Ports, S. Sparier, and I. Billings. "Changes in myocardial perfusion abnormalities by positron emission tomography after long-term, intense risk factor modification." *JAMA* 274:894–901 (1995).

Grundy, S. M. "Small LDL, atherogenic dyslipidemia, and the metabolic syndrome." *Circulation* 95:1–4 (1997).

Haffner, S. M., L. Mykkanen, M. P. Stern, R. Valdez, J. A. Heisserman, and R. R. Bowsher. "Relationship of proinsulin and insulin to cardiovascular risk factors in nondiabetic subjects." *Diabetes* 42:1297–1302 (1993).

Harker, L. A., A. B. Kelly, S. R. Hanson, W. Krupski, A. Bass, B. Osterud, G. A. FitzGerald, S. H. Goodnight, and W. E. Connor. "Interruption of vascular thrombus formation and vascular lesion formation by dietary n-3 fatty acids in fish oils in non-human primates." *Circulation* 87:1017–1029 (1993).

Harris, T. B., L. Ferrucci, R. P. Tracy, M. C. Corti, S. Wacholder, W. H. Ettinger, H. Heimovitz, H. J. Cohen, and R. Wallace. "Association of elevated interleukin-6 and C-reactive protein levels with mortality in the elderly." *Am J Med* 106:506–512 (1999).

Harris, W. S. "N-3 fatty acids and serum lipoproteins: Human studies." *Am J Clin Nutr* 65:1645S–1654S (1997).

———. "N-3 fatty acids and human lipoprotein metabolism: An update." *Lipids* 34:S257–S258 (1999).

Harris, W. S., H. N. Ginsberg, N. Arunakul, N. S. Shachter, S. L. Windsor, M. Adams, L. Berlund, and K. Osmundsen. "Safety and efficacy of Omacor in severe hypertriglyceridemia." *J Cardiovasc Risk* 4:385–392 (1997).

Harris, W. S., and W. L. Isley. "Clinical trial evidence for the cardioprotective effects of omega-3 fatty acids." *Curr Atheroscler Rep* 3:174–179 (2001).

Hegele, R. A. "Premature atherosclerosis associated with monogenic insulin resistance." *Circulation* 103:2225–2229 (2001).

Heller, R. F., S. Chinn, H. D. Tunstall-Pedoe, and G. Rose. "How well can we predict coronary heart disease?" *Br Med J* 288:1409–1411 (1984).

Harjai, K. J. "Potential new cardiovascular risk factors." *Ann Intern Med* 131:376–386 (1999).

Hirai, A., T. Terano, Y. Tamura, and S. Yoshida. "Eicosapentaenoic acid and adult disease in Japan." *J Intern Med* 225:69–75 (1989).

Hollenbeck, C., and G. M. Reaven. "Variations in insulin-stimulated glucose uptake in healthy individuals with normal glucose tolerance." *J Clin Endocrinol Metab* 64:1169–1173 (1987).

Horne, B. D., J. B. Muhlestein, J. F. Carlquist, T. L. Bair, T. E. Madsen, N. I. Hart, and J. L. Anderson. "Statin therapy, lipid levels, C-reactive protein, and the survival of patients with angiographically severe coronary artery disease." *J Am Coll Cardiol* 36:1774–1780 (2000).

Howard, B. V. "Insulin resistance and lipid metabolism." *Am J Cardiology* 84:28J–32J (1999).

Hu, F. B., M. J. Stampfer, J. E. Manson, E. Rimm, G. A. Colditz, F. E. Speizer, C. H. Hennekens, and W. C. Willett. "Dietary protein and risk of ischemic heart disease in women." *Am J Clin Nutr* 70:221–227 (1999).

Hu, F. B., J. E. Manson, and W. C. Willett. "Types of dietary fat and risk of coronary heart disease: a critical review." *J Am Coll Nutr* 20:5–19 (2001).

Hudgins, L. C., M. Hellerstein, C. Seidman, and J. Hirsch. "Human fatty acid synthesis is stimulated by a eucaloric low fat, high carbohydrate diet." *J Clin Invest* 97:2081–2091 (1996).

Jeppesen, J., H. O. Hein, P. Suadicani, and F. Gyntelberg. "Relation of high TG low HDL cholesterol and LDL cholesterol to the incidence of ischemic heart disease—An 8-year follow-up in the Copenhagen Male Study." *Arterioscler Thromb* Vasc Biol 17:1114–1120 (1997).

Jeppesen, J., F. Schaff, C. Jones, M-Y. Zhou, Y. D. Chen, and G. M. Reaven. "Effects of low-fat, high-carbohydrate diets on risk factors for ischemic heart disease in postmenopausal women." *Am J Clin Nutr* 65:1027–1033 (1997).

Jeppesen, J., H. O. Hein, F. Suadicani, and F. Gyntelberg. "Low triglycerides-high high-density lipoprotein cholesterol and risk of ischemic heart disease." *Arch Intern Med* 161:361–366 (2001).

Job, F. P., J. Wolfertz, R. Meyer, A. Hubinger, F. A. Gries, and H. Kuhn. "Hyperinsulinism in patients with coronary artery disease." *Coronary Artery Disease* 5:487–492 (1994).

Jones, P. M., and S. J. Persaud. "Arachidonic acid as a second messenger in glucose-induced insulin secretion from pancreatic beta cells." *J Endocrinol* 137:7–14 (1993).

Juhan-Vague, I., M. C. Alessi, and P. Vague. "Increased plasma plasminogen activator inhibitor 1 levels: A possible link between insulin resistance and atherothrombosis." *Diabetologia* 34:457–462 (1991).

Kagawa, Y., M. Nishizawa, M. Suzuki, T. Miyatake, I. Hamamoto, K. Goto, E. Motonaga, H. Izumikawa, H. Hirata, and A. Ebihara. "Eicosapolyenoic acid of serum lipids of Japanese islanders with low incidence of cardiovascular diseases." *J Nutr* Sci Vitaminol 28:441–453 (1982).

Kang, J. X., and A. Leaf. "The cardiac antiarrhythmic effects of polyunsaturated fatty acids." *Lipids* S541–S544 (1996).

Kano, H., T. Hayashi, D. Sumi, T. Esaki, Y. Asai, N. K. Thakur, M. Jayachandran, and A. Iguchi. "A HMG-CoA reductase inhibitor improved regression of atherosclerosis in the rabbit aorta without affecting serum lipid levels: Possible relevance of up-regulation of endothelial NO synthase mRNA." *Biochem Biophys Res Comm* 259:414–419 (1999).

Kaplan, N. "The deadly quartet: Upper body obesity, glucose intolerance, hypertriglyceridemia, and hypertension." *Arch Intern Med* 149:1514–1520 (1989).

Karhapaa, P., M. Malkki, and M. Laakso. "Isolated low HDL cholesterol: An insulin-resistant state." *Diabetes* 43:411–417 (1994).

Katan, M. B., S. M. Grundy, and W. C. Willett. "Beyond low-fat diets." *N Engl J Med* 337:563–566 (1997).

Kern, P. A., J. M. Ong, B. Soffan, and J. Carty. "The effects of weight loss on the activity and expression of adipose-tissue lipoprotein lipose in very obese individuals." *N Engl J Med* 322:1053–1059 (1990).

Kesaniemi, Y. A. "Relevance of the reduction of triglycerides in the prevention of coronary heart disease." Curr Opin Lipidol 9:571–574 (1998).

Knopp, R. H. "Serum lipids after a low-fat diet." *JAMA* 279:1345–1346 (1998).

Knopp, R. H., C. E. Walden, B. M. Retzlaff, B. S. McCann, A. A. Dowdy, J. J. Albers, G. O. Gey, and M. N. Cooper. "Long-term cholesterol-lowering effects of 4 fat-restricted diets in hypercholesterolemic and combined hyperlipidemic men: The dietary alternative study." *JAMA* 278:1509–1515 (1997).

Koh, K. K. "Effects of statins on vascular wall: Vasomotor function, inflammation, and plaque stability." *Cardiovas Res* 1:23–32 (2000)

Krauss, R. M., R. H. Eckel, B. Howard, L. J. Appel, S. R. Daniels, R. J. Deckelbaum, J. W. Erdman, P. Kris-Etherton, I. J. Goldberg, T. A. Kotchen, A. H. Lichtenstein, W. E. Mitch, R. Mullis, K. Robinson, J. Wylie-Rosett, S. St. Jeor, J. Suttie, D. L. Tribble, and T. L. Bazzarre. "American Heart Association Guidelines." *Circulation* 102:2284–2299 (2000).

Kris-Etherton, P. M., T. A. Pearson, Y. Wan, R. L. Hargrove, K. Moriarty, V. Fishell, and T. D. Etherton. "High-monounsaturated fatty acid diets lower both plasma cholesterol and triacylglycerol concentrations." *Am J Clin Nutr* 70:1009–1015 (1999).

Kromann, N., and A. Green. "Epidemiological studies in the Upernavik district, Greenland: Incidence of some chronic diseases 1950–1974." *Acta Med Scand* 208:401–406 (1980).

Kromhout, D., E. B. Bosscheter, and C. L. Coulander. "The inverse relationship between fish consumption and 20-year mortality from coronary heart disease." *N Engl J Med* 312:1205–1209 (1985).

Kuczmarski, R. J., K. M. Flegal, S. M. Campbell, and C. L. Johnson. "Increasing prevalence of overweight among U.S. adults." *JAMA* 272:205–211 (1994).

Lagrand, W. K., C. A. Visser, W. T. Hermens, H. W. M. Niessen, F. W. A. Verheugt, G-J. Wolbink, and E. H. Hack. "C-reactive protein as a cardiovascular risk factor." *Circulation* 100:96–102 (1999).

Laino, C. "Trans fatty acids in margarine can increase MI risk." *Circulation* 89:94–101 (1994).

Lakshmanan, M. R., C. M. Nepokroeff, G. C. Ness, R. E. Dugan, and J. W. Porter. "Stimulation by insulin of rat liver beta hydroxy methyl HMG-CoA and cholesterol synthesizing activities." *Biochem Biophys Res Comm* 50:704–710 (1973).

Lamarche, B., J–P. Despres, S. Moorjani, B. Cantin, G. R. Dagenais, and R. J. Lupien. "Triglycerides and HDL cholesterol as risk factors for ischemic heart disease: Results from the Quebec Cardiovascular Study." *Atherosclerosis* 119:235–245 (1996).

Lamarche, B., A. Tchernof, G. R. Dagenais, B. Cantin, P. J. Lupien, and J-P. Despres. "Small, dense LDL particles and the risk of ischemic heart disease: Prospective results from the Quebec Cardiovascular Study." *Circulation* 95:69–75 (1997).

Lamarche, B., A. Tchernof, P. Mauriege, B. Cantin, G. R. Gagenais, P. J. Lupien, and J-P. Despres. "Fasting insulin and apolipoprotein B levels and low-density particle size as risk factors for ischemic heart disease." *JAMA* 279:1955–1961 (1998).

Lamarche, B., I. Lemieux, and J.-P. Despres. "The small, dense LDL phenotype and the risk of coronary heart disease: Epidemiology, pathophysiology and therapeutic aspects." *Diabetes Metab* 25:199–211 (1999).

Lamarche, B., L. Rashid, and G. F. Lewis. "HDL metabolism in hypertriglyceridemic states: An overview." *Clin Chim Acta* 286:145–161 (1999).

Larsson, B., K. Svarsudd, L. Welin, L. Wilhelmssen, P. Bjorntorp, and G. Tilbin. "Abdominal adipose tissue distribution, obesity, and risk of cardiovascular disease and death." *Br Med J* 288:1401–1404 (1984).

Laws, A., A. C. King, W. L. Haskell, and G. M. Reaven. "Relation of fasting plasma insulin concentration to high density lipoprotein cholesterol and triglyceride concentration in men." *Arterioscler Thromb* Vasc Biol 11:1636–1642 (1991).

Laws, A., and G. M. Reaven. "Evidence for an independent relationship between insulin resistance and fasting: HDL-cholesterol, triglyceride, and insulin concentrations." *J Intern Med* 231:25–30 (1992).

Laws, A., and G. M. Reaven. "Insulin resistance and risk factors for coronary heart disease." *Clin Endocrinol Metab* 7:1063–1078 (1993).

Leaf, A., and P. C. Weber. "Cardiovascular effects of omega-3 fatty acids." *N Engl J Med* 318:549–557 (1988).

Leaf, A. "Dietary prevention of coronary heart disease: The Lyon diet heart study." *Circulation* 99:733–735 (1999).

Leaf, A., G. E. Billman, and H. Hallaq. "Prevention of ischemia-induced ventricular fibrillation by omega-3 fatty acids." *Proc Nat Acad Sci USA* 91:4427–4430 (1994).

Leaf, A., and J. X. Kang. "Dietary n-3 fatty acids in the prevention of lethal cardiac arrhythmias." *Curr Opin Lipidol* 8:4–6 (1997).

Leaf, A., J. X. Kang, Y. F. Xiao, and G. E. Billman. "Dietary n-3 fatty acids in the prevention of cardiac arrhythmias." *Curr Opin Clin Nutr Metab Care* 1:225–228 (1998).

Lefer, A. M. "Platelets: Unindicted coconspirators in inflammatory tissue injury." *Circ Res* 22:1077–1078 (2000).

Lefer, A. M., R. Scalia, and D. J. Lefer. "Vascular effect of HMG CoA-reductase inhibitors (statins) unrelated to cholesterol lowering: New concepts for cardiovascular disease." *Cardiovasc Res* 49:281–287 (2001).

Lichtenstein, A. H. "Trans fatty acids and cardiovascular disease risk." *Curr Opin Lipidol* 11:37–42 (2000).

Lichtenstein, A. H., and L. van Horn. "Very low fat diets." *Circulation* 98:935–939 (1998).

Liu, S., W. C. Willett, M. J. Stampfer, F. B. Hu, M. Franz, L. Sampson, C. H. Hennekens, and J. B. Manson. "A prospective study of dietary glycemic load, carbohydrate intake, and risk of coronary heart disease in U.S. women." *Am J Clin Nutr* 71:1455–1461 (2000).

Luostarinen, R., M. Bober, and T. Saldeen. "Fatty acid composition in total phospholipids of human coronary arteries in sudden cardiac death." *Athero* 99:187–189 (1993).

Mauch, D. H., K. Nagler, S. Schumacher, C. Goritz, E-C. Muller, A. Otto, and F. W. Pfieger. "CNS synaptogenesis promoted by glia-derived cholesterol." *Science* 294:1354–1357 (2001).

McLaughlin, T., F. Abbasi, C. Lamendola, H. Yen-Komshian, and G. Reaven. "Carbohydrate-induced hypertriglyceridemia: An insight into the link between plasma insulin and triglyceride concentrations." *J Clin Endocrinol Metab* 85:3085–3088 (2000).

McNamara, J. R., J. L. Jenner, Z. Li, P. W. Wilson, and E. J. Schaefer. "Change in LDL particle size is associated with change in plasma triglyceride concentration." *Arterioscler Thromb Vasc Biol* 12:1284–1290 (1992).

Meagher, E. A., O. P. Barry, J. A. Lawson, J. Rokach, and G. A. FitzGerald. "Effects of vitamin E on lipid peroxidation in healthy persons." *JAMA* 285:1178–1182 (2001).

Metz, S., W. Fujimoto, and R. O. Robertson. "Modulation of insulin secretion by cyclic AMP and prostaglandin E." *Metab* 31:1014–1033 (1982).

Metz, S., M. van Rollins, R. Strife, W. Fujimoto, and R. P. Robertson. "Lipoxygenase pathway in islet endocrine cells: Oxidative metabolism of arachidonic acid promotes insulin release." *J Clin Invest* 71:1191–1205 (1983).

Modan, M., J. Or, A. Karasik, Y. Drory, Z. Fuchs, A. Lusky, and A. Cherit. "Hyperinsulinemia, sex, and risk of atherosclerotic cardiovascular disease." *Circulation* 84:1165–1175 (1991).

Nair, S. S. D., J. W. Leitch, J. Falconer, and M. Garg. "Prevention of cardiac arrhythmia by dietary (n-3) polyunsaturated fatty acids and their mechanism of action." *J Nutr* 127:383–393 (1997).

Nieto, F. J. "Cardiovascular disease and risk factor epidemiology: A look back at the epidemic of the 20th century." *Am J Pub Health* 89:292–294 (1999).

O'Keefe, J. H., and W. S. Harris. "Omega-3 fatty acids: Time for clinical implementation?" *Am J Cardiol* 85:1239–1241 (2000).

Olszewski, A. J. "Fish oil decreases homocysteine in hyperlipidemic men." Coronary Artery Dis 4:53–60 (1993).

Oomen, C. M., E. J. M. Feskens, L. Rasaen, P. Fidanza, A. M. Nissinen, A. Menotti, F. J. Kok, and D. Kromhout. "Fish consumption and coronary heart disease mortality in Finland, Italy, and the Netherlands." *Am J Epidemiol* 151:999–1006 (2000).

Oparil, S., and A. Oberman. "Nontraditional cardiovascular risk factors." *Am J Med* Sci 317:193–207 (1999).

Orchard, T. J., D. J. Becker, M. Bates, L. H. Kuller, and A. L. Drash.

"Plasma insulin and lipoprotein concentrations: An atherogenic association?" *Am J Epidemiol* 118:326–337 (1983).

Ornish, D., S. E. Brown, L. W. Scherwitz, J. H. Billings, W. T. Armstrong, T. A. Ports, S. M. McLanahan, R. L. Kirkeeide, R. J. Brand, and K. L. Gould. "Can lifestyle changes reverse coronary heart disease?" *Lancet* 336:129–133 (1990).

Ornish, D., L. W. Scherwitz, J. H. Billings, K. L. Gould, T. A. Merritt, S. Sparler, W. T. Armstrong, T. A. Ports, R. L. Kirkeeide, C. Hogeboom, and R. J. Brand. "Intensive lifestyle changes for reversal of coronary heart disease." *JAMA* 280:2001–2007 (1998).

Osler, W. *Lectures on Angina Pectoris and Allied States*. New York: Appleton, 1897.

Palinski, W. "New evidence for beneficial effects of statins unrelated to lipid lowering." *Arterioscler Thromb Vasc Biol* 21:3–5 (2001).

Papanicolau, D. A., and A. N. Vgontzas. "Interleukin-6: The endocrine cytokine." *J Clin Endocrinol Metab* 85:1331–1332 (2000).

Pek, S. B., and M. F. Walsh. "Leukotrienes stimulate insulin released from rat pancreas." *Proc Nat Acad Sci USA* 82:2199–2202 (1984).

Pentikainen, M. O., K. Oorni, M. Ala-Korpela, and P. T. Kovaen. "Modified LDL-trigger of atherosclerosis and inflammation in the arterial intima." *J Intern Med* 247:359–370 (2000).

Perry, I. J., S. G. Wannamethee, P. H. Whincup, A. G. Shaper, M. K. Walker, and K. G. Alberti. "Serum insulin and incident coronary heart disease in middle-aged British men." *Am J Epidemiol* 144:224–234 (1996).

Pinkey, J. A., C. D. Stenhower, S. W. Coppack, and J. S. Yudkin. "Endothelial cell dysfunction: Cause of insulin resistance syndrome." *Diabetes* 46:S9–S13 (1997).

Pyorala, K. "Relationship of glucose tolerance and plasma insulin in the incidence of coronary heart disease: Results from two population studies in Finland." *Diabetes Care* 21:131–141 (1979).

Pyorala, K., E. Savolainen, S. Kaukula, and J. Haapakowski. "Plasma insulin as coronary heart disease risk factor." *Acta Med Scand* 701:38–52 (1985).

Pyorala, M., H. Miettinen, M. Laasko, and K. Pyorala. "Plasma insulin and all-cause, cardiovascular, and non-cardiovascular mortality." *Diabetes Care* 23:1097–1102 (2000).

Pyorala, M., H. Miettinen, P. Halonen, M. Laasko, and K. Pyorala. "Insulin resistance syndrome predicts the risk of coronary heart disease and stroke in healthy middle-aged men." *Arterioscler Thromb Vasc Biol* 20:538–544 (2000).

Radack, K., C. Deck, and G. Huster. "Dietary supplementation with low-dose fish oils lowers fibrinogen levels." *Ann Intern Med* 11:757–758 (1989).

Rader, D. J. "Inflammatory markers of coronary risk." *N Engl J Med* 343:1179–1182 (2000).

Reaven, G. M., and B. Hoffman. "Abnormalities of carbohydrate metabolism may play a role in the etiology and clinical course of hypertension." *TIPS* 9:78–79 (1988).

Reaven, G. M. "Role of insulin resistance in human disease." *Diabetes* 37:1595–1607 (1989).

———. "The role of insulin resistance and hyperinsulinemia in coronary heart disease." *Metab* 41:16–19 (1992).

———. "Syndrome X: 6 years later." *J Intern Med* 736:13–22 (1994).

Reaven, G. M., Y. D. Chen, J. Jeppesen, P. Maheux, and R. M. Krauss. "Insulin resistance and hyperinsulinemia in individuals with small, dense low density lipoprotein particles." *J Clin Invest* 92:141–146 (1993).

Ridker, P. M., M. Cushman, M. Stampfer, R. P. Tracy, and C. H. Hennekens. "Inflammation, aspirin, and the risk of cardiovascular disease in apparently healthy men." *N Engl J Med* 336:973–979 (1996).

Ridker, P. M., R. J. Glynn, and C. H. Hennekens. "C-reactive protein adds to the predictive value of total and HDL cholesterol in determining risk of first myocardial infarction." *Circulation* 97:2007–2011 (1997).

Ridker, P. M., C. H. Hennekens, N. Rifai, J. E. Buring, and J. E. Manson. "Hormone replacement therapy and increased plasma concentration of C-reactive protein." Circulation 100:713–716 (1999).

Ridker, P. M., C. H. Hennekens, J. E. Buring, and N. Rifai. "C-reactive protein and other markers of inflammation in the prediction of cardiovascular disease in women." *New Engl J Med* 42:836–843 (2000).

Ridker, P. M., N. Rifai, M. J. Stampfer, and C. H. Hennekens. "Plasma concentration of interleukin-6 and the risk of future myocardial infarction among apparently healthy men." *Circulation* 101:1767–1772 (2000).

Ridker, P. M., N. Rifai, M. Clearfield, J. R. Downs, S. E. Weis, and A. M. Gotto. "Measurement of C-reactive protein for the targeting of statin therapy in the primary prevention of acute coronary events." *N Engl J Med* 344:1959–1965 (2001).

Ridker, P. M. "High-sensitivity C-reactive protein." *Circulation* 103:1813–1818 (2001).

Rifai, N., and P. M. Ridker. "High-sensitivity C-reactive protein: A novel and promising marker of coronary heart disease." *Clin Chem* 47:403–411 (2001).

Rodwell, V. W., J. L. Nordstrom, and J. J. Mitschelen. "Regulation of HMG-CoA reductase." *Adv Lipid Res* 14:1–76 (1976).

Rohde, L. E. P., C. H. Hennekens, and P. M. Ridker. "Survey of C-reactive protein and cardiovascular risk factors in apparently healthy men." *Am J Cardiol* 84:1018–1022 (1999).

Rosamond, W. D., L. E. Chambless, A. R. Folsom, L. S. Cooper, D. E. Conwill, L. Legg, Ch-H. Wang, and G. Heiss. "Trends in the incidence of myocardial infarction and in mortality due to coronary heart disease, 1987 to 1994." *N Engl J Med* 339:861–867 (1998).

Rosenson, R. S., C. C. Tangney, and L. C. Casey. "Inhibition of proinflammatory cytokine production by pravastatin." *Lancet* 353:983 (1999).

Ross, R. "The pathogenesis of atherosclerosis: A perspective for the 1990s." *Nature* 362:801–809 (1993).

———. "*Atherosclerosis*: An inflammatory disease." *N Engl J Med* 340:115–126 (1999).

———. "*Atherosclerosis* is an inflammatory disease." *Am Heart J* 138:S419–S420 (1999).

Rouse, L. R., K. D. Hammel, and M. D. Jensen. "Effects of isoenergetic, low-fat diets on energy metabolism in lean and obese women." *Am J Clin Nutr* 60:470–475 (1994).

Rubins, H. B., S. J. Robins, D. Collins, A. Iranmanesh, T. J. Wilt, D. Mann, M. Mayo-Smith, F. H. Fass, M. R. Elam, and G. H. Rutan. "Distribution of lipids in 8,500 men with coronary heart disease." *Am J Cardiol* 75:1196–1201 (1995).

Ruderman, N., and C. Haudenschild. "*Diabetes* as an atherogenic factor." *Prog Cardio Dis* 26:373–412 (1984).

Salmeron, J., J. E. Manson, M. J. Stampfer, G. A. Colditz, A. L. Wing, and W. C. Willett. "Dietary fiber, glycemic load, and risk of coronary heart disease in women." *JAMA* 277:472–477 (1997).

Salonen, J. T., K. Seppanen, T. A. Lakka, R. Salonen, and G. A. Kaplan. "Mercury accumulation and accelerated progression of carotid atherosclerosis." *Athero* 148:265–273 (1999).

Scandinavian Simvastatin Survival Study Group. "Randomized trial of cholesterol lowering in 4444 patients with coronary heart disease: The Scandinavian simvastatin survival study (4S)." *Lancet* 344:1383–1389 (1994).

Sears, B. *The Zone*. New York: Regan Books, 1995.

———. *The Anti-Aging Zone*. New York: Regan Books, 1999.

See, J., W. Shell, O. Matthews, C. Canizales, M. Vargos, J. Giddings, and J. Cerrone. "Prostaglandin E1 infusion after angioplasty in humans inhibits abrupt occlusion and early restenosis." Adv Pros Throm Leuko Res 17:266–270 (1987).

Serhan, C. N. "Lipoxin biosynthesis and its impact in inflammatory and vascular events." *Biochim Biophys Acta* 1212:1–25 (1994).

————. "Lipoxins and novel aspirin-triggered 15-epi-lipoxins." *Prostaglandins* 53:107–137 (1997).

Serhan, C. N., C. B. Clish, J. Brannon, S. P. Colgan, N. Chiang, and K. Gronert. "Novel functional sets of lipid-derived mediators with anti-inflammatory actions generated from omega-3 fatty acids via cyclo-oxyogenase 2-nonsteroidal anti-inflammatory drugs and transcellular processing." *J Exp Med* 192:1197–1204 (2000).

Serhan, C. N., C. B. Clish, J. Brannon, S. P. Colgan, K. Gronert, and N. Chiang. "Anti-microinflammatory lipid signals generated from dietary N-3 fatty acids via cyclo-oxygenase-2 and transcellular processing: A novel mechanism for NSAID and N-3 PUFA therapeutic actions." *J Physiol Pharmacol* 51:643–654 (2000).

Serhan, C. N., and E. Oliw. "Unorthodox routes to prostanoid formation: New twists in cyclooxygenase-initiated pathways." *J Clin Invest* 107:1481–1489 (2001).

Simopoulos, A. P., and J. Robinson. *The Omega Plan.* New York: Harper-Collins, 1998.

Sinclair, A., and R. Gibson. Essential Fatty Acids and Eicosanoids. Champaign, Ill.: *American Oil Chemists Society,* 1992.

Sinclair, H. M. "Deficiency of essential fatty acids and atherosclerosis, et cetera." *Lancet* i:381–383 (1956).

Singh, R. B., M. A. Niaz, J. P. Sharma, R. Kumar, V. Rastogi, and M. Moshiri. "Randomized, double-blind, placebo-controlled trial of fish oil and mustard oil in patients with suspected acute myocardial infarction: The Indian Experiment of Infarct Survival-4." *Cardiovasc Drugs Ther* 11:485–491 (1997).

Sinzinger, H., and W. Rogatti, eds. Prostaglandin E1 in *Atherosclerosis.* New York: Springer-Verlag, 1986.

Siscovick, D. S., T. E. Raghunathan, I. King, S. Weinmann, K. G. Wicklund, J. Albright, V. Bovjerg, P. Arbogast, H. Smith, L. H. Hushi, L. A. Cobb, M. K. Copass, B. M. Pstay, R. Lemaire, B. Retzlaff, M. Childs, and R. H. Knopp. "Dietary intake and cell membrane levels of long-chain n-3 polyunsaturated fatty acids and risk of primary cardiac arrest." *JAMA* 274:1363–1367 (1995).

Sprecher, D. L. "Triglycerides as a risk factor for coronary artery disease." *Am J Cardiol* 82:49U–56U (1998).

Stampfer, M. J., F. B. Hu, J. E. Manson, E. B. Rimm, and W. O. Willett. "Primary prevention of coronary heart disease in women through diet and lifestyle." *N Engl J Med* 343:16–22 (2000).

Stephens, N. G., A. Parson, P. M. Schofield, F. Kelly, K. Cheeseman, and M. J. Mitchinson. "Randomized controlled trial of vitamin E in patients with coronary disease: Cambridge Heart Antioxidant Study (CHAOS)." *Lancet* 347:781–786 (1996).

Stern, M. P., and S. M. Haffner. "Body fat distribution and hyperinsulinemia as risk factors for diabetes and cardiovascular disease." *Arterioscler* 6:123–130 (1986).

Steering Committee of Physicans Health Study Research Group. "Preliminary Report: Findings for aspirin component of the ongoing physician health study." *N Engl J Med* 320:262–264 (1988).

Stolar, M. "*Atherosclerosis* in diabetes: The role of hyperinsulinemia." Metab 37:1–9 (1988).

Stout, R. "The relationship of abnormal circulating insulin levels to atherosclerosis." *Athero* 27:1–13 (1977).

———. "Insulin and atheroma: An update." *Lancet* i:1077–1079 (1987).

Stranberg, T. E., H. Vanhanen, and M. J. Tikkanen. "Effect of statins on C-reactive protein in patients with coronary artery disease." *Lancet* 353:118–119 (1999).

Tchernof, A., B. Lamarche, D. Prud'Homme, A. Nadeau, S. Moorjani, F. Labrie, P. J. Lupien, and J-P. Despres. "The dense LDL phenotype: Association with plasma lipoprotein levels, visceral obesity, and hyperinsulinemia in men." *Diabetes Care* 19:629–637 (1996).

Thompson, P. D. "More on low-fat diets." *N Engl J Med* 338:1623–1624 (1998).

Torjesen, P. A., K. J. Kirkeland, S. A. Andersson, I. Hjermann, I. Holme, and P. Urdal. "Lifestyle changes may reverse development of the insulin resistance syndrome." *Diabetes Care* 30:26–31 (1997).

Tracy, R. P. "Inflammation markers and coronary heart disease." *Curr Opinion Lipidol* 10:435–441 (1999).

Unger, R. H. "Glucagon and the insulin glucagon ratio in diabetes and other catabolic illnesses." *Diabetes* 20:834–838 (1971).

Unger, R. H., and P. J. Lefebvre. *Glucagon: Molecular Physiology, Clinical and Therapeutic Implications.* Oxford: Pergamon Press, 1972.

Visser, M. "Higher levels of inflammation in obese children." *Nutr* 17:480–484 (2001).

Volek, J. S., A. L. Gomez, and W. J. Kraemer. "Fasting lipoprotein and postprandial triacylglycerol responses to a low-carbohydrate diet supplemented with n-3 fatty acids." *J Am Coll Nutr* 19:383–391 (2000).

Von Lente, F. V. "Markers of inflammation as predictors in cardiovascular disease." *Clin Chim Acta* 293:31–52 (2000).

Von Schacky, C. "Prophylaxis of atherosclerosis with marine omega-3 fatty acids." *Ann Intern Med* 107:890–899 (1987).

———. "Omega-3 fatty acids: From Eskimos to clinical cardiology: What took us so long?" *World Rev Nutr Diet* 88:90–99 (2001).

Von Schacky, C., P. Angerer, W. Kothny, K. Theisen, and H. Mudra. "The effect of dietary omega-3 fatty acids on coronary atherosclerosis: A randomized, double-blind placebo-controlled trial." *Ann Intern Med* 130:554–562 (1999).

Weiner, B. H., I. S. Ockene, P. H. Levine, H. F. Cuenoud, M. Fisher, B. F. Johnson, A. S. Daoud, J. Jarmolych, D. Hosmer, and M. H. Johnson. "Inhibition of atherosclerosis by cod-liver oil in a hyperlipidemic swine model." *N Engl J Med* 315:841–846 (1986).

Wellborn, T. A., and K. Wearne. "Coronary heart disease incidence and cardiovascular mortality in Busselton with reference to glucose and insulin concentrations." *Diabetes Care* 2:154–160 (1979).

Westphal, S. A., M. C. Gannon, and F. Q. Nutrall. "Metabolic response to glucose ingested with various amounts of protein." *Am J Clin Nutr* 62:267–272 (1990).

Williams, P. T., and R. M. Krauss. "Low-fat diets, lipoprotein subclasses, and heart disease risk." *Am J Clin Nutr* 70:949–950 (1999).

Yarnell, J. W. G., P. M. Sweetnam, V. Marks, and J. D. Teale. "Insulin in ischaemic heart disease: Are associations explained by triglyceride concentrations? The Caerphilly prospective study." *Br Heart J* 171:293–296 (1994).

Yudkin, J. S., M. Kumari, S. E. Humphries, and V. Mohamed-Ali. "Inflammation, obesity, stress, and coronary heart disease: Is interleukin-6 the link?" *Athero* 148:209–214 (2000).

Yusuf, S., G. Dagenais, J. Pogue, J. Bosch, and P. Sleight. "Vitamin E supplementation and cardiovascular events in high-risk patients: The Heart Outcomes Prevention Evaluation Study (HOPE)." *N Eng J Med* 342:154–160 (2000).

Zaman, A. G., G. Helft, S. G. Worthley, and J. J. Badimon. "The role of plaque rupture and thrombosis in coronary artery disease." *Athero* 149:251–266 (2000).

Zavaroni, I., E. Dall'Aglio, O. Alpi, F. Brunschi, E. Bonora, A. Pezzarossa, and U. Butturini. "Evidence for an independent relationship between plasma insulin and concentrations of high density lipoproteins cholesterol and triglycerides." *Athero* 55:259–266 (1985).

Zavaroni, I., E. Bonora, M. Pagliara, E. Dall'Aglio, L. Luchetti, G. Buonnanno, P. A. Bonati, M. Bergonzani, L. Gnudi, M. Passeri, and

G. Reaven. "Risk factors for coronary artery disease in healthy persons with hyperinsulinemia and normal glucose tolerance." *N Engl J Med* 320:702–706 (1989).

Zavroni, I., L. Bonini, M. Fantuzzi, E. Dall'Aglio, M. Passeri, and G. M. Reaven. "Hyperinsulinemia, obesity, and syndrome X." *J Intern Med* 235:51–56 (1994).

Zimmet, P., and S. Baba. "Central obesity, glucose intolerance, and other cardiovascular risk factors." *Diabetes Res Clin Proc* 16:S167–S171 (1990).

Zipes, D. P., and H. J. J. Wellens. "Sudden cardiac death." *Circulation* 98:2334–2351 (1998).

Chapter 12 Cancer: Your Greatest Fear

Ablin, R. J., and M. W. Shaw. "Prostaglandin modulation of prostate tumor growth and metastases." *Anticancer Res* 6:327–388 (1986).

Akre, K., A. M. Ekstrom, L. B. Signorello, L. E. Hansson, and O. Nyren. "Aspirin and risk for gastric cancer." *Br J Cancer* 84:965–968 (2001).

Aronson, W. J., J. A. Glaspy, S. T. Reddy, D. Reese, D. Heber, and D. Bagga. "Modulation of omega-3/omega-6 polyunsaturated ratios with dietary fish oils in men with prostate cancer." *Urology* 58:283–288 (2001).

Attiga, F. A., P. M. Fernandez, A. T. Weeraratna, M. J. Manyak, and S. R. Patierno. "Inhibitors of prostaglandin synthesis inhibit human prostate tumor cell invasiveness and reduce the release of matrix metalloproteinases." *Cancer Res* 60:4629–4637 (2000).

Bagga, D., S. Capone, H. J. Wang, D. Heber, M. Lill, L. Chap, and J. A. Glaspy. "Dietary modulation of omega-3/omega-6 polyunsaturated fatty acid ratios in patients with breast cancer." *J Natl Cancer Inst* 89:1123–1131 (1997).

Bailar, J. C., and E. M. Smith. "Progress against cancer?" *N Engl J Med* 314:1226–1232 (1986).

Barber, M. D., J. A. Ross, and K. C. H. Fearon. "Changes in nutritional, functional, and inflammatory markers in advanced pancreatic cancer." *Nutr Cancer* 35:106–110 (1999).

Barber, M. D., J. A. Ross, A. C. Voss, M. J. Tisdale, and K. C. Fearon. "The effect of an oral nutritional supplement enriched with fish oil on weight-loss in patients with pancreatic cancer." *Br J Cancer* 81:80–86 (1999).

Barber, M. D., D. C. McMillan, T. Preston, J. A. Ross, and K. C. Fearon. "Metabolic response to feeding in weight-losing pancreatic cancer patients and its modulation by a fish-oil-enriched nutritional supplement." *Clin Sci* 98:389–399 (2000).

Barber, M. D., and K. C. H. Fearon. "Tolerance and incorporation of a high-dose eicosapentaenoic acid diester emulsion by patients with pancreatic cancer cachexia." *Lipids* 36:347–351 (2001).

Baron, J. A., and R. S. Sandler. "Nonsteroidal anti-inflammatory drugs and cancer prevention." *Ann Rev Med* 51:511–523 (2000).

Baronzio, G. F., F. Galante, A. Gramaglia, A. Barlocco, S. de Grandi, and I. Freitas. "Tumor microcirculation and its significance in therapy: Possible role of omega-3 fatty acids as rheological modifiers." *Med Hypotheses* 50:175–182 (1998).

Bartsch, H., J. Nair, and R. W. Owen. "Dietary polyunsaturated fatty acids and cancer of the breast and colorectum: Emerging evidence for their role as risk modifiers." *Carcinogenesis* 20:2209–2218 (1999).

Bougnoux, P. "N-3 polyunsaturated fatty acids and cancer." *Curr Opin Clin Nutr Metab Care* 2:121–126 (1999).

Bougnoux, P., E. Germain, V. Chajes, B. Hubert, C. Lhuillery, O. Le Floch, G. Body, and G. Calais. "Cytotoxic drugs efficacy correlates with adipose tissue docosahexaenoic acid level in locally advanced breast carcinoma." *Br J Cancer* 79:1765–1769 (1999).

Bruce, W. R., T. M. S. Wolever, and A. Giacca. "Mechanisms linking diet and colorectal cancer: The possible role of insulin resistance." *Nutr Cancer* 37:19–26 (2000).

Bruning, P. F., J. M. G. Bonfrer, P. A. H. van Noodr, A. A. M. Hart, M. de Jong-Bakker, and W. J. Nooijen. "Insulin resistance and breast cancer." *Int J Cancer* 52:511–516 (1992).

Burns, C. P., S. Halabi, G. H. Clamon, V. Hars, B. A. Wagner, R. J. Hohl, E. Lester, J. J. Kirshner, V. Vinciguerra, and E. Paskett. "Phase I clinical study of fish oil fatty acid capsules for patients with cancer cachexia: Cancer and leukemia group B study 9473." *Clin Cancer Res* 5:3942–3947 (1999).

Cannizzo, F., Jr., and S. A. Broitman. "Postpromotional effects of dietary marine or safflower oils on large bowel or pulmonary implants of CT-26 in mice." *Cancer Res* 49:4289–4294 (1989).

Capuron, L., A. Ravaud, and R. Dantzer. "Early depressive symptoms in cancer patients receiving interleukin 2 and/or interferon alpha-2b therapy." *J Clin Oncol* 18:2143–2151 (2000).

Chapkin, R. S., N. E. Hubbard, D. K. Buckman, and K. L. Erickson. "Linoleic acid metabolism in metastatic and nonmetastatic murine mammary tumor cells." *Cancer Res* 49:4724–4728 (1989).

Chatenoud, L., C. La Vecchia, S. Franceschi, A. Tavani, D. R. Jacobs, M. T. Parpinel, M. Soler, and E. Negri. "Refined-cereal intake and risk of selected cancers in Italy." *Am J Clin Nutr* 70:1107–1110 (1999).

Chen, Y. Q., B. Liu, D. G. Tang, and K. V. Honn. "Fatty acid modulation of tumor cell-platelet-vessel wall interaction." *Cancer Metastasis Rev* 11:389–409 (1992).

Chen, Y. Q., Z. M. Duniec, B. Liu, W. Hagmann, X. Gao, K. Shimoji, L. J. Marnett, C. R. Johnson, and K. V. Honn. "Endogenous 12(S)-HETE production by tumor cells and its role in metastasis." *Cancer Res* 15:1574–1579 (1994).

Claria, J., M. H. Lee, and C. N. Serhan. "Aspirin-triggered lipoxins are generated by human lung adrenocarcinoma cell (A549)–neutrophil interactions and are potent inhibitors of cell proliferation." *Mol Med* 2:583–596 (1996).

Connolly, J. M., X. H. Liu, and D. P. Rose. "Dietary linoleic acid–stimulated human breast cancer cell growth and metastasis in nude mice and their suppression by indomethacin, a cyclooxygenase inhibitor." *Nutr Cancer* 25:231–240 (1996).

Copeland, G. P., S. J. Leinster, J. C. Davis, and L. J. Hipkin. "Insulin resistance in patients with colorectal cancer." *Br J Surgery* 74:1031–1036 (1987).

Dailey, L. A., and P. Imming. "12-Lipoxygenase: Classification, possible therapeutic benefits from inhibition, and inhibitors." *Curr Med Chem* 6:389–398 (1998).

Damtew, B., and P. J. Spagnuolo. "Tumor cell–endothelial cell interactions: Evidence for roles for lipoxygenase products of arachidonic acid in metastasis." *Prostaglandins Leuko Essen Fatty Acids* 56:295–300 (1997).

Daneker, G. W., S. A. Lund, S. W. Caughman, C. A. Staley, and W. C. Wood. "Antimetastatic prostacyclins inhibit the adhesion of colon carcinoma to endothelial cells by blocking E-selectin expression." *Clin Exp Metastasis* 14:230–238 (1996).

DeLongeril, M., P. Salen, J. L. Martin, I. Monjaud, P. Boucher, and N. Mamelle. "Mediterranean dietary pattern in a randomized trial: Prolonged survival and possible reduced rate of cancer." *Arch Intern Med* 158:1181–1188 (1998).

DuBois, R. N., F. M. Giardiello, and W. E. Smalley. "Nonsteroidal anti-inflammatory drugs, eicosanoids, and colorectal cancer prevention." *Gastroenterol Clin North Am* 25:773–791 (1996).

Dunlop, R. J., and C. W. Campbell. "Cytokines and cancer." *J Pain Symptom* 20:214–232 (2000).

Ellis, L. M., E. M. Copeland, K. I. Bland, and H. S. Sitren. "Inhibition of tumor growth and metastasis by chronic intravenous infusion of prostaglandin E1." *Ann Surg* 212:45–50 (1990).

Form, D. M., and R. R. Auerbach. "PGE2 and angiogenesis." *Proc Soc Exp Biol Med* 172:214–218 (1983).

Fernandez, E., L. Chatenoud, C. La Vecchia, E. Negri, S. Franceschi. "Fish consumption and cancer risk." *Am J Clin Nutr* 70:85–90 (1999).

Franceschi, S., A. Favero, A. Decari, E. Negri, C. La Vecchia, M. Ferraroni, A. Russo, S. Salvini, D. Amadori, and E. Conti. "Intake of macronutrients and the risk of breast cancer." *Lancet* 347:1351–1356 (1996).

Franceschi, S., A. Favero, C. La Vecchia, E. Negri, E. Conti, M. Montella, A. Giacosa, O. Nanni, and A. Decarli. "Food groups and risk of colorectal cancer in Italy." *Int J Cancer* 72:56–61 (1997).

Franceschi, S., A. Favero, M. Parpinel, A. Giacosa, and C. La Vecchia. "Italian study of colorectal cancer with emphasis on influence of cereals." *Eur J Cancer Prev* 7:S19–S223 (1998).

Franceschi, S., C. La Vecchia, A. Russo, A. Favero, E. Negri, E. Conti, M. Montella, R. Filiberti, D. Amadori, and A. Decarli. "Macronutrient intake and risk of colorectal cancer in Italy." *Int J Cancer* 76:321–324 (1998).

Fuchs, C. S., E. L. Giovannucci, G. A. Colditz, D. Hunter, M. J. Stampfer, B. Rosner, F. E. Speizer, and W. C. Willett. "Dietary fiber and the risk of colorectal cancer and adenoma in women." *N Engl J Med* 340:169–176 (1999).

Fulton, A. M. "The role of eicosanoids in tumor metastasis." *Prostaglandins Leuko Essen Fatty Acids* 34:229–237 (1988).

Fulton, A. M., S. Z. Zhang, and Y. C. Chong. "Role of the prostaglandin E2 receptor in mammary tumor metastasis." *Cancer Res* 51:2047–2050 (1991).

Gao, X., and K. V. Honn. "Biological properties of 12(S)-HETE in cancer metastasis." *Adv Pros Thromb Leuko Res* 23:439–444 (1995).

Gao, X., W. Hagmann, A. Zacharek, N. Wu, M. Lee, A. T. Porter, and K. V. Honn. "Eicosanoids, cancer metastasis, and gene regulation: An overview." *Adv Exp Med Bio* 400A:545–555 (1997).

Garcia-Rodriguez, L. A., and C. Huerta-Alvarez. "Reduced risk of colorectal cancer among long-term users of aspirin and nonaspirin nonsteroidal anti-inflammatory drugs." *Epidemiology* 12:88–93 (2001).

Germain, E., V. Chajes, S. Cognault, C. Lhuillery, and P. Bougnoux. "Enhancement of doxorubicin cytotoxicity by polyunsaturated fatty acids in the human breast tumor cell line MDA-MB-231: Relationship to lipid peroxidation." *Int J Cancer* 75:578–583 (1998).

Germain, E., F. Lavandier, V. Chajes, V. Schubnel, P. Bonnet, C. Lhuillery, and P. Bougnoux. "Dietary n-3 polyunsaturated fatty acids and oxidants increase rat mammary tumor sensitivity to epirubicin without change in cardiac toxicity." *Lipids* 34:S203 (1999).

Ghost, J., and C. E. Myers. "Arachidonic acid stimulates prostate cancer cell growth: Critical role of 5-lipoxygenase." *Biochem Biophys Res Comm* 235:418–423 (1997).

Ghost, J., and C. E. Myers. "Arachidonic acid metabolism and cancer of the prostate." *Nutr* 14:48–57 (1998).

Giardiello, F. M., G. J. Offerhaus, and R. N. DuBois. "The role of nonsteroidal anti-inflammatory drugs in colorectal cancer prevention." *Eur J Cancer A*(7–8):1071–1076 (1995).

Giovannucci, E. "Insulin and colon cancer." *Cancer Causes and Control* 6:164–179 (1995).

Gogos, C. A., P. Ginopoulos, B. Salsa, E. Apostolidou, N. C. Zoumbos, and F. Kalfarentzos. "Dietary omega-3 polyunsaturated fatty acids plus vitamin E restore immunodeficiency and prolong survival for severely ill patients with generalized malignancy: A randomized control trial." *Cancer* 82:395–402 (1998).

Hansen-Petrik, M. B., M. F. McEntee, C-H. Chiu, and J. Whelan. "Antagonism of arachidonic acid is linked to the antitumorigenic effect of dietary eicosapentaenoic acid in APC mice." *J Nutr* 130:1153–1158 (2000).

Hardman, W. E., M. P. Moyer, and I. L. Cameron. "Dietary fish oil sensitizes A549 lung xenografts to doxorubicin chemotherapy." *Cancer Lett* 151:145–151 (2000).

Hardman, W. E., C. P. Avula, G. Fernandes, and I. L. Cameron. "Three percent dietary fish oil concentrate increased efficacy of doxorubicin against mda-mb 231 breast cancer xenografts." Clin *Cancer Res* 7:2041–2049 (2001).

Holmes, M. D., M. J. Stampfer, G. A. Colditz, B. Rosner, D. J. Hunter, and W. C. Willett. "Dietary factors and the survival of women with breast cancer." *Cancer* 86:751–753 (1999).

Honn, K. V., W. D. Busse, and B. F. Sloane. "Prostacyclin and thromboxanes: Implications for their role in tumor cell metastasis." *Biochem Pharmacol* 32:1–11 (1983).

Honn, K. V., I. M. Grossi, C. A. Diglio, M. Wojtukiewicz, and J. D. Taylor. "Enhanced tumor cell adhesion to the subendothelial matrix resulting from 12(S)-HETE-induced endothelial cell retraction." *FASEB J* 3:2285–2293 (1989).

Honn, K. V., I. M. Grossi, B. W. Steinert, H. Chopra, J. Onoda, K. K. Nelson, and J. D. Taylor. "Lipoxygenase regulation of membrane expression of tumor cell glycoproteins and subsequent metastasis." *Adv Pros Throm Leuko Res* 19:439–443 (1989).

Honn, K. V., K. K. Nelson, C. Renaud, R. Bazaz, C. A. Diglio, and J. Timar. "Fatty acid modulation of tumor cell adhesion to microvessel endothelium and experimental metastasis." *Prostaglandins* 44:413–429 (1992).

Honn, K. V., D. G. Tang, X. Gao, I. A. Butovich, B. Liu, J. Timar, and W. Hagmann. "12-lipoxygenases and 12(S)-HETE: Role in cancer metastasis." *Cancer Metastasis Rev* 13:365–396 (1994).

Honn, K. V., D. G. Tang, I. Grossi, Z. M. Duniec, J. Timar, C. Renaud, M. Leithauser, I. Blair, C. R. Johnson, and C. A. Diglio. "Tumor cell—derived 12(S)-hydroxyeicosatetraenoic acid induces microvascular endothelial cell retraction." *Cancer Res* 54:565–574 (1994).

Honn, K. V., D. G. Tang, I. M. Grossi, C. Renaud, Z. M. Duniec, C. R. Johnson, and C. A. Diglio. "Enhanced endothelial cell retraction mediated by 12(S)-HETE: A proposed mechanism for the role of platelets in tumor cell metastasis." *Exp Cell Res* 210:1–9 (1994).

Honn, K. V., and D. G. Tang. "Eicosanoid 12(S)-HETE upregulates endothelial cell alpha V beta 3 integrin expression and promotes tumor cell adhesion to vascular endothelium." *Adv Exp Med Bio* 400B:765–773 (1997).

Hu, F. B., J. E. Manson, S. Liu, D. Hunter, G. A. Colditz, K. B. Michels, F. E. Speizer, and E. Giovannucci. "Prospective study of adult onset diabetes mellitus (type 2) and risk of colorectal cancer in women." *J Natl Cancer Inst* 91:542–547 (1999).

Huang, Y. C., J. M. Jessup, and G. L. Blackburn. "N-3 fatty acids decrease colonic epithelial cell proliferation in high-risk bowel mucosa." *Lipids* 31:S313–S316 (1996).

Hubbar, N. E., D. Lim, and K. L. Erickson. "Alteration of murine mammary tumorigenesis by dietary enrichment with n-3 fatty acids in fish oil." *Cancer Lett* 124:1–7 (1998).

Hursting, S. D., and F. W. Kari. "The anticarcinogenic effects of dietary restriction: Mechanisms and future directions." *Mutation Res* 443:235–249 (1999).

Hussey, H. J., and M. H. Tidale. "Inhibition of tumour growth by lipoxygenase inhibitors." *Br J Cancer* 74:683–687 (1996).

Hwang, D., D. Scollard, J. Byrne, and E. Levine. "Expression of cyclooxygenase-1 and cyclooxygenase-2 in human breast cancer." *J Natl Cancer Inst* 90:455–460 (1998).

Kaizer, L., N. F. Boyd, V. Kriukov, and D. Trichler. "Fish consumption and breast cancer risk." *Nutr Cancer* 12:61–68 (1989).

Karmali, R. A. "Eicosanoids and cancer." *Prog Clin Biol Res* 222:687–697 (1986).

————. "N-3 fatty acids and cancer." *J Intern Med* 225:197–200 (1989).

————. "N-3 fatty acids: Biochemical actions in cancer." *J Nutr Sci Vitaminol* spec. no.:148–152 (1992).

————. "Historical perspective and potential use of n-3 fatty acids in therapy of cancer cachexia." *Nutr* 12:S2–S4 (1996).

Kinoshita, K., M. Noguchi, M. Earashi, M. Tanaka, and T. Sasaki. "Inhibitory effects of purified eicosapentaenoic acid and docosahexaenoic acid on growth and metastasis of murine transplantable mammary tumor." *In Vivo* 8:371–374 (1994).

Kort, W. J., I. M. Weijma, A. M. Bijma, W. P. van Schalkwijk, A. J. Vergroesen, and D. L. Westbroek. "Omega-3 fatty acids inhibiting the growth of a transplantable rat mammary adenocarcinoma." *J Natl Cancer Inst* 79:593–599 (1987).

Kritchevsky, D. "Caloric restriction and experimental Carcinogenesis." *Toxicological Sci* 52:13–16 (1999).

————. "Calorie restriction and cancer." *J Nutr Sci Vitaminol* 47:13–19 (2001).

Ledwozyw, A. "Phospholipids and fatty acids in human brain tumors." *Acta Physiol Hungarica* 79:381–387 (1992).

Liu, B., J. Timar, J. Howlett, C. A. Diglio, and K. V. Honn. "Lipoxygenase metabolites of arachidonic and linoleic acids modulate the adhesion of tumor cells to endothelium via regulation of protein kinase C." *Cell Regul* 2:1045–1055 (1991).

Liu, B., R. J. Maher, Y. A. Hannum, A. T. Porter, and K. V. Honn. "12-HETE enhancement of prostate tumor cell invasion: Selective role of PKC alpha." *J Natl Cancer Inst* 86:1145–1151 (1994).

Liu, B., L. J. Marnett, A. Chaudhary, C. Ji, I. A. Blair, C. R. Johnson, C. A. Diglio, and K. V. Honn. "Biosynthesis of 12-hydroxy eicosatetraenoic acid by B16 amelanotic melanoma cells is a determinant of their metastatic potential." *Lab Invest* 70:314–323 (1994).

Liu, X. H., J. M. Connolly, and D. P. Rose. "Eicosanoids as mediators of linoleic acid—stimulated invasion and type IV collagenase production by a metastatic human breast cancer cell line." *Clin Exp Metastasis* 14:145–152 (1996).

Lundholm, K., G. Holm, and T. Schersten. "Insulin resistance in patients with cancer." *Cancer Res* 38:4665–4670 (1978).

Marcus, A. J. "Aspirin as prophylaxis against colorectal cancer." *N Engl J Med* 333:656–658 (1995).

Marks, F., K. Muller-Decker, and G. Furstenberger. "A causal relationship between unscheduled eicosanoid signaling and tumor development:

Cancer chemoprevention by inhibitors of arachidonic acid metabolism." *Toxicology* 153:11–26 (2000).

Martin, D. D., M. E. C. Robbins, A. A. Spector, B. Chen Wen, and D. H. Hussey. "The fatty acid composition of human gliomas differs from that found in nonmalignant brain tissue." *Lipids* 31:1283–1288 (1996).

Martinez, M. E., D. Heddens, D. L. Earnest, C. L. Bogert, D. Roe, J. Einspahr, J. R. Marshall, and D. S. Alberts. "Physical activity, body mass index, and prostaglandin E2 levels in rectal mucosa." *J Natl Cancer Inst* 91:950–953 (1999).

McCarty, M. F. "Fish oil may impede tumour angiogenesis and invasiveness by down-regulating protein kinase C and modulating eicosanoid production." *Med Hypotheses* 46:107–115 (1996).

McKeown-Eyssen, G. "Epidemiology of colorectal cancer revisited: Are serum triglycerides and/or plasma glucose associated with risk?" *Cancer Epidemiol Biomarkers Prev* 3:687–695 (1994).

Mori, H., Y. Takada, H. Kondoh, and T. Tamaya. "Augmentation of antiproliferative activity of recombinant human tumor necrosis factor by delta 12-prostaglandin J2." *J Biol Response Mod* 9:260–263 (1990).

Moysich, K. B., C. Mettlin, M. S. Piver, N. Natarajan, R. J. Menezes, and H. Swede. "Regular use of analgesic drugs and ovarian cancer risk." *Cancer Epidemiol Biomarkers Prev* 10:903–906 (2001).

Mukutmoni-Norris, M., N. E. Hubbard, and K. L. Erickson. "Modulation of murine mammary tumor vasculature by dietary n-3 fatty acids in fish oil." *Cancer Lett* 150:101–109 (2000).

Murota, S., T. Kanayasu, J. Nakano-Hayashi, and I. Morita. "Involvement of eicosanoids in angiogenesis." *Adv Pros Throm Leuko Res* 21:623–625 (1990).

Narisawa, T., H. Kusaka, Y. Yamazaki, M. Takahashi, H. Koyama, K. Koyama, Y. Fukaura, and A. Wakizaka. "Relationship between blood plasma prostaglandin E2 and liver and lung metastases in colorectal cancer." *Dis Colon Rectum* 33:840–845 (1990).

Natarajan, R., and J. Nadler. "Role of lipoxygenases in breast cancer." *Front Biosci* 3:E81–E88. (1998).

Nie, D., G. G. Hillman, T. Geddes, K. Tang, C. Pierson, D. J. Grignon, and K. V. Honn. "Platelet-type 12-lipoxygenase in a human prostate carcinoma stimulates angiogenesis and tumor growth." *Cancer Res* 58:4047–4051 (1998).

Nie, D., M. Lamberti, A. Zacharek, L. Li, K. Szekeres, K. Tang, Y. Chen, and K. V. Honn. "Thromboxane A2 regulation of endothelial cell migration, angiogenesis, and tumor metastasis." *Biochem Biophys Res Comm* 267:245–251 (2000).

Nie, D., K. Tang, C. Diglio, and K. V. Honn. "Eicosanoid regulation of angiogenesis: Role of endothelial arachidonate 12-lipoxygenase." *Blood* 95:2304–2311 (2000).

Nie, D., K. Tang, K. Szekeres, M. Trikha, and K. V. Honn. "The role of eicosanoids in tumor growth and metastasis." *Ernst Schering Res Foundation Workshop* 31:201–217 (2000).

Noguchi, M., D. P. Rose, M. Earashi, and I. Miyazaki. "The role of fatty acids and eicosanoid synthesis inhibitors in breast carcinoma." *Oncology* 52:265–271 (1995).

Noguchi, Y., T. Yoskikawa, D. Marat, C. Doi, T. Makin, K. Fukuzawa, A. Tsuburaya, S. Staoh, T. Ito, and S. Mitsuse. "Insulin resistance in cancer patients is associated with enhanced tumor necrosis factor expression in skeletal muscle." *Biochem Biophys Res Comm* 253:887–892 (1998).

Norrish, A. E., C. M. Skeaff, G. L. Arribas, S. J. Sharpe, and R. T. Jackson. "Prostate cancer risk and consumption of fish oils: A dietary biomarker-based case-control study." *Br J Cancer* 81:1238–1242 (1999).

Ogilvie, G. K., M. J. Fettman, C. H. Mallinckrodt, J. A. Walton, R. A. Hansen, D. J. Davenport, K. L. Gross, K. L. Richardson, Q. Rogers, and M. S. Hand. "Effect of fish oil, arginine, and doxorubicin chemotherapy on remission and survival time for dogs with lymphoma: A double-blind, randomized placebo-controlled study." *Cancer* 88:1916–1928 (2000).

Okuno, K., H. Jinnai, Y. S. Lee, K. Nakamura, T. Hirohata, H. Shigeoka, and M. Yasutomi. "A high level of prostaglandin E2 (PGE2) in the portal vein suppresses liver-associated immunity and promotes liver metastases." *Surg Today* 25:954–958 (1995).

Powles, T. J., P. J. Dady, J. Williams, G. C. Easty, and R. C. Coombes. "Use of inhibitors of prostaglandin synthesis in patients with breast cancer." *Adv Pros Throm Leuko Res* 6:511–516 (1980).

Prescott, S. M., and F. A. Fitzpatrick. "Cyclooxygenase-2 and *Carcinogenesis*." *Biochim Biophys Acta* 1470:M69–M78 (2000).

Radisky, D., C. Hagios, and M. J. Bissell. "Tumors are unique organs defined by abnormal signaling and context." *Cancer Biol* 11:87–95 (2001).

Reich, R., and G. R. Martin. "Identification of arachidonic acid pathways required for the invasive and metastatic activity of malignant tumor cells." *Prostaglandins* 51:1–17 (1996).

Rice, R. L., D. G. Tang, M. Haddad, K. V. Honn, and J. D. Taylor. "12(S)-hydroxyeicosatetraenoic acid increases the actin microfilament content in B16a melanoma cells: A protein kinase-dependent process." *Int J Cancer* 77:271–278 (1998).

Rigas, B., I. S. Goldman, and L. Levine. "Altered eicosanoid levels in human colon cancer." J Lab Clin Med 122:518–523 (1993).

Rioux, N., and A. Castonguay. "Inhibitors of lipoxygenase: A new class of cancer chemopreventive inhibitors." *Carcinogenesis* 19:1393–1400 (1998).

Rohdeburg, G. L., A. Bernhard, and O. Krehniel. "Sugar tolerance in cancer." *JAMA* 72:1528 (1919).

Rolland, P. H., M. Martin, and M. Toga. "Prostaglandin in human breast cancer: Evidence suggesting the elevated prostaglandin production is a marker of high metastatic potential." *J Nat Cancer Inst* 64:1061–1070 (1980).

Romero, L. M., K. M. Raley-Susman, D. M. Redish, S. M. Brooke, and R. Sapolsky. "Possible mechanism by which stress accelerates growth of virally derived tumors." *Proc Natl Acad Sci USA* 89:11084–11087 (1992).

Rose, D. P., and M. A. Hatala. "Dietary fatty acids and breast cancer invasion and metastasis." *Nutr Cancer* 21:103–111 (1994).

Rose, D. P., J. M. Connolly, J. Rayburn, and M. Coleman. "Influence of diets containing eicosapentaenoic or docosahexaenoic acid on growth and metastasis of breast cancer cells in nude mice." *J Natl Cancer Inst* 87:587–592 (1995).

Rose, D. P., J. M. Connolly, and M. Coleman. "Effect of omega-3 fatty acids on the progression of metastases after the surgical excision of human breast cancer cell solid tumors growing in nude mice." Clin *Cancer Res* 2:1751–1756 (1996).

Rose, D. P. "Dietary fat, fatty acids, and breast cancer." *Breast Cancer* 4:7–16 (1997).

———. "Dietary fatty acids and cancer." *Am J Clin Nutr* 66:998S–1003S (1997).

———. "Dietary fatty acids and prevention of hormone-responsive cancer." *Proc Soc Exp Biol Med* 216:224–233 (1997).

———. "Effects of dietary fatty acids on breast and prostate cancers: Evidence from in vitro experiments and animal studies." *Am J Clin Nutr* 66:1513S–1522S (1997).

Rose, D. P., and J. M. Connolly. "Effects of dietary omega-3 fatty acids on human breast cancer growth and metastases in nude mice." *J Natl Cancer Inst* 85:1743–1747 (1993).

———. "Antiangiogenicity of docosahexaenoic acid and its role in the suppression of breast cancer cell growth in nude mice." *Int J Oncol* 15:1011–1015 (1999).

———. "Omega-3 fatty acids as cancer chemopreventive agents." *Pharmacol Therap* 83:217–244 (1999).

———. "Regulation of tumor angiogenesis by dietary fatty acids and eicosanoids." *Nutr Cancer* 37:119–127 (2000).

Rose, D. P., J. M. Connolly, and X. H. Liu. "Diet and breast cancer: Opportunities for prevention and intervention." *Prog Clin Biol Res* 396:147–158 (1997).

———. "Fatty acid regulation of breast cancer cell growth and invasion." *Adv Exp Med Bio* 422:47–55 (1997).

Rudra, P. K., and H. E. Krokan. "Cell-specific enhancement of doxorubicin toxicity in human tumour cells by docosahexaenoic acid." *Anticancer Res* 21(1A):29–38 (2001).

Sakanoue, Y., T. Hatada, M. Kusunoki, H. Yanage, T. Yamamura, and J. Utsunomiya. "Protein kinase C activity as marker for colorectal cancer." *Int J Cancer* 48:803–806 (1991).

Sasaki, S., M. Horacsek, and H. Kesteloot. "An ecological study of the relationship between dietary fat and breast cancer mortality." *Prev Med* 22:187–202 (1993).

Sauer, L. A., R. T. Dauchy, and D. E. Blask. "Mechanism for the antitumor and anticachectic effects of n-3 fatty acids." *Cancer Res* 60:5289–5295 (2000).

Sawaoka, H., S. Tsuji, M. Tsuji, E. S. Gunawan, Y. Sasaki, S. Kawano, and M. Hori. "Cyclooxygenase inhibitors suppress angiogenesis and reduce tumor growth In Vivo." *Lab Invest* 79:1469–1477 (1999).

Schapira, D. V., N. B. Kumar, G. H. Lyman, and C. E. Cox. "Abdominal obesity and breast cancer risk." *Ann Intern Med* 112:182–186 (1990).

Schirner, M., R. B. Lichtner, and M. R. Schneider. "The stable prostacyclin analogue Cicaprost inhibits metastasis to lungs and lymph nodes in the 13762NF MTLn3 rat mammary carcinoma." *Clin Exp Metastasis* 12:24–30 (1994).

Schneider, M. R., D. G. Tang, M. Schirner, and K. V. Honn. "Prostacyclin and its analogues: Antimetastatic effects and mechanisms of action." *Cancer Metastasis Rev* 13:349–364 (1994).

Schoen, R. E., C. M. Tengen, L. H. Kuller, G. L. Burke, M. Cushman, R. P. Tracy, A. Dops, and P. J. Savage. "Increased blood glucose and insulin, body size, and incidence of colorectal cancer." *J Natl Cancer Inst* 91:1147–1154 (1999).

Shao, Y., L. Pardini, and R. S. Pardini. "Dietary menhaden oil enhances mitomycin C antitumor activity toward human mammary carcinoma MX-1." *Lipids* 30:1035–1045 (1995).

Sheehan, K. M., K. Sherhan, D. P. O'Donoghue, F. MacSweeney, R. M.

Conroy, D. J. Fitzgerald, and F. E. Murray. "The relationship between cyclooxygenase-2 expression and colorectal cancer." *JAMA* 282:1254–1257 (1999).

Shiff, S. J., and B. Rigas. "Nonsteroidal anti-inflammatory drugs and colorectal cancer: Evolving concepts of their chemopreventive actions." *Gastroenterology* 113:1992–1998 (1997).

———. "Aspirin for cancer." Nature Medicine 5:1348–1349 (1999).

Silletti, S., J. Timar, K. V. Honn, and A. Raz. "Autocrine motility factor induces differential 12-lipoxygenase expression and activity in high- and low-metastatic K1735 melanoma cell variants." *Cancer Res* 54:5752–5766 (1994).

Singh, J., R. Hamid, and B. S. Reddy. "Dietary fat and colon cancer: Modulation of cyclooxygenase-2 by types and amount of dietary fat during the postinitiation stage of colon Carcinogenesis." *Cancer Res* 57:3465–3470 (1997).

Stark, L. A., F. V. N. Din, R. M. Zwacka, and M. G. Dunlop. "Aspirin-induced activation of the NF kappa B signaling pathway: A novel mechanism for aspirin-mediated apoptosis in colon cancer cells." *FASEB J* 15:1273–1275 (2001).

Steele, V. E., C. A. Holmes, E. T. Hawk, L. Kipelovich, R. A. Lubet, J. A. Crowell, C. C. Sigman, and G. J. Kelloff. "Lipoxygenase inhibitors as potential cancer chemopreventives." *Cancer Epidemiol Biomarkers Prev* 8:467–483 (1999).

Stoll, B. A. "Essential fatty acids, insulin resistance, and breast cancer risk." *Nutr Cancer* 31:72–77 (1998).

———. "Western nutrition and the insulin resistance syndrome: A link to breast cancer." *Eur J Clin Nutr* 53:83–87 (1999).

Takahata, K., M. Tada, K. Yazawa, and T. Tamaki. "Protection from chemotherapy-induced alopecia by docosahexaenoic acid." *Lipids* 34:S105 (1999).

Taketo, M. M. "Cyclooxygenase-2 inhibitors in tumorigenesis." *J Natl Cancer Inst* 90:1609–1620 (1998).

Tang, D. G., and K. V. Honn. "12-Lipoxygenase, 12(S)-HETE, and cancer metastasis." *Ann NY Acad Sci* 744:199–215 (1994).

Tang, D. G., C. Renaud, S. Stojakovic, C. A. Diglio, A. Porter, and K. V. Honn. "12-HETE is a mitogenic factor for microvascular endothelial cells: Its potential role in angiogenesis." *Biochem Biophys Res Comm* 211:462–468 (1995).

———. "Adhesion molecules and tumor cell–vasculature interactions: Modulation by bioactive lipid molecules." *Curr Top Microbiol Immunol* 213:69–88 (1996).

Tang, K., and K. V. Honn. "Lipoxygenase metabolites and cancer metasta-sis." *Adv Exp Med Bio* 422:71–84 (1997).

———. "12(S)-HETE in cancer metastasis." *Adv Exp Med Bio* 447:181–191 (1999).

Terry, P., P. Lichtenstein, M. Feychting, A. Ahlbom, and A. Wolk. "Fatty fish consumption and risk of prostate cancer." *Lancet* 357:1764–1766 (2001).

Thaler-Dao, H., A. Crastes de Paulet, and R. Paoletti. *Eicosanoids and Cancer.* New York: Raven Press, 1984.

Thun, M. J. "NSAID use and decreased risk of gastrointestinal cancers." *Gastroenterol Clin North Am* 25:333–348 (1996).

Tran, T. T., A. Medline, and W. R. Bruce. "Insulin promotion of colon tumors in rats." *Cancer Epidemiol Biomarkers Prev* 5:1013–1015 (1996).

Tsujii, M., S. Kawano, and R. N. DuBois. "Cyclooxygenase-2 expression in human colon cancer cells increases metastatic potential." *Proc Nat Acad Sci USA* 94:3336–3340 (1997).

Uefuji, K., T. Ichikura, and H. Mochizuki. "Cyclooxygenase-2 expression is related to prostaglandin biosynthesis and angiogenesis in human gastric cancer." Clin *Cancer Res* 6:135–138 (2000).

Vartak, S., M. E. Robbins, and A. A. Spector. "Polyunsaturated fatty acids increase the sensitivity of 36B10 rat astrocytoma cells to radiation-induced cell kill." *Lipids* 332:283–292 (1997).

Vergote, I. B., P. A. van Dam, G. M. Laekeman, G. H. Keersmaeckers, F. L. Uyttenbroeck, and A. G. Herman. "Prostacyclin/thromboxane ratio in human breast cancer." *Tumor Biol* 12:261–266 (1991).

Welch, H. G., L. M. Schwartz, and S. Woloshin. "Are increasing 5-year sur-vival rates evidence of success against cancer?" *JAMA* 283:2975–2978 (2000).

Wigmore, S. J., M. D. Barber, J. A. Ross, M. J. Tisdale, and K. C. Fearon. "Effect of oral eicosapentaenoic acid on weight loss in patients with pancreatic cancer." *Nutr Cancer* 36:177–814 (2000).

Williams, C. S., M. Mann, and R. N. DuBois. "The role of cyclooxyge-nases in inflammation, cancer, and development." *Oncogene* 18:7980–7916 (1999).

Xia, X., S. Yang, J. Kowalski, and M. E. Gerritsen. "Peroxisome proliferator–activated receptor gamma ligands are potent inhibitors of angiogenesis in vitro and In Vivo."" *J Biol Chem* 274:9916–9121 (1999).

Yam, D. "Insulin-cancer relationships: Possible dietary implications." *Med Hypotheses* 38:111–117 (1992).

Yam, D., H. Ben-Hur, A. Fink, R. Dgani, A. Shani, A. Eliraz, V. Insler, and E. M. Berry. "Insulin and glucose status, tissue and plasma lipids in patients with tumours of the ovary or endometrium: Possible dietary implications." *Br J Cancer* 70:1186–1187 (1994).

Yam, D., A. Peled, and M. Shinitzky. "Suppression of tumor growth and metastasis by dietary fish oil combined with vitamins E and C and cisplatin." *Cancer Chemother Pharmacol* 47:34–40 (2001).

Yokoyama, I., S. Hayashi, T. Kobayashi, M. Negita, M. Yasutomi, K. Uchida, and H. Takagi. "Prevention of experimental hepatic metastasis with thromboxane synthase inhibitor." *Res Exp Med* (Berl) 195:209–215 (1995).

Yoshikawa, T., Y. Noguchi, C. Doi, T. Makino, and K. Noruma. "Insulin resistance in patients with cancer: Relationships with tumor site, tumor stage, body-weight loss, acute-phase response, and energy expenditure." *Nutr* 17:590–593 (2001).

Zimmermann, K.C., M. Sarbia, A-A. Weber, F. Borchard, H. E. Gabbert, and K. Schor. "Cyclooxygenase-2 expression in human esophageal carcinoma." *Cancer Res* 59:198–204 (1999).

Chapter 13 Obesity and *Diabetes*: The Twin Epidemics

Agus, M. S. D., J. F. Swain, C. L. Larson, E. A. Eckert, and D. S. Ludwig. "Dietary composition and physiological adaptations to energy restriction." *Am J Clin Nutr* 71:901–907 (2000).

Allison, D. B., R. Zannolli, M. S. Faith, M. Heo, A. Pietrobelli, T. B. Van Itallie, F. X. Pi-Sunyer, and S. B. Heymsfield. "Weight loss increases and fat loss decreases all-cause mortality rate." *Int J Obesity* 23:603–611 (1999).

American Diabetes Association. "Diabetes: 1996 Vital Statistics" (1996).

———. "Economic consequences of diabetes mellitus in the U.S. in 1997" (1997).

Barzlai, N., L. She, B-O. Liu, P. Vuguin, P. Cohen, J. Wang, and L. Rossetti. "Surgical removal of visceral fat reverses hepatic insulin resistance." *Diabetes* 48:94–98 (1999).

Blair, S. N., and S. Brodney. "Effects of physical inactivity and obesity on morbidity and mortality." *Med Sci Sports Exerc* 31:S642–S662 (1999).

Bleich, D., S. Chen, J. L. Gu, and J. L. Nadler. "The role of 12-lipoxygenase in pancreatic cells." *Int J Mol Med*1:265–272 (1998).

Boizel, R., P. Y. Behhamou, B. Lardy, P. Laporte, T. Foulon, and S. Halimi. "Ratio of triglycerides to HDL cholesterol is an indicator of LDL particle size in patients with type 2 diabetes and normal HDL cholesterol levels." *Diabetes Care* 23:1679–1685 (2000).

Bonora, E., J. Willeit, S. Kicchi, F. Oberhollenzer, G. Egger, R. Bonadonna, and M. Muggeo. "Relationship between insulin and carotid atherosclerosis in the general population: The Bruneck Study." *Stroke* 28:1147–1152 (1997).

Borkman, M., L. H. Storlien, D. A. Pan, A. B. Jenkins, D. J. Chisholm, and L. V. Campbell. "The relation between insulin sensitivity and the fatty acid composition of skeletal-muscle phospholipids." *N Engl J Med* 328:911–917 (1993).

Botion, L. M., and A. Green. "Long-term regulation of lipolysis and hormone-sensitive lipase by insulin and glucose." *Diabetes* 48:1691–1697 (1999).

Brandes, J. "Insulin induced overeating in the rat." *Physiol Rev* 18:1095–1102 (1977).

Campbell, L. V., P. E. Marmot, J. A. Dyer, M. Borkman, and L. H. Storlien. "The high-monounsaturated fat diet as a practical alternative for non-insulin dependent diabetes mellitus." *Diabetes Care* 17:177–182 (1994).

Challem, J., B. Berkson, and M. D. Smith. *Syndrome X*. New York: John Wiley and Sons, 2000.

Chatzipanteli, K., S. Rudolph, and L. Axelrod. "Coordinate control of lipolysis by prostaglandin E_2 and prostacyclin in rat adipose tissue." *Diabetes* 41:927–935 (1992).

Chen, Y. D., A. M. Coulston, Z. Ming-Yue, C. B. Hollenbeck, and G. M. Reaven. "Why do low-fat high-carbohydrate diets accentuate postprandial lipemia in patients with NIDDM?" *Diabetes Care* 18:10–16 (1995).

Cincott, A. H., E. Tozzo, and P. W. D. Scislowski. "Bromocriptine/SKF 38393 treatment ameliorates obesity and associated metabolic dysfunction in obese (ob/ob) mice." *Life Sci* 61:951–956 (1997).

Cshe, K., G. Winkler, Z. Melczer, and E. Baranyi. "The role of tumor necrosis factor resistance in obesity and insulin resistance." *Diabetologia* 43:525 (2000).

Dek, S. B., and M. F. Walsh. "Leukotrienes stimulate insulin release from rat pancreas." *Proc Nat Acad Sci USA* 81:2199–2202 (1985).

Del Aguila, L. F., K. P. Calffey, and J. P. Kirwan. "TNF alpha impairs insulin signaling and insulin stimulation of glucose uptake in C_2C_{12} muscle cells." *Am J Physiol* 276:E849–E855 (1999).

Despres, J-P., I. Lemieux, and D. Prud'Homme. "Treatment of obesity: Need to focus on high-risk abdominally obese patients." *Br J Med* 22:716–720 (2001).

Drewnowski, A. "Nutrition transition and global dietary trends." *Nutr* 16:486–487 (2000).

Ducimetiere, P., J. L. Richard, and I. Cambrien. "The pattern of subcutaneous fat distribution in middle-aged men and risk of coronary heart disease." *Int J Obesity* 10:229–240 (1986).

Fernandez-Real, J-M., M. Vayreda, C. Richart, C. Gutierrez, M. Broch, J. Vendrell, and W. Ricart. "Circulating interleukin-6 levels, blood pressure, and insulin sensitivity in apparently healthy men and women." *J Clin Endocrinol Metab* 86:1154–1159 (2001).

Festa, A., R. D'Agostino, G. Howard, L. Mykkanen, R. P. Tracy, and S. M. Haffner. "Chronic subclinical inflammation as part of the insulin resistance syndrome." *Circulation* 102:42–47 (2000).

Folsom, A. R., J. Ma, P. G. McGovern, and H. Eckfeldt. "Relationship between plasma phospholipid saturated fatty acids and hyperinsulinemia." *Metab* 45:223–228 (1996).

Fruhbeck, G., J. Gomez-Ambrosi, F. J. Muruzabal, and M. A. Burrell. "The adipocyte: A model for integration of endocrine and metabolic signaling in energy metabolism regulation." *Am J Physiol Endocrinol Metab* 280:E827–E847 (2001).

Garg, A., S. M. Grudy, and R. H. Unger. "Comparison of effects of high and low carbohydrate diets on plasma lipoproteins and insulin sensitivity in patients with mild NIDDM." *Diabetes* 41:1278–1285 (1992).

Garg, A., J. P. Bantle, R. R. Henry, A. M. Coulston, K. A. Griven, S. K. Raatz, L. Brinkley, I. Chen, S. M. Grundy, B. A. Huet, and G. M. Reaven. "Effects of varying carbohydrate content of diet in patients with non-insulin-dependent diabetes mellitus." *JAMA* 271:1421–1428 (1994).

Garg, A. "High-monounsaturated fat diets for patients with diabetes mellitus: A meta analysis." *Am J Clin Nutr* 67:577S–582S (1998).

Gaudet, D., M. C. Vohl, P. Perron, G. Tremblay, C. Gagne, D. Lesiege, J. Bergeron, S. Moorjani, and J-P. Despres. "Relationships of abdominal obesity and hyperinsulinemia to angiographically assessed coronary artery disease in men with known mutations in the LDL receptor gene." *Circulation* 97:871–877 (1998).

Gerbi, A., J-M. Maxient, J-L. Ansaldi, M. Pierlovisi, T. Coste, J-F. Pelissier, P. Vague, and D. Raccah. "Fish oil supplementation prevents diabetes-induced nerve conduction velocity and neuroanatomical changes in rats." *J Nutr* 129:207–213 (1999).

Gerbi, A., J-M. Maxient, O. Barbey, I. Jamme, M. Pierlovishi, T. Coste, G. Pieroni, A. Nouvelot, P. Vague, and D. Raccah. "Neuroprotective effect of fish oil in diabetic neuropathy." *Lipids* 34:S93–S94 (1999).

Gumbiner, B., C. C. Low, and P. D. Reaven. "Effects of a monounsaturated fatty acid enriched hypocaloric diet on cardiovascular risk factors in obese patients with type 2 diabetes." *Diabetes Care* 21:9–15 (1998).

Haffner, S. M., S. Lehto, T. Ronnemaa, K. Pyorala, and M. Laakso. "Mortality from coronary heart disease in subjects with type 2 diabetes and in nondiabetic subjects with and without prior myocardial infarction." *N Engl J Med* 339:229–234 (1998).

Hayden, J. M., and P. D. Reaven. "Cardiovascular disease in diabetes mellitus type 2: A potential for novel cardiovascular risk factors." *Curr Opin Lipidol* 11:519–528 (2000).

Hopkins, K. D. "Ways of changing sensitivity to insulin." *Lancet* 350:341 (1997).

Hostens, K., D. Pavlovic, Y. Zambre, Z. Ling, C. van Schravendijk, D. L. Eizirik, and D. G. Pipeleers. "Exposure of human islets to cytokines can result in the disproportionately elevated proinsulin release." *J Clin Invest* 104:67–72 (1999).

Hotamisligil, G. S., and B. M. Spiegelman. "Tumor necrosis factor: A key component of the obesity-diabetes link." *Diabetes* 43:1271–1278 (1994).

Hotamisligil, G. S., P. Arner, J. F. Caro, R. L. Atkinson, and B. M. Spegelman. "Increased adipose tissue expression of tumor necrosis factor in human obesity and insulin resistance." *J Clin Invest* 95:2409–2415 (1995).

Hotamisligil, G. S. "Mechanisms of TNF induced insulin resistance." *Exp Clin Endocrinol Diabetes* 107:119–125 (1999).

Hu, F. B., M. J. Stampfer, C. G. Solomon, S. Liu, W. C. Willett, F. E. Speizer, D. M. Nathan, and J. E. Manson. "The impact of diabetes mellitus on mortality from all causes and coronary heart disease in women: 20 years of follow-up." *Arch Intern Med* 161:1717–1723 (2001).

Itani, S. I., Q. Zhou, W. J. Pories, K. G. MacDonald, and G. L. Dohm. "Involvement of protein kinase C in human skeletal muscle insulin resistance and obesity." *Diabetes* 49:1353–1358 (2000).

Jain, S. K., K. Kannan, and G. Lim. "Ketosis can generate oxygen radicals and cause increased peroxidation and growth inhibition in human endothelial cells." *Free Radical Biol Med* 25:1083–1088 (1998).

Jensen, T., S. Stender, K. Goldstein, G. Holmer, and T. Deckert. "Partial normalization by dietary cod liver oil of increased microvascular albumin leakage in patients with insulin-dependent diabetes and albuminuria." *N Engl J Med* 321:1572–1577 (1989).

Jones, D. R., and I. Varel-Nieto. "*Diabetes* and the role of inositol-containing lipids in insulin signaling." *Mol Med* 5:505–514 (1999).

Kahn, B. B., and J. S. Flier. "Obesity and insulin resistance." *J Clin Invest* 106:473–481 (2000).

Katan, M. B., S. M. Grundy, and W. C. Willett. "Should a low-fat, high-carbohydrate diet be recommended for everyone? Beyond low-fat diets." *N Engl J Med* 337:563–567 (1997).

Kemnitz, J. W., E. B. Roecker, R. Weindruch, D. F. Elson, S. T. Baum, and R. N. Bergman. "Dietary restriction increases insulin sensitivity and lowers blood glucose in rhesus monkeys." *Am J Physiol* 266:E540–E547 (1994).

Kern, P. A., S. Ranganathan, C. Li, L. Wood, and G. Ranganathan. "Adipose tissue tumor necrosis factor and interleukin-6 expression in human obesity and insulin resistance." *Am J Physiol Endocrinol Metab* 280:E745–E751 (2001).

Khan, L. K., and B. A. Bowman. "Obesity: A major global public health problem." Ann Rev Nutr 19: xii–xvii (1999).

Kim, S., and N. Moustaid-Moussa. "Secretory, endocrine, and autocrine/paracrine function of the adipocyte." *J Nutr* 130:3110S–3115S (2000).

King, G. L., and H. Wakasaki. "Theoretical mechanisms by which hyperglycemia and insulin resistance could cause cardiovascular diseases in diabetes." *Diabetes Care* 23:C31–C37 (1999).

Koya, D., and G. L. King. "Protein kinase C activation and the development of diabetic complications." *Diabetes* 47:859–866 (1998).

Lee, C. D., S. N. Blair, and A. S. Jackson. "Cardiorespiratory fitness, body composition, and all-cause and cardiovascular disease mortality in men." *Am J Clin Nutr* 69:373–380 (1999).

Levin, B. E., A. A. Dunn-Meynell, and V. H. Routh. "Brain glucose sensing and body energy homeostasis: Role in obesity and diabetes." *Am J Physiol* 276:R1223–R1231 (1999).

Lotufo, P. A., J. M. Gaziano, Cu Chae, U. A. Ajani, G. Moreno-John, J. E. Buring, and J. E. Manson. "*Diabetes* and all-cause and coronary heart disease mortality among U.S. male physicians." *Arch Intern Med* 161:242–247 (2001).

Low, C. C., E. B. Grossman, and B. Gumbiner. "Potentiation of effects of weight loss by monounsaturated fatty acids in obese NIDDM patients." *Diabetes* 45:569–575 (1996).

Luo, J., S. W. Rizkalla, J. Boillot, C. Alamowitch, H. Chaib, F. Bruzzo, N. Desplanque, A. M. Dalix, G. Durand, and G. Slama. "Dietary (n-3) polyunsaturated fatty acids improve adipocyte insulin action and glucose metabolism in insulin-resistant rats: Relationship to membrane fatty acids." *J Nutr* 126:1951–1958 (1996).

Ludwig, D. S., J. A Majzoub, A. Al-Zahrami, G.E. Dallal, J. Blanco, and S. B. Roberts. "High glycemic foods, overeating, and obesity." *Pediatrics* 103:E26 (1999).

Luzi, R. L., A. Caumo, A. C. Andreotti, M. F. Manzone, M. E. Malighetti, L. P. Sereni, and A. E. Pontiroli. "Elevated insulin levels contribute to reduced growth hormone response to GH-releasing hormone in obese subjects." *Metab* 48:1152–1156 (1999).

Markovic, T. P., A. C. Fleury, L. V. Campbell, L. A. Simons, S. Balasubramanian, D. J. Chisholm, and A. B. Jenkins. "Beneficial effect on average lipid levels from energy restriction and fat loss in obese individuals with or without type 2 diabetes." *Diabetes Care* 21:695–700 (1998).

Markovic, T. P., A. B. Jenkins, L. V. Campbell, S. M. Furler, E. W. Kragen, and D. J. Chisholm. "The determinants of glycemic responses to diet restriction and weight loss in obesity and NIDDM." *Diabetes Care* 21:687–694 (1998).

Meguid, M. M., S. O. Fetissov, M. Varma, T. Sato, L. Zhang, A. Lavian, and F. Rossi-Fanelli. "Hypothalamic dopamine and serotonin in the regulation of food intake." *Nutr* 16:843–857 (2000).

Mobbs, C. V. "Genetic influences on glucose neurotoxicity, aging, and diabetes: A possible role for glucose hysteresis." *Genetica* 91:239–253 (1993).

Mokdad, A. H., E. S. Ford, B. A. Bowman, D. E. Nelson, M. M. Engelgau, F. Vinicor, and J. S. Marks. "*Diabetes trends in the U.S., 1990–1998.*" *Diabetes Care* 23:1278–1283 (2000).

Mokdad, A. H., M. K. Serdula, W. H. Dietz, B. A. Bowman, J. S. Marks, and J. P. Kaplan. "The spread of the obesity epidemic in the United States, 1991–1998." *JAMA* 282:1519–1522 (1999).

Montague, C. T., and S. O'Rahilly. "The perils of portliness: Causes and consequences of visceral adiposity." *Diabetes* 49:883–888 (2000).

Montori, V. M., A. Farmer, P. C. Wollan, and S. F. Dinneen. "Fish oil supplementation in type 2 diabetes: A quantitative systematic review." *Diabetes Care* 23:1407–1415 (2000).

Moran, T. H. "Cholecystolkinin and satiety." Nutr 16:858–865 (2000).

Mori, T. A., D. Q. Bao, V. Burke, I. B. Puddey, G. F. Watts, and L. J. Beilin. "Dietary fish as a major component of a weight-loss diet: Effect on serum lipids, glucose, and insulin metabolism in overweight hypertensive subjects." *Am J Clin Nutr* 70:817–825 (1999).

Mori, Y., Y. Murakawa, J. Yohoyama, N. Tajima, Y. Ikeda, H. Nobukata, T. Ishikawa, and Y. Shibutani. "Effect of highly purified eicosapentaenoic acid ethyl ester on insulin resistance and hypertension in Dahl salt-sensitive rats." *Metab* 48:1089–1095 (1999).

Nichols, G. A., H. S. Glauber, and J. B. Brown. "Type 2 diabetes: Incremental medical care costs during the 8 years preceding diagnosis." *Diabetes Care* 23:1654–1659 (2000).

Ofei, F., S. Hurel, J. Newkirk, M. Sopwith, and R. Taylor. "Effects of an engineered human anti-TNF alpha antibody on insulin sensitivity and glycemic control in patients with NIDDM." *Diabetes* 45:881–885 (1996).

Parillo, M., A. A. Rivellese, A. V. Ciardullo, B. Capaldo, A. Giacco, S. Genovese, and G. Riccardi. "A high-monounsaturated-fat/low-carbohydrate diet improves peripheral insulin sensitivity in non-insulin dependent diabetic patients." *Metab* 41:1373–1378 (1992).

Peraldi, P., and B. Spiegelman. "TNF and insulin resistance: Summary and future prospects." *Mol Cell Biochem* 182:169–175 (1998).

Qi, C., and P. H. Pekala. "Tumor necrosis factor alpha induced insulin resistance in adipocytes." *Proc Soc Exp Biol Med* 223:128–135 (2000).

Raheja, B. S., S. M. Sakidot, R. B. Phatak, and M. B. Rao. "Significance of the N-6/N-3 ratio for insulin action in diabetics." *Ann NY Acad Sci* 983:258–271 (1993).

Rasmussen, O. W., C. Thomsen, K. W. Hansen, M. Vesterlund, E. Winther, and K. Hermansen. "Effects on blood pressure, glucose, and lipid levels of a high-monounsaturated fat diet compared with a high-carbohydrate diet in non-insulin dependent subjects." *Diabetes Care* 16:1565–1571 (1993).

Reaven, G. M., and A. Laws. *Insulin Resistance: The Metabolic Syndrome X.* Totowa, N.J.: Humana Press, 1999.

Rivellese, A., A. Maffettone, C. Iovine, L. Di Marino, G. Annuzzi, M. Mancini, and G. Riccardi. "Long-term effects of fish oil on insulin resistance and plasma lipoprotein in NIDDM patients with hypertriglyceridemia." *Diabetes Care* 19:1207–1213 (1996).

Roberts, S. B. "High glycemic index foods, hunger, and obesity: Is there a connection?" *Nutr Rev* 58:163–169 (2000).

Robertson, R. P., D. J. Gavarenski, D. Porte, and E. L. Bierman. "Inhibition of In Vivo insulin secretion by prostaglandin E1." *J Clin Invest* 54:310–315 (1974).

Robertson, R. P. "Prostaglandins, glucose homeostasis, and diabetes mellitus." *Ann Rev Med* 34:1–12 (1983).

Robin, R. J., W. M. Altman, and D. N. Mendelson. "Health care expenditures for people with diabetes mellitus." *J Clin Endocrinol Metab* 78:809A–809F (1992).

Rosenbloom, A. L., J. R. Joe, R. S. Young, and W. E. Winter. "Emerging epidemic of type 2 diabetes in youth." *Diabetes Care* 22:345–354 (1999).

Ruderman, N., and C. Haudenschild. "Diabetes as an atherogenic factor." *Prog Cardio Dis* 26:373–412 (1984).

Sacca, L., G. Perez, F. Pengo, I. Pascucci, and M. Conorelli. "Reduction of circulating insulin levels during the infusion of different prostaglandins in the rat." Acta Endocrinol 79:266–274 (1975).

Sadur, C. N., and R. H. Eckel. "Insulin stimulation of adipose tissue lipoprotein lipase." *J Clin Invest* 69:1119–1123 (1982).

Salmeron, J., A. Ascherio, E. B. Rimm, G. A. Colditz, D. Spiegelman, D. J. Jenkins, M. J. Stampfer, A. L. Wing, and W. C. Willett. "Dietary fiber, glycemic load, and risk of NIDDM in men." *Diabetes Care* 20:545–550 (1997).

Salmeron, J., J. E. Manson, and W. C. Willett. "Dietary fiber, glycemic load, and risk of non-insulin dependent diabetes mellitus in women." *JAMA* 277:472–477 (1997).

Samaras, K., and L. V. Campbell. "Increasing incidence of type 2 diabetes in the third millennium." *Diabetes Care* 23:441–442 (2000).

Schwartz, M. W. "Staying slim with insulin in mind." *Science* 289:2066–2067 (2000).

Schwartz, M. W., D. F. Figlewicz, D. G. Baskin, S. C. Woods, and D. Porte. "Insulin in the brain: A hormonal regulation of energy balance." *Endocrine Rev* 43:387–414 (1992).

Seidell, J. C. "Obesity, insulin resistance, and diabetes: A worldwide epidemic." Br *J Nutr* 83:S5-S8 (2000).

Skolnik, E., and J. Marcusohn. "Inhibition of insulin receptor signaling by TNF: Potential role in obesity and non-insulin dependent diabetes mellitus." *Cytokine Growth Factor Rev* 7:161–173 (1996).

Skov, A. R., S. Toubro, B. Renn, I. Holm, and A. Astrup. "Randomized trial on protein vs. carbohydrate in ad libitum fat reduced diet for the treatment of obesity." *Int J Obes Relat Metab Disorders* 23:528–536 (1999).

Steinberg, H. O., H. Chaker, R. Learning, A. Johnson, G. Brechtel, and A. D. Baron. "Obesity/insulin resistance is associated with endothelial dysfunction: Implications for the syndrome of insulin resistance." *J Clin Invest* 97:2601–2610 (1996).

Stene, L. C., J. Ulriksen, P. Magnus, and G. Joner. "Use of cod liver oil during pregnancy associated with lower risk of type 1 diabetes in the offspring." *Diabetologia* 42:1093–1098 (2000).

Storlien, L. H., E. W. Kraegen, D. J. Chisholm, G. L. Ford, D. G. Bruce, and W. S. Pascoe. "Fish oil prevents insulin resistance induced by high-fat feeding in rats." *Science* 237:885–888 (1987).

Storlien, L. H., A. B. Jenkins, D. J. Chisholm, W. S. Pascoe, S. Khour, and E. W. Kraegen. "Influence of dietary fat composition on development of insulin resistance in rats: Relationship to muscle triglycerides and omega-3 fatty acids in muscle phospholipids." *Diabetes* 40:280–289 (1991).

Storlien, L. H., D. A. Pan, A. D. Kriketos, J. O'Connor, I. D. Caterson, G. J. Cooney, A. B. Jenkins, and L. A. Baur. "Skeletal muscle membrane lipids and insulin resistance." *Lipids* 31:S261–S265 (1996).

Taubes, G. "The soft science of dietary fat." *Science* 291:2536–2545 (2001).

Unger, R. H., and P. J. Lefebvre. *Glucagon: Molecular Physiology, Clinical and Therapeutic Implications.* Oxford: Pergamon Press, 1972.

Van Liew, J. B., F. B. David, P. J. Davis, B. Noble, and L. L. Bernardis. "Calorie restriction decreases microalbuminuria associated with aging in barrier-raised Fischer 344 rats." *Am J Physiol* 263: F554–F561 (1992).

Vessby, B., S. Tengblad, and H. Lithell. "Insulin sensitivity is related to the fatty acid composition of serum lipids and skeletal muscle phospholipids in 70-year-old men." *Diabetologia* 37:1044–1050 (1994).

Vinik, A. I., T. S. Park, K. B. Stansberry, and G. L. Pittenger. "Diabetic neuropathies." *Diabetologia* 43:957–973 (2000).

Visser, M., L. M. Bouter, G. M. McQuillan, M. H. Wener, and T. B. Harris. "Elevated C-reactive protein levels in overweight and obese adults." *JAMA* 282:2131–2315 (1999).

Wagner, E. H., N. Sandhu, K. M. Newton, D. K. McCulloch, S. D. Ramsey, and L. C. Grothaus. "Effect of improved glycemic control on health care costs and utilization." *JAMA* 285:182–189 (2001).

Willett, W. C. "Dietary fat and obesity: An unconvincing relation." *Am J Clin Nutr* 68:1149–1150 (1998).

———. "Is dietary fat a major source of body fat?" *Am J Clin Nutr* 67:556S–562S (1998).

Wojtaszewski, J. R. P., B. F. Hansen, J. Gade, B. Kiena, J. F. Markuna, L. J. Goodyear, and E. A. Richter. "Insulin signaling and insulin sensitivity after exercise in human skeletal muscle." *Diabetes* 49:325–331 (2000).

Wolfe, B. M., and L. A. Diche. "Replacement of carbohydrate by protein in a conventional-fat diet reduces cholesterol and triglyceride concentrations in normalipidemic subjects." *Clin Invest Med* 22:140–148 (1999).

Yost, T. J., and R. H. Eckel. "Fat calories may be preferentially stored in reduced-obese women: A permissive pathway for resumption of the obese state." *J Clin Endocrinol* 67:259–264 (1988).

Yudkin, J. S., M. Kumari, S. E. Humphries, and V. Mohamed-Ali. "Inflammation, obesity, stress, and coronary heart disease: Is interleukin-6 the link?" *Athero* 148:209–214 (2000).

Yudkin, J. S., C. D. A. Stehouwer, J. J. Emeis, and S. W. Coppack. "C-reactive protein in healthy subjects: Associations with obesity, insulin resistance, and endothelial dysfunction: A potential role for cytokines originating from adipose tissue?" *Arterioscler Thromb Vasc Biol* 19:972–978 (1999).

Chapter 14 Why It Hurts: Pain and Inflammation

American Academy of Allergy. *Asthma* (1997).

Arend, W. P. "Cytokines and cellular interactions in inflammatory synovitis." *J Clin Invest* 107:1081–1082 (2001).

Ariza-Ariza, R., M. Peralta-Mestanza, and M. H. Cardiel. "Omega-3 fatty acids in rheumatoid arthritis: An overview." *Sem Arthr Rheum* 27:366–370 (1998).

Babcok, T., W. S. Helton, and N. J. Espat. "Eicosapentaenoic acid: An anti-inflammatory omega-3 fat with potential clinical applications." *Nutr* 16:1116–1118 (2000).

Bechoua, S., M. Dubois, G Nemoz, P. Chapy, E. Vericel, M. Lagarde, and A. F. Prigent. "Very low dietary intake of n-3 fatty acids affects the immune function of healthy elderly people." *Lipids* 34:S143 (1999).

Belluzzi, A., C. Brignola, M. Campieri, A. Pera, S. Boschi, and M. Miglioli. "Effect of an enteric-coated fish-oil preparation on relapses in Crohn's disease." *N Engl J Med* 354:1557–1560 (1996).

Belluzzi, A., S. Boschi, C. Brignola, A. Munarini, G. Cariani, and F. Miglio. "Polyunsaturated fatty acids and inflammatory bowel disease." *Am J Clin Nutr* 71:339S–342S (2000).

Black, P. N., and S. Sharpe. "Dietary fat and asthma: Is there a connection?" *Eur Respir J* 10:6–12 (1997).

Blok, W. L., M. B. Katan, and J. W. van der Meer. "Modulation of inflammation and cytokine production by dietary (n-3) fatty acids." *J Nutr* 126:1515–1533 (1996).

Broughton, K. S., C. S. Johnson, B. K. Pace, M. Liebman, and K. M. Kleppinger. "Reduced asthma symptoms with n-3 fatty acid ingestion are related to 5-series leukotriene production." *Am J Clin Nutr* 65:1011–1017 (1997).

Brown, S. A., C. A. Brown, W. A. Crowell, J. A. Barsanti, T. Allen, C. Cowell, and D. R. Finco. "Beneficial effects of chronic administration of dietary omega-3 polyunsaturated fatty acids in dogs with renal insufficiency." *J Clin Lab Med* 131:447–455 (1998).

Brown, S. A., C. A. Brown, W. A. Crowell, J. A. Barsanti, C-W. Kang, T. Allen, C. Cowell, and D. R. Finco. "Effects of dietary polyunsaturated fatty acids supplementation in early renal insufficiency in dogs." *J Lab Clin Med* 135:275–286 (2000).

Calder, P. C. "N-3 polyunsaturated fatty acids and cytokine production in health and disease." *Ann Nutr Metab* 41:203–234 (1997).

———. "N-3 polyunsaturated fatty acids, inflammation, and immunity." *Nutr Res* 21:309–341 (2001).

Chandrasekar, B., and G. Fernandes. "Decreased pro-inflammatory cytokines and increased antioxidant enzyme gene expression by omega-3 lipids in murine lupus nephritis." *Biochem Biophys Res Commun* 200(2):893–898 (1994).

Cho, Y., and V. A. Ziboh. "A novel 15-hydroxyeicosatrienoic acid-substituted diacylglycerol selectively inhibits epidermal protein kinase C-beta." *Biochim Biophys Acta* 1349:67–71 (1997).

Clark, W. F., A. Parbtani, C. D. Naylor, C. M. Levinton, N. Muirhead, E. Spanner, M. W. Huff, D. J. Philbrick, and B. J. Holub. "Fish oil in lupus nephritis: Clinical findings and methodological implications." *Kidney Int* 44:75–86 (1993).

Cleland, L. G., J. K. French, W. H. Betts, G. A. Murphy, and M. J. Elliott. "Clinical and biochemical effects of dietary fish oil supplements in rheumatoid arthritis." *J Rheumatol* 15:1471–1475 (1988).

Das, U. N. "Beneficial effects of eicosapentaenoic and docosahexanenoic acids in the management of systemic erythematosus and its relationship to the cytokine network." *Prostaglandins Leuko Essen Fatty Acids* 51:207–213 (1994).

DeLuca, P., R. G. Rossetti, C. Alavian, P. Karim, and R. B. Zurier. "Effects of gamma linolenic acid on interleukin-1 beta and tumor necrosis factor alpha secretion by stimulated human peripheral blood monocytes: Studies in vitro and *In Vivo*." *J Invest Med* 47:246–250 (1999).

Donadio, J. V., E. J. Bergstralh, K. P. Offord, D. C. Spencer, and K. E. Holley. "A controlled trial of fish oil in IgA nephropathy." *N Engl J Med* 331:1194–1199 (1994).

Donadio, J. V., J. P. Grande, E. J. Bergstralh, R. A. Dart, T. S. Larson, and D. C. Spencer. "The long-term outcome of patients with IgA nephropathy treated with fish oil in a controlled trial." *J Am Soc Nephrol* 10:1772–1777 (1999).

Endres, S., R. Ghorbani, V. E. Kelley, K. Georgilis, G. Lonnemann, J. W. van der Meer, J. G. Cannon, T. S. Rogers, M. S. Klempner, P. C. Weber, et al. "The effect of dietary supplementation with n-3 polyunsaturated fatty acids on the synthesis of interleukin-1 and tumor necrosis factor by mononuclear cells." *N Engl J Med* 320:265–271 (1989).

Endres, S. "Messengers and mediators: Interactions among lipids, eicosanoids, and cytokines." *Am J Clin Nutr* 57:798S–800S (1993).

Endres, S., B. Sinha, and T. Eisenhut. "Omega-3 fatty acids in the regulation of cytokine synthesis." *World Rev Nutr Diet* 76:89–94 (1994).

Endres, S. "N-3 polyunsaturated fatty acids and human cytokine synthesis." *Lipids* 31:S239–S242 (1996).

Endres, S., and C. von Schacky. "N-3 polyunsaturated fatty acids and human cytokine synthesis." *Curr Opin Lipidol* 7:48–52 (1996).

Endres, S., R. Lorenz, and K. Loeschke. "Lipid treatment of inflammatory bowel disease." *Curr Opin Clin Nutr Metab Care* 2:117–120 (1999).

Espersen, G. T., N. Grunnet, H. H. Lervang, G. L. Nielsen, B. S. Thomsen, K. L. Faarvang, J. Dyerberg, and E. Ernst. "Decreased interleukin-1 beta levels in plasma from rheumatoid arthritis patients after dietary supplementation with n-3 polyunsaturated fatty acids." *Clin Rheumatol* 11:393–395 (1992).

Fernandes, G., P. Friend, E. J. Yunis, and R. A. Good. "Influence of dietary restriction on immunologic function and renal disease in (NZB×NZW) F1 mice." *Proc Nat Acad Sci USA* 75:1500–1504 (1978).

Fogh, K., and K. Krabballe. "Eicosanoids in inflammatory skin diseases." *Prostaglandins Other Lipid Mediat* 63:43–54 (2000).

Fox, D. A. "Cytokine blockade as a new strategy to treat rheumatoid arthritis: Inhibition of tumor necrosis factor." *Arch Intern Med* 160:437–444 (2000).

Gennuso, J., L. H. Epstein, R. Paluch, and F. Cerny. "The relationship between asthma and obesity in urban minority children and adolescents." *Arch Pediatri Adolesc* 152:1197–1200 (1998).

Geusens, P., C. Wouters, J. Nijs, Y. Jiang, and J. Dequeker. "Long-term effect of omega-3 fatty acid supplementation in active rheumatoid arthritis: A 12-month, double-blind, controlled study." *Arthritis Rheum* 37:824–829 (1994).

Goldberg, D. L. "Fibromyalgia syndrome a decade later: What have we learned?" *Arch Intern Med* 159:777–785 (1999).

Goldyne, M. E. "Cyclooxygenase isoforms in human skin." *Prostaglandins Other Lipid Mediat* 63:15–23 (2000).

Hodge, L., C. M. Salome, J. M. Hughes, D. Liu-Brennan, J. Rimmer, M. Allman, D. Pang, C. Armour, and A. J. Woolcock. "Effect of dietary intake of omega-3 and omega-6 fatty acids on severity of asthma in children." *Eur Respir* J 11:361–365 (1998).

Hodge, L., C. M. Salome, J. K. Peat, M. M. Haby, W. Xuan, and A. J. Woolcock. "Consumption of oily fish and childhood asthma risk." *Med J Austr* 164:137–140 (1996).

Holgate, S. T., and A. P. Sampson. "Antileukotriene therapy." *Am J Respir Critical Care Med* 161:S147–S153 (2000).

Inversen, L., and K. Kragballe. "Arachidonic acid metabolism in skin health and disease." *Prostaglandins Other Lipid Mediat* 63:25–42 (2000).

Kelley, D. S., P. C. Taylor, G. J. Nelson, P. C. Schmidt, A. Ferretti, K. L. Erickson, R. Yu, R. K. Chandra, B. E. Mackey. "Docosahexaenoic acid ingestion inhibits natural killer cell activity and production of inflammatory mediators in young healthy men." *Lipids* 34:317–324 (1999).

Kremer, J. M., D. A. Lawrence, W. Jubiz, R. DiGiacomo, R. Rynes, L. F. Bartholomew, and M. Sherman. "Dietary fish oil and olive oil supplementation in patients with rheumatoid arthritis: Clinical and immunologic effects." *Arthritis Rheum* 33:810–820 (1990).

Kremer, J. M., D. A. Lawrence, G. F. Petrillo, L. L. Litts, P. M. Mullaly, R. J. Rynes, R. P. Stocker, N. Parhami, N. S. Greenstein, and B. R. Fuchs. "Effects of high-dose fish oil on rheumatoid arthritis after stopping nonsteroidal anti-inflammatory drugs: Clinical and immune correlates." *Arthritis Rheum* 38:1107–1114 (1995).

Kremer, J. M. "N-3 fatty acid supplements in rheumatoid arthritis." *Am J Clin Nutr* 71:349S–351S (2000).

Lam, B. K., and F. Austen. "Leukotriene C4 synthase: A pivotal enzyme in the biosynthesis of the cysteinyl leukotrienes." *Am J Respir Critical Care Med* 161:S16–S19 (1999).

Lee, T. H., R. L. Hoover, J. D. Williams, R. I. Sperling, J. Ravalese, B. W. Spur, D. R. Robinson, E. J. Corey, R. A. Lewis, and K. P. Austen. "Effect of dietary enrichment with eicosapentaenoic acid and docosahexaenoic acid on in vitro neurophil and monocyte leukotriene generation and neurophil function." *N Engl J Med* 312:1217–1224 (1985).

Leung, K. H., and H. S. Koren. "Regulation of human natural killing: Protective effect of interferon on NK cells and suppression by PGE2." *J Immunol* 129:1742–1747 (1982).

Lo, C. J., K. C. Chiu, M. Fu, R. Lo, and S. Helton. "Fish oil decreases macrophage tumor necrosis factor gene transcription by altering the NF kappa B activity." *J Surg Res* 82:216–221 (1999).

Meydani, S. N. "Effect of n-3 polyunsaturated fatty acid on cytokine production and their biological action." *Nutr* 12:S8–S14 (1996).

Nagakura, T., S. Matsuda, K. Shichijyo, H. Sugimoto, and K. Hata. "Dietary supplementation with fish oil rich in omega-3 polyunsaturated fatty acids in children with bronchial asthma." *Eur Respir J*:861–865 (2000).

Ninnemam, J. L. *Prostaglandins, Leukotrienes, and the Immune Response.* New York: Cambridge University Press, 1998.

Ozgocmen, S., S. A. Catal, O. Ardicoglu, and A. Kamanli. "Effect of omega-3 fatty acids in the management of fibromyalgia syndrome." *Int J Clin Pharmacol Ther* 38:362–363 (2000).

Pisetsky, D. S. "Tumor necrosis factor blockers in rheumatoid arthritis." *N Engl J Med* 342:810–811 (2000).

Prickett, J. D., D. R. Robinson, and A. D. Steinberg. "Dietary enrichment with polyunsaturated acid eicosapentaenoic acid prevents proteinuria and prolongs survival in NZB×NZW F1 mice." *J Clin Invest* 68:556–559 (1981).

Purba, M., A. Kouris-Blazos, N. Wattanapenpaiboon, W. Lukito, E. M. Rothenberg, B. C. Steen, and M. L. Wahlqvist. "Skin wrinkling: Can food make a difference?" *J Am Coll Nutr* 20:71–80 (2001).

Reilly, D. M., R. Parslew, G. R. Sharpe, S. Powell, and M. R. Green. "Inflammatory mediators in normal, sensitive, and diseased skin types." *Acta Derm Venerol* 80:171–174 (2000).

Robinson, D. R. "Alleviation of autoimmune disease by dietary lipids containing omega-3 fatty acids." *Rheum Dis Clin North Am* 17:213–222 (1991).

Robinson, D. R., L. L. Xu, S. Tateno, M. Guo, and R. E. Colvin. "Suppression of autoimmune disease by dietary n-3 fatty acids." *J Lipid Res* 34:1435–1444 (1993).

Ross, E. "The role of marine fish oils in the treatment of ulcerative colitis." *Nutr Rev* 51:47–49 (1993).

Ruzicka, R. *Eicosanoids and the Skin.* Boca Raton, Fla.: CRC Press, 1990.

Sperling, R. I. "The effects of dietary n-3 polyunsaturated fatty acids on neutrophils." *Proc Nutr Soc* 57:527–534 (1998).

Szczeklik, A., R. J. Gryglewski, and J. R. Vane. *Eicosanoids, Aspirin, and Asthma.* New York: Marcel Dekker, 1998.

Tak, P. P., and G. S. Firestein. "NF kappa B: A key role in inflammatory diseases." *J Clin Invest* 107:7–11 (2001).

Teitelbaum, J. E., and W. Allan Walker. "The role of omega-3 fatty acids in intestinal inflammation." *J Nutr Biochem* 12:21–32 (2001).

Walton, A. J., M. L. Snaith, M. Locniskar, A. G. Cumberland, W. J. Morrow, and D. A. Isenberg. "Dietary fish oil and the severity of symptoms in patients with systemic lupus erythematosus." *Ann Rheum Dis* 50:463–466 (1991).

Watkins, L. R., K. T. Nguyen, J. E. Lee, and S. F. Maier. "Dynamic regulation of proinflammatory cytokines." *Adv Exp Med Bio* 461:153–178 (1999).

Wolfe, F., K. Ross, J. Anderson, I. J. Russel, and L. Hebert. "The prevalence and characteristics of fibromyalgia in the general population." *Arthritis Rheum* 38:19–28 (1995).

Xi, S., H. Pham, and V. A. Ziboh. "15-hydroxyeicosatrienoic acid (15-HeTrE) suppresses epidermal hyperproliferation via the modulation of nuclear transcription factor (AP-1) and apoptosis." *Arch Dermatol Res* 292:397–403 (2000).

Ziboh, V. A., C. C. Miller, and Y. Cho. "Significance of lipoxygenase-derived monohydroxy fatty acids in cutaneous biology." *Prostaglandins Other Lipid Mediat* 63:3–13 (2000).

Zukerman, E., and J. R. Ingelfinger. *Coping with Prednisone.* New York: St. Martin's Press, 1997.

Zurier, R. B. "Prostaglandins, immune response, and murine lupus." *Arthritis Rheum* 25:804–809 (1982).

———. "Eicosanoids and inflammation." In *Prostaglandins in Clinical Practice,* ed. W. D. Watkins, M. B. Peterson, and J. R. Fletcher, pp. 79–96. New York: Raven Press, 1989.

———. "*Lipids* and lupus." In *Lupus: Molecular and Cellular Pathogenesis,* ed. G. M. Kammer and G. C. Tsokos, pp. 599–611. Totowan, N.J.: Humana Press, 1998.

Chapter 15 Women's Health Concerns: Infertility, Menopause, and Beyond

Adachi, J. D., and G. Joannidis. "Glucocorticoid-induced osteoporosis." *Drug Development Res* 49:120–134 (2000).

Al, M. D., A. C. van Houwelingen, and G. Hornstra. "Relation between birth order and the maternal and neonatal docosahexaenoic acid status." *Eur J Clin Nutr* 51:548–553 (1997).

———. "Long-chain polyunsaturated fatty acids, pregnancy, and pregnancy outcome." *Am J Clin Nutr* 71:285S–291S (2000).

Allen, K. G., and M. A. Harris. "The role of n-3 fatty acids in gestation and parturition." *Exp Bio Med* 226:498–506 (2001).

Anderson, J. W., B. M. Johnsstone, and D. T. Remlley. "Breast feeding and cognitive development: A meta-analysis." *Am J Clin Nutr* 70:535–535 (1999).

Bitman, J., L. Wood, M. Hamosh, P. Hamosh, and R. Mehta. "Comparison of the lipid composition of breast milk from mothers of term and preterm infants." *Am J Clin Nutr* 38:300–312 (1983).

Brush, M. G., S. J. Watson, D. F. Horrobin, and M. S. Manku. "Abnormal essential fatty acid levels in plasma of women with premenstrual syndrome." *Am J Obstet Gynecol* 150:363–366 (1984).

Cerin, A., A. Collins, B. M. Landgren, and P. Eneroth. "Hormonal and biochemical profiles of premenstrual syndrome: Treatment with essential fatty acids." *Acta Obstet Gynecol Scand* 72:337–343 (1993).

Cibula, D., R. Cifova, M. Fanta, R. Poledne, J. Livny, and J. Skibova. "Increased risk of non-insulin dependent diabetes mellitus, arterial hypertension, and coronary disease in perimenopausal women with a history of the polycystic ovary syndrome." *Human Reproduction* 15:785–789 (2000).

Cushman, M., C. Legault, E. Barrett-Connor, M. L. Stefanick, C. Kessler, H. L. Judd, P. A. Sakkinen, and R. P. Tracy. "Effect of postmenopausal hormones on inflammation-sensitive proteins: The Postmenopausal Estrogen/Progestin Interventions (PEPI) study." *Circulation* 100:717–722 (1999).

Deutch, B., E. B. Jorgensen, and J. C. Hansen. "Menstrual discomfort in Danish women reduced by dietary supplements of omega-3 PUFA and B12." *Nutr Res* 20:621–631 (2000).

Dewey, K. G., R. J. Cohen, K. H. Brown, and L. L. Rivera. "Effects of exclusive breastfeeding for four versus six months on maternal nutritional status and infant motor development: Results of two randomized trials in Honduras." *J Nutr* 131:262–267 (2001).

Eggelmeijer, F. "Prevention and treatment of glucocorticoid-induced osteoporosis." *Pharm World Sci* 20:193–197 (1998).

Gibson, R. A., and G. M. Kneebone. "Fatty acid composition of human colostrum and mature human milk." *Am J Clin Nutr* 34:252–256 (1981).

Glueck, C. J., P. Wang, R. Fontaine, T. Tracy, and L. Sieve-Smith. "Metformin-induced resumption of normal menses in 39 of 43 (91%) previously amenorrheic women with the polycystic ovary syndrome." *Metab* 48:511–519 (1999).

Glueck, C. J., H. Phillips, D. Cameron, L. Sieve-Smith, and L. Wang. "Continuing metformin throughout pregnancy in women with polycystic ovary syndrome appears to safely reduce first-trimester spontaneous abortion: A pilot study." *Fert Steril* 75:46–52 (2001).

Haynes, P., and B. L. Parry. "Mood disorders and the reproductive cycle: Affective disorders during the menopause and premenstrual dysphoric disorder." *Psychopharmacology Bull* 34:313–318 (1998).

Heart and Estrogen/Progestin Replacement Study (HERS) Group. "Randomized trial of estrogen/progestin for secondary prevention of coronary heart disease in postmenopausal women." *JAMA* 280:605–613 (1998).

Holman, R. T., S. B. Johnson, and P. L. Ogburn. "Deficiency of essential fatty acids and membrane fluidity during pregnancy and lactation." *Proc Nat Acad Sci USA* 88:4835–4839 (1991).

Horwood, L. J., and D. M. Fergusson. "Breast feeding and later cognitive and academic outcomes." *Pediatrics* 101:E9 (1998).

Jensen, R. G. *The Lipids of Human Milk.* Boca Raton, Fla.: CRC Press, 1989.

————. "Lipids in human milk." *Lipids* 34:1243–1271 (1999).

Johnson, D. L., P. R. Swank, V. M. Howie, C. D. Baldwin, and M. Owen. "Breast feeding and children's intelligence." *Psychol Reports* 79:1179–1185 (1996).

Kerstetter, J. E., A. C. Looker, and K. L. Insogna. "Low dietary protein and low bone density." *Calcif Tissue Int* 66:313 (2000).

Kerstetter, J. E., C. M. Svastisalee, D. M. Casseria, M. E. Mitnick, and K. L. Insogna. "A threshold for low-protein-diet-induced elevations in parathyroid hormone." *Am J Clin Nutr* 72:168–173 (2000).

Kettler, D. B. "Can manipulation of the ratios of essential fatty acids slow the rapid rate of postmenopausal bone loss?" *Altern Med Rev* 6:61–77 (2001).

Kiddy, D. S., D. Hamilton-Fairley, A. Bush, F. Short, V. Anyaoku, M. J. Reed, and S. Franks. "Improvement in endocrine and ovarian function during dietary treatment of obese women with polycystic ovary syndrome." *Clin Endocrinol* 36:105–111 (1992).

Kiddy, D. S., D. Hamilton-Fairley, M. Seppala, R. Koistinem, V. H. Jones, M. J. Reed, and S. Franks. "Diet-induced changes in sex hormone binding globulin and free testosterone in women with normal or polycystic ovaries: Correlation with serum insulin and insulin-like growth factor." *Clin Endocrinol* 31:757–763 (1989).

Kramer, M. S., K. Demisse, H. Yang, R. W. Platt, R. Sauve, and R. Liston. "The contribution of mild and moderate preterm birth to infant mortality." *JAMA* 284:843–849 (2000).

Lane, M. A., A. Z. Reznick, E. M. Tilmont, A. Lanir, S. S. Ball, V. Read, D. K. Ingram, R. G. Cutler, and G. S. Roth. "Aging and food restriction alter some indices of bone metabolism in male rhesus monkeys." *J Nutr* 125:1600–1610 (1995).

Legro, R. S. "Insulin resistance in polycystic ovary syndrome." *Mol Cell Endocrinol* 143:103–110 (1998).

Lindheim, S. R., S. C. Presser, E. C. Ditkoff, M. A. Vijod, F. Z. Stanczyk, and R. A. Lobo. "A possible bimodal effect of estrogen on insulin sensitivity in postmenopausal women and the attenuating effect of added progestin." *Fert Steril* 60:664–667 (1993).

Lucas, A., R. Morley, T. J. Cole, G. Lister, and C. Leeson-Payne. "Breast milk and subsequent intelligence quotient in children born preterm." *Lancet* 339:261–264 (1992).

Makrides, M., K. Simmer, M. Goggin, and R. A. Gibson. "Erythrocyte docosahexaenoic acid correlates with the visual response of healthy, term infants." *Pediatr Res* 33:425–427 (1993).

Makrides, M., M. A. Neumann, R. W. Byard, K. Simmer, and R. A. Gibson.

"Fatty acid composition of brain, retina, and erythrocytes in breast-fed and formula-fed infants." *Am J Clin Nutr* 60:189–194 (1994).

Makrides, M., M. A. Neumann, K. Simmer, J. Pater, and R. A. Gibson. "Are long-chain polyunsaturated fatty acids essential nutrients in infancy?" *Lancet* 345:1463–1468 (1995).

Makrides, M., M. A. Neumann, and R. A. Gibson. "Is dietary docosahexaenoic acid essential for term infants?" *Lipids* 31:115–119 (1996).

Manelli, F., and A. Giustina. "Glucocorticoid-induced osteoporosis." *TEM* 11:79–85 (2000).

McGregor, J. A., K. G. Allen, M. A. Harris, M. Reece, M. Wheeler, J. I. French, and J. Morrison. "The omega-3 story: Nutritional prevention of preterm birth and other adverse pregnancy outcomes." *Obstet Gynecol Surv* 56:S1–S13 (2001).

Mills, J. L., R. DerSimonian, J. D. Morrow, L. J. Roberts, J. D. Clemens, J. C. Hauth, P. Catalano, B. Sibai, L. B. Curet, and R. J. Levine. "Prostacyclin and thromboxane changes predating clinical onset of preeclampsia." *JAMA* 282:356–362 (1999).

Moriguchi, T., S. Greiner, and N. Salem. "Behavioral deficits associated with dietary induction of decreased brain docosahexaenoic acid concentration." *J Neurochem* 75:2563–2573 (2000).

Munger, R. G., J. R. Cerhan, and B. Chiu. "Prospective study of dietary protein intake and risk of hip fracture in postmenopausal women." *Am J Clin Nutr* 69:147–152 (1999).

Nestler, J. E., and D. J. Jakubowicz. "Decreases in ovarian cyctochrone P450c17α activity and serum free testosterone after reduction of insulin secretion in polycystic ovary syndrome." *N Engl J Med* 335:617–623 (1996).

Nestler, J. E., D. J. Jakubowicz, W. S. Evans, and R. Pasquali. "Effects of metformin on spontaneous and clomiphene-induced ovulation in the polycystic ovary syndrome." *N Engl J Med* 338:1876–1880 (1998).

Neuringer, M., G. J. Anderson, and W. E. Connor. "Cerebral cortex docosahexaenoic acid is lower in formula-fed than in breast-fed infants." *Nutr Rev* 51:238–241 (1993).

Olsen, S. F., H. S. Hansen, N. J. Secher, B. Jensen, and B. Sandstrom. "Gestation length and birth weight in relation to intake of marine n-3 fatty acids." *Br J Nutr* 73:397–404 (1995).

Olsen, S. F., N. J. Secher, A. Tabor, T. Weber, J. J. Walker, and C. Gluud. "Randomized clinical trials of fish oil supplementation in high risk pregnancies." *Br J Obstet Gynecol* 107:382–395 (2000).

Otto, S. J., A. C. van Houwelingen, A. Badart-Smook, and G. Hornstra. "Comparison of the peripartum and postpartum phospholipid polyunsaturated fatty acid profiles of lactating and nonlactating women." *Am J Clin Nutr* 73:1074–1079 (2001).

Phinney, S. "Potential risk of prolonged gamma-linolenic acid use." *Ann Intern Med* 120:692 (1994).

Pulido, J. M. E., and M. A. Salazar. "Changes in insulin sensitivity, secretion, and glucose effectiveness during menstrual cycle." *Arch Med Res* 30:19–22 (1999).

Puolakka, J., L. Makarainen, L. Viinikka, and O. Ylikorkala. "Biochemical and clinical effects of treating the premenstrual syndrome with prostaglandin synthesis precursors." *J Reprod Med* 30:149–153 (1985).

Rubinstein, M., A. Marazzi, and E. P. de Fried. "Low-dose aspirin treatment improves ovarian responsiveness, uterine and ovarian blood flow velocity, implantation, and pregnancy rates in patients undergoing in vitro fertilization: A prospective, randomized double-blind placebo-controlled assay." *Fert Steril* 71:825–829 (1999).

Stark, K. D., E. J. Park, V. A. Maines, and B. J. Holub. "Effect of a fish-oil concentrate on serum lipids in postmenopausal women receiving and not receiving hormone replacement therapy in a placebo-controlled, double-blind trial." *Am J Clin Nutr* 72:389–394 (2000).

Terano, T. "Effect of omega-3 polyunsaturated fatty acid ingestion on bone metabolism and osteoporosis." *World Rev Nutr Diet* 88:141–147 (2001).

Thatcher, S. S. Polycystic Ovary Syndrome. Indianapolis, Ind.: Perspectives Press, 2000.

Trujillo, E. P., and K. S. Broughton. "Ingestion of n-3 polyunsaturated fatty acids and ovulation in rats." *J Reprod Fertil* 105:197–203 (1995).

Velazquez, E. M., S. Mendoza, T. Hamer, E. Sosa, and C. J. Glueck. "Metformin therapy in polycystic ovary syndrome reduces hyperinsulinemia, insulin resistance, hyperandrogenemia, and systolic blood pressure, while facilitating normal menses and pregnancy." *Metab* 43:647–654 (1994).

Watkins, B. A., M. F. Seifert, and K. G. Allen. "Importance of dietary fat in modulating PGE2, responses and influence of vitamin E on bone morphometry." *World Rev Nutr Diet* 82:250–259 (1997).

Watkins, B. A., Y. Li, H. E. Lippman, and M. F. Seifert. "Omega-3 polyunsaturated fatty acids and skeletal health." *Exp Bio Med* 226:485–497 (2001).

Watkins, B. A., Y. Li, and M. F. Seifert. "Lipids as modulators of bone remodeling." *Curr Opin Clin Nutr Metab Care* 4:105–110 (2001).

Watkins, B. A., H. E. Lippman, L. Le Bouteiller, Y. Li, and M. F. Seifert. "Bioactive fatty acids: Role in bone biology and bone cell function." *Prog Lipid Res* 40:125–148 (2001).

Willatts, P., J. S. Forsyth, M. K. DiModugno, S. Varma, and M. Colvin. "Effect of long-chain polyunsaturated fatty acids in infant formula on problem solving at 10 months of age." *Lancet* 352:688–691 (1998).

Yeh, Y. Y., M. F. Gehman, and S. M. Yeh. "Maternal dietary fish oil enriches docosahexaenoate levels in brain subcellular fractions of offspring." *J Neurosci Res* 35:218–226 (1993).

Chapter 16 Building a Better Brain

Al, M. D. M., A. C. van Houwelingen, and G. Hornstra. "Relation between birth order and the maternal and neonatal docosahexaenoic acid status." *Eur J Clin Nutr* 51:548–553 (1997).

———. "Long-chain polyunsaturated fatty acids, pregnancy, and pregnancy outcome." *Am J Clin Nutr* 71:285S–291S (2000).

Anderson, J. W., B. M. Johnsstone, and D. T. Remlley. "Breast-feeding and cognitive development: A meta-analysis." *Am J Clin Nutr* 70:535–535 (1999).

Benson, H. *The Relaxation Response.* New York: William Morrow, 1975.

Bertoni-Freddari, C. L., P. Fattoretti, U. Caselli, T. Casoi, G. Di Stefano, and S. Algeri. "Dietary restriction modulates synaptic structural dynamics in the aging hippocampus." *Age* 22:107–113 (1999).

Bitman, J., L. Wood, M. Hamosh, P. Hamosh, and R. Mehta. "Comparison of the lipid composition of breast milk from mothers of term and preterm infants." *Am J Clin Nutr* 38:300–312 (1983).

Bowen, D. M., C. B. Smith, and A. N. Davidson. "Molecular changes in senile dementia." *Brain* 96:849–856 (1973).

Bruce-Keller, A. J., G. Umberger, R. McFall, and M. P. Mattson. "Food restriction reduces brain damage and improves behavioral outcome following excitotoxic and metabolic insults." *Ann Neurology* 45:8–15 (1999).

Connor, W. E., M. Neuringer, and D. S. Lin. "Dietary effects on brain fatty acid composition: The reversibility of the n-3 fatty acid deficiency and turnover of docosahexaenoic acid in the brain, erythrocytes, and plasma of rhesus monkeys." *J Lipid Res* 31:237–247 (1990).

DeKosy, S., S. Scheef, and C. Cotman. "Elevated corticosterone levels: A possible cause of reduced axon sprouting in aged animals." *Neuroendocrinology* 38:33–38 (1984).

Dewey, K. G., R. J. Cohen, K. H. Brown, and L. L. Rivera. "Effects of exclusive breastfeeding for four versus six months on maternal nutritional status and infant motor development: Results of two randomized trials in Honduras." *J Nutr* 131:262–267 (2001).

Gage, F. H. "Mammalian neural stem cells." *Science* 287:1433–1438 (2000).

Gamoh, S., M. Hashimoto, K. Sugioka, S. Hossain, N. Hata, Y. Misawa, and S. Masumura. "Chronic administration of docosahexaenoic acid improves reference memory-related learning ability in young rats." *Neurosci* 93:237–241 (1999).

Gibson, R. A., and G. M. Kneebone. "Fatty acid composition of human colostrum and mature human milk." *Am J Clin Nutr* 34:252–256 (1981).

Francois, C. A., S. L. Connor, R. C. Wander, and W. E. Connor. "Acute effects of dietary fatty acids on the fatty acids of human milk." *Am J Clin Nutr* 67:301–308 (1998).

Fuchs, E., and G. Fluge. "Stress, glucocorticoids, and structural plasticity of the hippocampus." *Neurosci Biobehav Rev* 23:295–300 (1998).

Holman, R. T., S. B. Johnson, and P. L. Ogburn. "Deficiency of essential fatty acids and membrane fluidity during pregnancy and lactation." *Proc Nat Acad Sci USA* 88:4835–4839 (1991).

Homer, H., D. Packan, and R. M. Sapolsky. "Glucocorticoids inhibit glucose transport in cultured hippocampal neurons and glia." *Neuroendocrinology* 52:57–63 (1990).

Horner, P. J., and F. H. Gage. "Regenerating the damaged central nervous system." *Nature* 407:963–970 (2000).

Horwood, L. J., and D. M. Fergusson. "Breast feeding and later cognitive and academic outcomes." *Pediatrics* 101:E9 (1998).

Hughes, J., T. W. Smith, H. W. Kosterlitz, L. A. Fothergill, B. A. Morgan, and H. R. Morris. "Identification of two related pentapeptides from the brain with potent opiate agonist activity." *Nature* 258:577–580 (1975).

Ikemoto, A., A. Nitta, S. Furukawa, M. Ohishi, A. Nakamura, Y. Fujii, and H. Okuyama. "Dietary n-3 fatty acid deficiency decreases nerve growth factor content in rat hippocampus." *Neurosci Lett* 285:99–102 (2000).

Jensen, R. G. *The Lipids of Human Milk.* Boca Raton, Fla.: CRC Press, 1989.

———. "Lipids in human milk." *Lipids* 34:1243–1271 (1999).

Johnson, D. L., P. R. Swank, V. M. Howie, C. D. Baldwin, and M. Owen. "Breast feeding and children's intelligence." *Psychol Reports* 79:1179–1185 (1996).

Jones, C. R., T. Aria, and S. I. Rapoport. "Evidence for the involvement of docosahexaenoic acid in cholinergic simulated signal transduction at the synapse." *J Neurochem Res* 22:663–670 (1997).

Kamei, T., Y. Toriumi, H. Kimura, S. Ohno, H. Kumano, and K. Kimura. "Decrease in serum cortisol during yoga exercise is correlated with alpha wave activation." *Percept Mot Skills* 90:1027–1032 (2000).

Keen, P. A., and T. W. Kuhn. "Do glucocorticoids have adverse effects on brain function?" *CNS Drugs* 11:245–251 (1999).

Kempermann, G., and F. H. Gage. "New nerve cells for the adult brain." *Sci Am* 280:48–53 (1999).

Kerr, D., L. Campbell, M. Applegate, A. Brodish, and P. W. Landfield. "Chronic stress-induced acceleration of electrophysiologic and morphometric biomarkers of hippocampal aging." *J Neurosci* 11:1316–1324 (1991).

Khalsa, D. S. *Brain Longevity.* New York: Warner Books, 1997.

Khalsa, D. S., and C. Stauth. *Meditation as Medicine.* New York: Pocket Books, 2001.

Kirschbaum, C., O. T. Wolf, M. May, W. Wippich, and D. H. Hellhammer. "Stress and treatment induced elevations of cortisol levels associated with impaired declarative memory in healthy adults." *Life Sci* 58:1475–1483 (1996).

Kneebone, G. M., R. Kneebone, and R. A. Gibson. "Fatty acid composition of breast milk from three racial groups from Penang, Malaysia." *Am J Clin Nutr* 41:765–769 (1985).

Kraemer, W. J., J. E. Dziados, L. J. Marchitelli, S. E. Gordon, E. A. Harman, R. Mello, S. J. Fleck, P. N. Frykman, and N. T. Triplett. "Effects of different heavy-resistance exercise protocols on plasma beta-endorphin concentration." *J Appl Physiol* 74:450–459 (1993).

Lee, J., W. Duen, J. M. Long, D. K. Ingram, and M. P. Mattson. "Dietary restriction increases the number of newly generated neural cells, and induces BDNF expression in the dentate gyrus of rats." *J Mol Neurosci* 15:99–108 (2000).

Lim, S., and H. Suzuki. "Effect of dietary docosahexaenoic acid and phosphatidylcholine on maze behavior and fatty acid composition of plasma and brain lipids in mice." *Int J Vitam Nutr Res* 70:251–259 (2000).

———. "Intakes of dietary docosahexaenoic acid ethyl ester and egg phosphatidylcholine improve maze-learning ability in young and old mice." *J Nutr* 130:1629–1632 (2000).

———. "Changes in maze behavior of mice occur after sufficient accumulation of docosahexaenoic acid in brain." *J Nutr* 131:319–324 (2001).

Lucas, A., R. Morley, T. J. Cole, G. Lister, and C. Leeson-Payne. "Breast milk and subsequent intelligence quotient in children born preterm." *Lancet* 339:261–264 (1992).

Lupien, S. J., M. deLeon, S. deStanti, A. Covit, C. Tarshish, N. P. V. Nair, M. Thakur, B. S. McEwen, R. L. Hauger, and M. J. Meaney. "Cortisol levels during human aging predict hippocampal atrophy and memory deficits." *Nature Neurosci* 1:69–73 (1998).

Lynch, C. D., P. T. Cooney, S. A. Bennett, P. L. Thornton, A. S. Khan, R. L. Ingram, and W. E. Sonntag. "Effects of moderate caloric restriction on cortical microvascular density and local cerebral blood flow in aged rats." *Neurobiol Aging* 20:191–200 (1999).

Maes, M., A. Christophe, E. Bosmans, A. Lin, and H. Neels. "In humans, serum polyunsaturated fatty acid levels predict the response of proinflammatory cytokines to psychologic stress." *Bio Psychiatry* 47:910–920 (2000).

Makrides, M., K. Simmer, M. Goggin, and R. A. Gibson. "Erythrocyte docosahexaenoic acid correlates with the visual response of healthy, term infants." *Pediatr Res* 33:425–427 (1993).

Makrides, M., M. A. Neumann, R. W. Byard, K. Simmer, and R. A. Gibson. "Fatty acid composition of brain, retina, and erythrocytes in breast-fed and formula-fed infants." *Am J Clin Nutr* 60:189–194 (1994).

Makrides, M., M. A. Neumann, and R. A. Gibson. "Is dietary docosahexaenoic acid essential for term infants?" *Lipids* 31:115–119 (1996).

Mauch, D. H., K. Nagler, S. Schumacher, C. Goritz, E-C. Muller, A. Otto, and F. W. Pfieger. "CNS synaptogenesis promoted by glia-derived cholesterol." *Science* 294:1354–1357 (2001).

McEwen, B. S. "Stress and hippocampal plasticity." *Ann Rev Neurosci* 22:105–122 (1999).

McKittrick, C. R., A. M. Magarinos, D. C. Blanchard, R. J. Blanchard, B. S. McEwen, and R. R. Sakai. "Chronic social stress reduces dendritic arbors in CA3 of hippocampus and decreases binding to serotonin transporter sites." *Synapse* 36:85–94 (2000).

Means, L. W., J. L. Higgins, and T. J. Fernandez. "Mid-life onset of dietary restriction extends life and prolongs cognitive functioning." *Physiol Behav* 54:503–508 (1993).

Moriguchi, T., S. Greiner, and N. Salem. "Behavioral deficits associated with dietary induction of decreased brain docosahexaenoic acid concentration." *J Neurochem* 75:2563–2573 (2000).

Moriguchi, T., J. Loeke, M. Garrison, J. N. Catalan, and N. Salem. "Reversal of docosahexaenoic acid deficiency in the rat brain, retina, liver, and serum." *J Lipid Res* 42:419–427 (2001).

Myer, T., L. Schwarz, and W. Kindermann. "Exercise and endogenous opiates." In *Contemporary Endocrinology: Sports Endocrinology,* ed. M. P. Warren and N. W. Constantini, pp. 31–42. Totowa, N. J.: Humana Press, 2000.

Neuringer, M., G. J. Anderson, and W. E. Connor. "Cerebral cortex docosahexaenoic acid is lower in formula-fed than in breast-fed infants." *Nutr Rev* 51:238–241 (1993).

Newcomer, J. W., S. Craft, T. Hershey, K. Askins, and M. E. Bardgett. "-Glucocorticoid-induced impairment in declarative memory performance in adult humans." *J Neurosci* 14:2047–2053 (1994).

Norden, M. Beyond Prozac. New York: Regan Books, 1995.

Oliff, H. S., N. C. Berchtold, P. Isackson, and C. W. Cotman. "Exercise-induced regulation of brain-derived neurotrophic factor (BDNF) transcripts in the rat hippocampus." *Brain Res* Mol *Brain Res* 61:147–153 (1998).

Otto, S. J., A. C. van Houwelingen, A. Badart-Smook, and G. Hornstra. "Comparison of the peripartum and postpartum phospholipid polyunsaturated fatty acid profiles of lactating and nonlactating women." *Am J Clin Nutr* 73:1074–1079 (2001).

Sapolsky, R. M., L. Krey, and B. S. McEwen. "Prolonged glucocorticoid exposure reduces hippocampal neuron number: Implications for aging." *J Neurosci* 5:1222–1227 (1985).

Sapolsky, R. M., D. R. Packan, and W. W. Vale. "Glucocorticoid toxicity in the hippocampus: In vitro demonstration." *Brain Res* 453:367–371 (1988).

Sapolsky, R. M. *Stress, the Aging Brain, and the Mechanisms of Neuron Death. Cambridge,* Mass.: MIT Press, 1992.

Schmidt, L. A., N. A. Fox, M. C. Goldberg, C. C. Smith, and J. Schulkin. "Effects of acute prenidsone administration on memory, attention, and emotion in healthy human adults." *Psychoneuroendocrinology* 24:461–483 (1999).

Schmidt, M. A. Smart Fats. Berkeley, Calif.: Frog, Ltd., 1997.

Simopoulos, A. P., and J. Robinson. *The Omega Plan.* New York: Harper-Collins, 1998.

Sinclair, A. J., and M. A. Crawford. "The effect of a low fat maternal diet on neonatal rats." *Br J Nutr* 29:127–137 (1973).

Smith, E. N., E. A. Oelen, E. Seerat, F. A. Muskiet, and E. R. Boersma. "Breast milk docosahexaenoic acid (DHA) correlates with DHA status of malnourished infants." *Arch Dis Child* 82:493–494 (2000).

Smith, D. E., J. Roberts, F. H. Gage, and M. H. Tuszynski. "Age-associated neuronal atrophy occurs in the primate brain and is reversible by growth factor gene therapy." *Proc Nat Acad Sci USA* 96:10893–10898 (1999).

Solfrizzi, V., F. Panza, F. Torres, F. Mastroianni, A. Del Parigi, A. Venezia, and A. Capurso. "High monounsaturated fatty acids intake protects against age-related cognitive decline." *Neurology* 52:1563–1569 (1999).

Sonderberg, M., C. Edlund, K. Kristensson, and G. Dallner. "Fatty acid composition of brain phospholipids in aging and Alzheimer's disease." *Lipids* 26:421–423 (1991).

Starkman, M., B. Giordani, S. Gebarski, S. Berent, M. Schork, and D. Schteingart. "Decrease in cortisol reverses human hippocampal atrophy following treatment of Cushing's disease." *Bio Psychiatry* 46:1595–1602 (1999).

Stoll, A. L. *The Omega-3 Connection.* New York: Simon and Schuster, 2001.

Suzuki, H., S. Hayakawa, and S. Wada. "Effect of age on modification of brain polyunsaturated fatty acids and enzyme activities by fish oil diet in rats." *Mech Ageing Dev* 50:17–25 (1989).

Suzuki, H., S. Manabe, O. Wado, and M. A. Crawford. "Rapid incorporation of docosahexaenoic acid from dietary sources into brain microsomal, synaptosomal, and mitochrondria membranes in adult mice." *Int J Vitam Nutr Res* 67:272–278 (1987).

Suzuki, H., S. J. Park, M. Tamura, and S. Ando. "Effect of the long-term feeding of dietary lipids on the learning ability, fatty acid composition of brain stem phospholipids, and synaptic membrane fluidity in adult mice: A comparison of sardine oil diet with palm oil diet." *Mech Ageing Dev* 101:119–128 (1998).

Urquiza, A. M., de, S. Liu, M. Sjoberg, R. H. Zetterstrom, W. Griffiths, J. Sjovall, and T. Perlmann. "Docosahexaenoic acid, a ligand for the retinoid X receptor in mouse brain." *Science* 290:2140–2144 (2000).

Vance, H. E., R. B. Campenot, and D. E. Vance. "The synthesis and transport of lipids for axonal growth and nerve regeneration." *Biochim Biophys Acta* 1486:84–96 (2000).

van Houwelingen, A. C., E. C. Ham, and G. Hornstra. "The female docosahexaenoic acid status related to the number of completed pregnancies." *Lipids* 34:S229 (1999).

Van Praag, H., G. Kempermann, and F. H. Gage. "Running increases cell proliferation and neurogenesis in the adult mouse dentate gyrus." *Nature Neurosci* 2:266–270 (1999).

Weisinger, H. S., A. J. Vingrs, B. V. Bui, and A. J. Sinclair. "Effect of dietary n-3 deficiency and repletion in the guinea pig retina." *Invest Ophthalmol Vis Sci* 40:327–338 (1999).

Willatts, P., and J. S. Forsyth. "The role of long-chain polyunsaturated fatty acids in infant cognitive development." *Prostaglandins Leuko Essen Fatty Acids* 63:95–100 (2000).

Willatts, P., J. S. Forsyth, M. K. DiModugno, S. Varma, and M. Colvin. "Effect of long-chain polyunsaturated fatty acids in infant formula on problem solving at 10 months of age." *Lancet* 352:688–691 (1998).

Xiang, M., S. Lei, and R. Zetterstrom. "Composition of long-chain polyun-saturated fatty acids in human milk and growth of young infants in rural areas of northern China." *Acta Paediatr* 88:126–131 (1999).

Yeh, Y. Y., M. F. Gehman, and S. M. Yeh. "Maternal dietary fish oil enriches docosahexaenoate levels in brain subcellular fractions of off-spring." *J Neurosci Res* 35:218–226 (1993).

Yermakova, A., and M. K. O'Banion. "Cyclooxygenases in the central nervous system: Implication for treatment of neurological disorders." *Curr Pharma Design* 6:1755–1776 (2000).

Yonekubo, A., S. Honda, T. Kanno, K. Takahashi, and Y. Yamamoto. "Physiological role of docosahexaenoic acid in mother's milk and infant formulas." *In Essential Fatty Acids and Eicosanoids,* ed. A. Sin-clair and R. Gibson, pp. 214–217. Champaign, Ill.: American Oil Chemists Press, 1992.

Chapter 17 Emotions: The Mind-Body-Diet Connection

Anton, P. A. "Stress and mind-body impact on the course of inflammatory bowel diseases." *Sem Gastrointest Dis* 10:14–19 (1999).

Benson, H. *The Relaxation Response.* New York: William Morrow, 1975.

———. *Timeless Healing.* New York: Scribner, 1996.

Blok, W. L., M. B. Katan, and J. W. van der Meer. "Modulation of inflam-mation and cytokine production by dietary (n-3) fatty acids." *J Nutr* 126:1515–1533 (1996).

Brambilla, F., L. Bellodi, G. Perna, A. Bertani, A. Panerai, and P. Sacer-dote. "Plasma interleukin-1 beta concentrations in panic disorder." *Psychiatry Res* 54:135–142 (1994).

Carrington, P. *The Book of Meditation.* Boston, Mass.: Element Books, 1998.

Chrousos, G. P., and P. W. Gold. "A healthy body in a healthy mind—and vice versa: The damaging owner of 'uncontrollable' stress." *J Clin Endocrinol Metab* 83:1842–1845 (1998).

Cousins, N. *Anatomy of an Illness.* New York: Bantam Books, 1983.

Cupps, T. R., and A. S. Fauci. "Corticosteroid-mediated immunoregulation in man." *Immunol Rev* 65:133–155 (1982).

Decker, S. A. "Salivary cortisol and social status among Dominican men." Hormones Behav 38:29–38 (2000).

DeKosy, S., S. Scheef, and C. Cotman. "Elevated corticosterone levels: A possible cause of reduced axon sprouting in aged animals." *Neuroen-docrinology* 38:33–38 (1984).

Fauci, A. S., and D. C. Dale. "The effect of *In Vivo* hydrocortisone on sub-population of human lymphocytes." *J Clin Invest* 53:240–246 (1974).

Fife, A., P. J. Beasley, and D. L. Fertig. "Psychoneuroimmunology and cancer: Historical perspectives and current research." *Adv Neuroimmunol* 6:179–190 (1996).

Fuchs, E., and G. Fluge. "Stress, glucocorticoids, and structural plasticity of the hippocampus." *Neurosci Biobehav Rev* 23:295–300 (1998).

Goya, L., R. Rivero, and A. M. Pascual-Leone. "Glucocorticoids, stress, and aging." In *Hormones and Aging*, ed. P. S. Timiras, W. B. Quay, and A. Vernadakis, pp. 249–266. Boca Raton, Fla.: CRC Press, 1995.

Hamazaki, T., S. Sawazaki, T. Nagasawa, Y. Nagao, Y. Kanagawa, and K. Yazawa. "Administration of docosahexaenoic acid influences behavior and plasma catecholamine levels at times of psychological stress." *Lipids* 34:S33–S37 (1999).

Hamazaki, T., M. Itomura, S. Sawazaki, and Y. Nagao. "Anti-stress effects of D. H. A." *Biofactors* 13:41–45 (2000).

Haynes, B. F., and A. S. Fauci. "The differential effects of In Vivo hydrocortisone on kinetics of subpopulations of human peripheral blood thymus-derived lymphocytes." *J Clin Invest* 61:703–707 (1978).

Hibbeln, J. R., J. C. Umhau, D. T. George, and N. Salem. "Do plasma polyunsaturates predict hostility and depression?" *World Rev Nutr Diet* 82:175–186 (1997).

Hirano, D., M. Nagashima, R. Ogawa, and S. Yoshino. "Serum levels of interleukin-6 and stress-related substances indicate mental stress condition in patients with rheumatoid arthritis." *J Rheumatol* 28:490–495 (2001).

Holliday, R. "Human ageing and the origins of religion." *Biogerontology* 2:73–77 (2001).

Holsboer, F. "Stress, hypercortisolism, and corticosteroid receptors in depression." *J Affect Dis* 62:77–91 (2001).

Homer, H., D. Packan, and R. M. Sapolsky. "Glucocorticoids inhibit glucose transport in cultured hippocampal neurons and glia." *Neuroendocrinology* 52:57–63 (1990).

Infante, J. R., F. Peran, M. Martinez, A. Roldan, R. Poyatos, C. Ruiz, F. Samaniego, and F. Garrido. "ACTH and beta-endorphin in transcendental meditation." *Physiol Behav* 64:311–315 (1998).

Jacobson, L., and R. M. Sapolsky. "The role of the hippocampus in feedback regulation of the hypothalamic-pituitary-adrenocortical axis." *Endocrine Rev* 12:118–134 (1991).

Jefferies, W. *Safe Uses of Cortisone*. Springfield, Ill.: Charles C. Thomas, 1981.

Kamei, T., Y. Toriumi, H. Kimura, S. Ohno, H. Kumano, and K. Kimura. "Decrease in serum cortisol during yoga exercise is correlated with alpha wave activation." *Percept Mot Skills* 90:1027–1032 (2000).

Katzman, R., and J. E. Jackson. "Alzheimer disease: Basic and clinical advances." *J Am Geriatrics Soc* 39:516–525 (1991).

Keen, P. A., and T. W. Kuhn. "Do glucocorticoids have adverse effects on brain function?" *CNS Drugs* 11:245–251 (1999).

Kerr, D., L. Campbell, M. Applegate, A. Brodish, and P. W. Landfield. "Chronic stress-induced acceleration of electrophysiologic and mor-phometric biomarkers of hippocampal aging." *J Neurosci* 11:1316–1324 (1991).

Khalsa, D. S. *Brain Longevity*. New York: Warner Books, 1997.

Khalsa, D. S., and C. Stauth. *Meditation as Medicine*. New York: Pocket Books, 2001.

Kirschbaum, C., O. T. Wolf, M. May, W. Wippich, and D. H. Hellhammer. "Stress and treatment induced elevations of cortisol levels associated with impaired declarative memory in healthy adults." *Life Sci* 58:1475–1483 (1996).

Landfield, P. W., J. C. Waymire, and G. Lynch. "Hippocampal aging and adrenocorticoids: A quantitative correlation." *Science* 202:1098–1102 (1978).

Leonard, B. E., and C. Song. "Stress and the immune system in the etiol-ogy of anxiety and depression." *Pharmacol Biochem Behav* 54:299–303 (1996).

Lupien, S. J., M. deLeon, S. deStanti, A. Covit, C. Tarshish, N. P. V. Nair, M. Thakur, B. S. McEwen, R. L. Hauger, and M. I. Meaney. "Cortisol levels during human aging predict hippocampal atrophy and memory deficits." *Nature Neurosci* 1:69–73 (1998).

MacLean, C. R., K. G. Walton, S. R. Wenneberg, D. K. Levitsky, J. P. Man-darino, R. Waziri, S. L. Hillis, and R. H. Schneider. "Effects of the Transcendental Meditation program on adaptive mechanisms: Changes in hormone levels and responses to stress after 4 months of practice." *Psychoneuroendocrinology* 22:277–295 (1997).

Maes, M., C. Song, A. Lin, R. De Jongh, A. Van Gastel, G. Kenis, E. Bosmans, I. De Meester, I. I. Benoy, H. Neels, P. Demedts, A. Janca, S. Scharpe, and R. S. Smith. "The effects of psychological stress on humans: Increased production of pro-inflammatory cytokines and a Th1-like response in stress-induced anxiety." *Cytokine* 10:313–331 (1998)

Maes, M., A. Christophe, E. Bosmans, A. Lin, and H. Neels. "In humans, serum polyunsaturated fatty acid levels predict the response of proin-flammatory cytokines to psychologic stress." *Bio Psychiatry* 47:910–920 (2000).

Maier, S. F., and L. R. Watkins. "Cytokines for psychologists: Implications of bidirectional immune-to-brain communication for understanding behavior, mood, and cognition." *Psychol Rev* 105:83–107 (1998).

Mastorakos, G., G. P. Chrousos, and J. S. Weber. "Recombinant interleukin-6 activates the hypothalamo-pituitary adrenal axis in humans." *J Clin Endocrinol Metab* 77:1690–1694 (1993).

McEwen, B. S. "Stress and hippocampal plasticity." *Ann Rev Neurosci* 22:105–122 (1999).

McKittrick, C. R., A. M. Magarinos, D. C. Blanchard, R. J. Blanchard, B. S. McEwen, and R. R. Sakai. "Chronic social stress reduces dendritic arbors in CA3 of hippocampus and decreases binding to serotonin transporter sites." *Synapse* 36:85–94 (2000).

Mittwoch-Jaffe, T., F. Shalit, B. Srendi, and S. Yehuda. "Modification of cytokine secretion following mild emotional stimuli." *Neuroreport* 6:789–792 (1995).

Munch, A., and G. R. Crabtree. "Glucocorticoid-induced lymphocyte death." In *Cell Death in Biology and Pathology,* ed. I. D. Bower and R. A. Lockskin, pp. 329–357. New York: Chapman and Hall, 1981.

Nemeroff, C. B., and D. L. Musselman. "Are platelets the link between depression and ischemic heart disease?" *Am Heart J* 140:S57–S62 (2000).

Newcomer, J. W., S. Craft, T. Hershey, K. Askins, and M. E. Bardgett. "-Glucocorticoid-induced impairment in declarative memory performance in adult humans." *J Neurosci* 14:2047–2053 (1994).

Norman, A. W., and G. Litwack. *Hormones.* 2d edition. New York: Academic Press, 1997.

Olff, M. "Stress, depression, and immunity." *Psychiatry Res* 85:7–15 (1999).

Orth, D. N. "Cushing's syndrome." *N Engl J Med* 332:791–803 (1995).

Pert, C., and S. H. Snyder. "Opiate receptor: Demonstration in nervous tissue." *Science* 179:1011–1014 (1973).

Pert, C., and H. Dienstfrey. "The neuropeptide network." *Ann NY Acad Sci* 521:189–194 (1988).

Pert, C. *Molecules of Emotion.* New York: Scribner, 1997.

Pert, C. B., H. E. Dreher, and M. R. Ruff. "The psychosomatic network: Foundations of mind-body medicine." *Altern Ther Health Med* 4:30–41 (1998).

Polnikoff, N. P., R. E. Faith, A. J. Murgo, and R. A. Good, eds. *Cytokines: Stress and Immunity.* Boca Raton, Fla.: CRC Press, 1999.

Reichenberg, A., R. Yirmiya, A. Schuld, T. Kraus, M. Haack, A. Morag, and T. Pollmacher. "Cytokine-associated emotional and cognitive disturbances in humans." *Arch Gen Psychiatry* 58:445–452 (2001).

Romero, L. M., K. M. Raley-Susman, D. M. Redish, S. M. Brooke, and R. Sapolsky. "Possible mechanism by which stress accelerates growth of virally derived tumors." *Proc Nat Acad Sci USA* 89:11084–11087 (1992).

Roses, A. D., W. J. Strittmatter, M. A. Pericak-Vance, E. H. Corden, A. M. Saunders, and D. E. Schmechel. "Clinical application of apoplipoprotein E genotyping to Alzheimer's disease." *Lancet* 343:1564–1565 (1994).

Sapolsky, R. M., L. Krey, and B. S. McEwen. "Glucocorticoid-sensitive hippocampal neurons are involved in terminating the adrenocorticol stress response." *Proc Nat Acad Sci USA* 81:6174–6177 (1984).

———. "Stress down regulates corticosterone receptors in a site-specific manner in the brain." *Endocrinology* 114:287–292 (1984).

———. "Prolonged glucocorticoid exposure reduces hippocampal neuron number: Implications for aging." *J Neurosci* 5:1222–1227 (1985).

Sapolsky, R. M., D. R. Packan, and W. W. Vale. "Glucocorticoid toxicity in the hippocampus: In vitro demonstration." *Brain Res* 453:367–371 (1988).

Sapolsky, R. M., H. Uno, C. S. Rebert, and C. E. Finch. "Hippocampal damage associated with prolonged glucocorticoid exposure in primates." *J Neurosci* 10:2897–2902 (1990).

Sapolsky, R. M. *Stress, the Aging Brain, and the Mechanisms of Neuron Death.* Cambridge, Mass.: MIT Press, 1992.

———. "Atrophy of the hippocampus in posttraumatic stress disorder." *Hippocampus* 11:90–91 (2001).

Schmidt, L. A., N. A. Fox, M. C. Goldberg, C. C. Smith, and J. Schulkin. "Effects of acute prednisone administration on memory, attention, and emotion in healthy human adults." *Psychoneuroendocrinology* 24:461–483 (1999).

Selye, H. "Studies on adaptation." Endocrinology 21:169–188 (1937).

Sheline, Y., P. W. Wang, M. H. Godo, J. B. Csernansky, and M. W. Vannier. "Hippocampal atrophy in recurrent major depression." *Proc Nat Acad Sci USA* 93:3908–3913 (1996).

Starkman, M., B. Giordani, S. Gebarski, S. Berent, M. Schork, and D. Schteingart. "Decrease in cortisol reverses human hippocampal atrophy following treatment of Cushing's disease." *Bio Psychiatry* 46:1595–1602 (1999).

Stein, M., C. Koverola, C. Hanna, M. Torchia, and B. McClarty. "Hippocampal volume in women victimized by childhood sexual abuse." *Psychol Med* 27:951–959 (1997).

Stein-Behrens, B. A., E. M. Elliott, C. A. Miller, J. W. Schilling, R. New-combe, and R. M. Sapolsky. "Glucocorticoids exacerbate kainic acid–induced extracellular accumulation of excitatory amino acids in the rat hippocampus." *J Neurochem* 58:1730–1735 (1992).

Sternberg, E. M. The Balance Within. New York: W. H. Freeman, 2000.

Sudsuang, R., V. Chentanez, and K. Veluvan. "Effect of Buddhist medita-tion on serum cortisol and total protein levels, blood pressure, pulse rate, lung volume, and reaction time." *Physiol Behav* 50:543–548 (1991).

Terry, R. D., R. DeTeresa, and L. A. Hansen. "Neocortical cell counts in the normal adult aging." *Ann Neurology* 21:530–539 (1987).

van Eekelen, J. A., and E. R. De Kloet. "Co-localization of brain corticos-teroid receptors in the rat hippocampus." *Prog Histochem Cytochem* 6:250–258 (1992).

Vernadakis, A. "Effects of hormones on neural tissue: *In Vivo* and in vitro studies." *In Hormones and Aging,* ed. P. S. Timiras, W. B. Quay, and A. Vernadakis, pp. 291–314. Boca Raton, Fla.: CRC Press, 1995.

Virgin, C. E., T. P. Hu, D. R. Packan, G. C. Tombaugh, S. H. Yang, H. C. Horner, and R. M. Sapolsky. "Glucocortoids inhibit glucose transport and glutamate uptake in hippocampal astrocytes: Implications for glu-cocorticoid toxicity." *J Neurochem* 57:1422–1428 (1991).

Vitkovic, L., J. P. Konsman, J. Bockaert, R. Dantzer, V. Homburger, and C. Jacque. "Cytokine signals propagate through the brain." *Mol Psychia-try* 5:604–615 (2000).

Weizman, R., N. Laor, Z. Wiener, L. Wolmer, and H. Bessler. "Cytokine production in panic disorder patients." *Clin Neuropharmacol* 22:107–109 (1999).

Wooley, C., E. Gould, and B. S. McEwen. "Exposure to excess glucocorti-coids alters dendritic morphology of adult hippocampal pyramidal neurons." *Brain Res* 531:225–231 (1990).

Yudkin, J. S., C. S. Yajnik, V. Mohamed-Ali, and K. Bulmer. "High levels of circulating pro-inflammatory cytokines and leptin in urban, but not rural, Asian Indians: A potential explanation for increased risk of dia-betes and coronary heart disease." *Diabetes Care* 22:363–364 (1999).

Zhou, D., A. W. Kusnecov, M. R. Shurin, M. DePaoli, and B. S. Rabin. "Exposure to physical and psychological stressors elevates plasma interleukin-6: Relationship to the activation of the hypothalamic-pituitary-adrenal axis." *Endocrinology* 133:2523–2530 (1993).

Chapter 18 How to Build a Better Athlete

Ainsworth, B. E., W. L. Haskell, A. S. Leon, D. R. Jacobs, H. J. Montoye, J. F. Sallis, and R. S. Paffenbarger. "Compendium of physical activities: Classification of energy costs of human physical effort." *Med Sci Sports Exerc* 25:71–80 (1993).

Alessio, H. M. "Exercise-induced oxidative stress." *Med Sci Sports Exerc* 25:218–224 (1993).

Bassett, D. R., and E. T. Howley. "Limiting factors for maximum uptake and determinants of endurance performance." *Med Sci Sports Exerc* 32:70–84 (2000).

Bergstrom, J., L. Hermannsen, E. Hultman, and B. Saltin. "Diet, muscle glycogen, and physical performance." *Acta Physiol Scan* 71:140–150 (1967).

Bernstein, L., B. E. Henderson, R. Hanisch, J. Sullivan-Halley, and R. K. Ross. "Physical exercise and reduced risk of breast cancer in young women." *J Natl Cancer Inst* 86:1403–1408 (1994).

Blair, S. N., H. W. Kohl, N. F. Gordon, and R. S. Paffenbarger. "How much physical activity is good for health?" *Ann Rev Public Health* 13:99–126 (1992).

Blair, S. N., H. W. Kohl, R. S. Paffenbarger, D. G. Clark, K. H. Cooper, and L. W. Gibbons. "Physical fitness and all-cause mortality: A prospective study of healthy men and women." *JAMA* 262:2395–2401 (1989).

Bruckner, G., P. Webb, L. Greenwell, C. Chow, and D. Richardson. "Fish oil increases peripheral capillary blood cell velocity in humans." *Atherosclerosis* 66:237–245 (1987).

Clark, V. R., W. G. Hopkins, J. A. Hawley, and L. M. Burke. "Placebo effect of carbohydrate feedings during a 40-km cycling time trial." *Med Sci Sports Exerc* 32:1642–1647 (2000).

Colker, C. M., M. A. Swain, B. Fabrucini, Q. Shi, and D. S. Kalman. "Effects of supplemental protein on body composition and muscular strength in healthy athletic male adults." *Curr Ther Res Clin Exp* 61:19–28 (2000).

Conlee, R. K., R. L. Hammer, W. W. Winder, M. L. Bracken, A. G. Nelson, and D. W. Barnett. "Glycogen repletion and exercise endurance in rats adapted to a high-fat diet." *Metab* 39(3):289–294 (1990).

Cordain, L., R. W. Gothshall, and S. B. Eaton. "Physical activity, energy expenditure, and fitness: An evolutionary perspective." *Int J Sports Med* 19:328–335 (1998).

Cumming, D. C. "Hormones and athletic performance." In *Endocrinology and Metabolism*. 3rd edition. Edited by P. Felig, J. D. Baxter, and L. A. Frohman. New York: McGraw-Hill, 1995.

D'Avanzo, B., O. Nanni, C. La Vecchia, S. Franceschi, E. Negri, A. Giacosa, E. Conti, M. Montella, R. Talamini, and A. Cecarli. "Physical activity and breast cancer risk." *Cancer Epidemiol Biomarkers Prev* 5:155–160 (1996).

DeMarco, H. M., K. P. Sucher, C. J. Cisar, and G. E. Butterfield. "Pre-exercise carbohydrate meals: Application of glycemic index." *Med Sci Sports Exerc* 31:164–170 (1999).

Felig, P., and J. Wahren. "Fuel homeostasis in exercise." *N Engl J Med* 293:1078–1084 (1975).

Fiatarone, M. A., E. C. Marks, N. D. Ryan, C. N. Meredith, L. A. Lipsitz, and W. J. Evans. "High-intensity strength training in nonagenarians: Effects on skeletal muscle." *JAMA* 263:3029–3034 (1990).

Folsom, A. R., D. R. Jacobs, L. E. Wagenknecht, S. P. Winkart, C. Yunis, J. E. Hilner, P. J. Savage, D. E. Smith, and J. M. Flack. "Increase in fasting insulin and glucose over seven years with increasing weight and inactivity of young adults." *Am J Epidemiol* 144:235–246 (1996).

Friedenreich, C. M., and T. E. Rohan. "Physical activity and risk of breast cancer." *Eur J Canc Prev* 4:145–151 (1995).

Frontera, W. R., C. Meredith, K. O'Reilly, H. Knuttgen, and W. Evans. "Strength conditioning in older men: Skeletal muscle hypertrophy and improved function." *J Appl Physiol* 64:1038–1044 (1988).

Fry, R. W., J. R. Grove, A. R. Morton, P. M. Zeroni, S. Gaudieri, and D. Keast. "Psychological and immunological correlates of acute overtraining." *Br J Sports Med* 28:241–246 (1994).

Galbo, H., J. J. Holst, and N. J. Christensen. "Glucagon and plasma catecholamine response to graded and prolonged exercise in man." *J Appl Physiol* 38:70–76 (1975).

———. "The effect of different diets of insulin on the hormonal response to prolonged exercise." *Acta Physiol Scan* 107:19–32 (1979).

Goedecke, J. H., C. Christie, G. Wilson, S. C. Dennis, T. D. Noakes, W. G. Hopkins, and E. V. Lambert. "Metabolic adaptations to a high-fat diet in endurance cyclists." *Metab* 48:1509–1517 (1999).

Goldbourt, U. "Physical activity, long-term CHD mortality, and longevity: A review of studies over the last 30 years." In *Nutrition and Fitness: Metabolic and Behavioral Aspects to Health and Disease,* ed. A. P. Simopoulos and K. N. Pavlou, pp. 229–239.

Goldfarb, A. H., and A. Z. Jamurtas. "Beta-endorphin response to exercise: An update." *Sports Med* 24:8–16 (1997).

Hein, H. O., P. Saudicani, and F. Gyntelberg. "Physical fitness or physical activity as a predictor of ischaemic heart disease: A 17-year follow-up in the Copenhagen Male Study." *J Int Med* 232:471–479 (1992).

Helmrich, S. P., D. R. Ragland, R. W. Leung, and R. S. Paffenbarger. "Physical activity and reduced occurrence of non-insulin dependent diabetes mellitus." *N Engl J Med* 325:147–152 (1991).

Holloszy, J. O., J. Schultz, J. Kusnierkiewica, J. M. Hagberg, and A. A. Ehsani. "Effects of exercise on glucose tolerance and insulin resistance." *Acta Med Scand* 711:55–65 (1996).

Hoppeler, H., R. Billeter, P. J. Horvath, J. J. Leddy, and D. R. Pendergast. "Muscle structure with low- and high-fat diets in well-trained male runners." *Int J Sports Med* 20:522–526 (1999).

Horvath, P. J., C. K. Eagen, N. M. Fisher, J. J. Leddy, and D. R. Pendergast. "The effects of varying dietary fat on performance and metabolism in trained male and female runners." *J Am Coll Nutr* 19:52–60 (2000).

Jeukendrup, A. E., W. H. M. Saris, and A. J. M. Wagenmakers. "Fat metabolism during exercise: A review. Part I. Fatty acid mobilization and muscle metabolism." *Int J Sports Med* 19:231–244 (1998).

————— "Fat metabolism during exercise: A review. Part II. Regulation of metabolism and the effects of training." *Int J Sports Med* 19:293–302 (1998).

—————. Wagenmakers. "Fat metabolism during exercise: A review. Part III. Effects of nutritional interventions." *Int J Sports Med* 19:371–379 (1998).

Kraemer, W. J. "Influence of the endocrine system on resistance training adaptations." *National Strength and Conditioning Association Journal* 14:47–53 (1992).

Lambert, E. V., D. P. Speechly, S. C. Dennis, and T. D. Noakes. "Enhanced endurance in trained cyclists during moderate intensity exercise following 2 weeks adaptation to a high-fat diet." *Eur J Appl Physiol Occup Physiol* 69:287–293 (1994).

Laron, Z., and A. D. Rogal, eds. *Hormones and Sports.* New York: Raven Press, 1989.

Leddy, J., P. Horvath, J. Rowland, and D. Pendergast. "Effect of a high- or a low-fat diet on cardiovascular risk factors in male and female runners." *Med Sci Sports Exerc* 29:17–25 (1997).

Lee, I. M., C-C. Hsieh, and R. S. Paffenbarger. "Chronic disease in former college students: Exercise intensity and longevity in men." *JAMA* 273:1179–1184 (1995).

Lee, I. M., J. E. Manson, C. H. Hennekens, and R. S. Paffenbarger. "Chronic disease in former college students: Body weight and mortality—A 27-year follow-up of middle-aged men." *JAMA* 270:2823–2828 (1990).

Lee, I. M., and R. S. Paffenbarger. "Change in body weight and longevity." *JAMA* 268:2045–2049 (1992).

Lemon, P. "Do athletes need more dietary protein and amino acids?" *Int J Sports Nutr* 5:S39–S61 (1995).

Leon, A. S., J. Connett, D. R. Jacobs, and R. Rauramaa. "Leisure-time physical activity levels and risk of coronary heart disease and death: The Multiple Risk Factor Intervention Trial." *JAMA* 258:2388–2395 (1987).

Manson, J. E., G. A. Colditz, and M. J. Stampfer. "Parity, ponderosity, and the paradox of a weight-preoccupied society." *JAMA* 271:1788–1790 (1994).

Manson, J. E., E. B. Rimm, M. J. Stampfer, G. A. Colditz, W. C. Willett, A. S. Krolewski, B. Rosner, C. H. Hennekens, and F. E. Speizer. "Physical activity and incidence of non-insulin dependent diabetes mellitus in women." *Lancet* 338:774–778 (1991).

Mayer-Davis, E. J., R. D'Agostino, A. J. Darter, S. M. Haffner, M. J. Rewers, M. Saad, and R. N. Bergman. "Intensity and amount of physical activity in relation to insulin sensitivity." *JAMA* 279:669–674 (1998).

Meydani, M., and W. J. Evans. "Free radicals, exercise, and aging." In *Free Radicals in Aging,* ed. B. P. Yu, pp. 183–204. Boca Raton, Fla.: CRC Press, 1993.

Mulla, N. A., L. Simonsen, and J. Bulow. "Postexercise adipose tissue and skeletal muscle lipid metabolism in humans." *J Physiol* 524:919–928 (2000).

Muoio, D. M., J. J. Leddy, P. J. Horvath, A. B. Awad, and D. R. Pendergast. "Effect of dietary fat on metabolic adjustments to maximal VO_2 and endurance in runners." *Med Sci Sports Exerc* 26:81–88 (1994).

Myer, T., L. Schwarz, and W. Kindermann. "Exercise and endogenous opiates." In *Contemporary Endocrinology: Sports Endocrinology,* ed. M. P. Warren and N. W. Constantini, pp. 31–42. Totowa, N. J.: Humana Press, 1999.

Paffenbarger, R. S., and W. E. Hale. "Work activity and coronary heart mortality." *N Engl J Med* 292:1109–1114 (1970).

Paffenbarger, R. S., A. L. Wing, and R. T. Hyde. "Physical activity as an index of heart attack risk in college alumni." *Am J Epidemio* 108:161–175 (1978).

Paffenbarger, R. S., R. T. Hyde, A. L. Wing, and C-C. Hsieh. "Physical activity, all-cause mortality, and longevity of college alumni." *N Engl J Med* 314:605–614 (1986).

Paffenbarger, R. S., R. T. Hyde, and A. L. Wing. "Physical activity and incidence of cancer in diverse populations: A preliminary report." *Am J Clin Nutr* 45:312–317 (1987).

Paffenbarger, R. S., and E. Olsen. *Lifefit.* Champaign, Ill.: Human Kinetics, 1996.

Papadakis, M. A., D. Grady, D. Black, M. J. Tierney, G. A. W. Gooding, M. Schambelan, and C. Grunfeld. "Growth hormone replacement in healthy older men improves body composition but not functional ability." *Ann Intern Med* 124:708–716 (1996).

Paul, G. L., J. T. Rokusek, G. L. Dykstra, R. A. Boileau, and D. K. Layman. "Preexercise meal composition alters plasma large neutral amino acid responses during exercise and recovery." *Am J Clin Nutr* 64:778–786 (1996).

Pendergast, D. R., P. J. Horvath, J. J. Leddy, and J. T. Venkatraman. "The role of dietary fat in performance, metabolism, and health." *Am J Sports Med* 24:S53–S58 (1996).

Phinney, S. "Potential risk of prolonged gamma-linolenic acid use." *Ann Intern Med* 120:692 (1994).

Pitsiladis, Y. P., I. Smith, and R. J. Maughan. "Increased fat availability enhances the capacity of trained individuals to perform prolonged exercise." *Med Sci Sports Exerc* 31:1570–1579 (1999).

Rauramaa, R., J. T. Salonen, K. Seppanen, R. Salonen, J. M. Venalainen, M. Ihanaien, and V. Rissanen. "Inhibition of platelet aggregability by moderate-intensity physical exercise: A randomized clinical trial in overweight men." *Circulation* 74:939–944 (1986).

Rico-Sanz, J., M. Moosavi, E. L. Thomas, J. McCarthy, G. A. Coutts, N. Saeed, and J. D. Bell. "In vivo evaluation of the effects of continuous exercise on skeletal muscle triglycerides in trained humans." *Lipids* 35:1313–1318 (2000).

Rogozkin, V. A. *Metabolism of Anabolic Androgenic Steroids.* Boca Raton, Fla.: CRC Press, 1991.

Schofield, J. G. "Prostaglandin E1 and the release of growth hormone in vitro." *Nature* 228:179 (1970).

Smith, L. L. "Cytokine hypothesis of overtraining: A physiological adaptation to excessive stress?" *Med Sci Sports Exerc* 32:317–331 (2000).

Thune, I., T. Brenn, E. Lund, and M. Garrd. "Physical activity and the risk of breast cancer." *N Engl J Med* 336:1269–1275 (1997).

Venkatraman, J. T., and D. Pendergast. "Effects of the level of dietary fat intake and endurance exercise on plasma cytokines in runners." *Med Sci Sports Exerc* 30:1198–1204 (1998).

Viru, A. *Hormones in Muscular Activity.* Volume 1, *Hormonal Ensemble in Exercise.* Boca Raton, Fla.: CRC Press, 1983.

————. *Hormones in Muscular Activity.* Volume 2, *Adaptive Effects of Hormones in Exercise.* Boca Raton, Fla.: CRC Press, 1983.

————. *Adaptation in Sports Training.* Boca Raton, Fla.: CRC Press, 1995.

Weltman, A., J. Y. Weltman, R. Schurrer, W. S. Evans, J. D. Veldhuis, and A. D. Rogal. "Endurance training amplifies the pulsatile release of growth hormone: Effects of training intensity." *J Appl Physiol* 72:2188–2196 (1992).

Willett, W. C., J. E. Manson, M. J. Stampfer, G. A. Colditz, B. Rosner, F. E. Spelzar, and C. H. Hennekens. "Weight, weight change, and coronary heart disease in women: Risk within the 'normal' weight range." *JAMA* 273:461–465 (1995).

Wood, P. D., and W. L. Haskell. "The effect of exercise on plasma high-density lipoproteins." *Lipids* 14:417–427 (1979).

Wood, P. D., M. L. Stefanick, P. T. Williams, and W. T. Haskell. "The effects on plasma lipoproteins of a prudent weight-reducing diet, with or without exercise, in overweight men and women." *N Engl J Med* 319:461–466 (1991).

Yamanouchi, K., T. Shinozaki, K. Chidada, T. Nishidawa, K. Ito, S. Shimizu, N. Ozawa, Y. Suzuki, H. Maeno, and K. Kato. "Daily walking combined with diet therapy is useful means for obese NIDDM patients not only to reduce body weight but also to improve insulin sensitivity." *Diabetes Care* 18:775–778 (1995).

Zawadzki, K. M., B. B. Yaspelkis, and J. L. Ivy. "Carbohydrate-protein complex increases the rate of muscle glycogen storage after exercise." *J Appl Physiol* 72:1854–1859 (1992).

Appendix C Your Biological Internet

Adjei, A. A. "Signal transduction pathway targets for anticancer drug discovery." *Curr Pharma Design* 6:361–378 (2000).

Baeuerle, P. A. "Pro-inflammatory signaling: Last pieces in the NF-kappa B puzzle?" *Curr Biol* 8:R19–R22 (1998).

Cohen, P. "Identification of a protein kinase cascade of major importance in insulin signal transduction." *Philos Trans R Soc Lond Biol Sci* 354:485–495 (1999).

Cooper, D. R., and O. Hanson-Painton. "Protein kinases: Receptors of external signals." *J Clin Ligand Assay* 23:50–56 (2000).

De Groot, L. J., M. Besser, H. G. Burger, J. L. Jameson, D. L. Loriaux, J. C. Marshall, W. D. Odell, J. T. Potts, and A. H. Rubenstein, eds.

Endocrinology. 3rd edition. Philadelphia, Pa.: W. B. Saunders Company, 1995.

Felig, P., J. D. Baxter, and L. A. Frohman. *Endocrinology and Metabolism.* 3rd edition. New York: McGraw-Hill, 1995.

Frisch, S. M. "cAMP takes control." *Nature Cell Bio* 2:E167–E168 (2000).

Gamet-Payrastre, L., S. Manenti, M-P. Gratacap, J. Tulliez, H. Chap, and B. Payrastre. "Flavonoids and the inhibition of PKC and PI 3-kinase." *Gen Pharmacol* 32:279–286 (1999).

Ghosh, S., M. J. May, and E. B. Kopp. "NF-kappa B and Rel proteins: Evolutionarily conserved mediators of immune responses." *Ann Rev Immunol* 16:225–260 (1998).

Hurley, J. H. "Structure, mechanism, and regulation of mammalian adenyl cyclase." *J Biol Chem* 274:7599–7602 (1999).

Johnson, H., J. K. Russell, and B. A. Torres. "Structural basis for arachidonic acid second messenger signal in gamma interferon induction." *Ann NY Acad Sci* 524:208–217 (1988).

Meier, R., and B. A. Hemmings. "Regulation of protein kinase B." *J Recept Signal Transduc Res* 19:121–128 (1999).

Mirnikjoo, B., S. E. Brown, H. F. Kim, L. B. Marangell, J. D. Sweatt, and E. J. Weeber. "Protein kinase inhibition by omega-3 fatty acids." *J Biol Chem* 276:10888–10896 (2001).

Norman, A. W., and G. Litwack. *Hormones.* 2d edition. New York: Academic Press, 1997.

Ottensmeyer, F. P., D. R. Beniac, R. Luo, and C. C. Yip. "Mechanism of transmembrane signaling: Insulin binding and insulin receptor." *Biochemistry* 39:12103–12112 (2000).

Renard, P., and M. Raes. "The proinflammatory transcription factor NF kappa B: A potential target for novel therapeutical strategies." *Cell Biol Toxicol* 15:341–344 (1999).

Sawin, C. T. "How does a hormone act inside a cell?" *Endocrinologist* 10:139–144 (1999).

Schmedtje, J. F., Y-S. Ji, W-L. Liu, R. N. DuBois, and M. S. Runge. "Hypoxia induces cyclooxygenase-2 via the NF-kappa B p65 transcription factor in human vascular endothelial cells." *J Biol Chem* 272:601–608 (1997).

Sears, B. *The Zone.* New York: Regan Books, 1995.

———. *The Anti-Aging Zone.* New York: Regan Books, 1999.

Seung Kim, H. F., E. J. Weeber, J. D. Sweatt, A. L. Stoll, and L. B. Marangell. "Inhibitory effects of omega-3 fatty acids on protein kinase C activity in vitro." *Mol Psychiatry* 6:246–248 (2001).

Wang, X. J., and D. M. Stocco. "Cyclic AMP and arachidonic acid: A tale of two pathways." *Mol Cell Endocrinol* 158:7–12 (1999).

Wilson, J. D., and D. W. Foster, eds. *Williams Textbook of Endocrinology.* 8th edition. Philadelphia, Pa.: W. B. Saunders Company, 1992.

Yamamoto, K., T. Arakawa, N. Ueda, and S. Yamamoto. "Transcriptional roles of nuclear factor kappa B and nuclear factor interleukin-6 in the tumor necrosis factor alpha-dependent induction of cyclooxygenase-2 in MC3T3-E1 cells." *J Biol Chem* 270:33157–33160 (1995).

Yin, Y., P. D. Allen, L. Jia, M. G. Macey, S. M. Kelsey, and A. C. Newland. "Constitutive levels of cAMP-dependent protein kinase activity determine sensitivity of human multi-drug resistant leukaemic cell lines to growth inhibition and apoptosis by forskolin and tumor necrosis factor alpha." *Br J Haematology* 108:565–573 (2000).

Zidek, Z. "Role of cytokines in the modulation of nitric oxide production by cyclic AMP." *Eur Cytokine Netw* 12:22–32 (2001).

Appendix D Eicosanoids

Abramovitz, M., M. Adam, Y. Boie, M-C. Carriere, D. Denis, C. Godbout, S. Lamontagne, C. Rochette, N. Sawyer, N. M. Tremblay, M. Belley, M. Gallant, C. Dufresne, Y. Gareau, R. Ruel, H. Juteau, M. Labelle, N. Ouimet, and K. M. Metters. "The utilization of recombinant prostanoid receptors to determine the affinities and selectivities of prostaglandins and related analogs." *Biochim Biophys Acta* 1483:285–293 (2000).

Adam, O. "Polyenoic fatty acid metabolism and effects on prostaglandin biosynthesis in adults and aged persons." In *Polyunsaturated Fatty Acids and Eicosanoids,* pp. 213–219. Champaign, Ill.: *American Oil Chemists Society Press,* 1987.

Aki, T., Y. Shimada, K. Inagaski, H. Higashimoto, S. Kawamoto, K. Shigeta, K. Ono, and O. Suzuki. "Molecular cloning and functional characterization of rat delta-6 fatty acid desaturase." *Biochem Biophys Res Commun* 255:575–579 (1999).

Ankel, H., O. Turriziani, and G. Antonelli. "Prostaglandin A inhibits replication of human immunodeficiency virus during acute infection." *J Gen Virol* 72:2997–2800 (1991).

Barham, J. B., M. B. Edens, A. N. Fonteh, M. M. Johnson, L. Easter, and F. H. Chilton. "Addition of eicosapentaenoic acid to gamma-linolenic-acid-supplemented diets prevents serum arachidonic acid accumulation in humans." *J Nutr* 130:1925–1931 (2000).

Barry, O. P., G. Kazanietz, K. Pratico, and G. A. FitzGerald. "Arachidonic acid in platelet microparticles up-regulates cyclooxygenase-2-dependent prostaglandin formation via a protein kinase C/mitogen-activated protein kinase-dependent pathway." *J Biol Chem* 274:7545–7556 (1999).

Bergstrom, S., R. Rhyhage, B. Samuelsson, and J. Sorval. "The structure of prostaglandins E_1, $E_{1\alpha}$ and $F_{1\beta}$." *J Biol Chem* 238:3555–3565 (1963).

Blond, J. P., and P. Lemarchel. "A study of the effect of alpha linolenic acid on the desaturation of dihomo gamma linolenic acid using rat liver homogenates." *Reprod Nutr Dev* 24:1–10 (1984).

Boie, Y., R. Stocco, N. Sawyer, D. M. Slipetz, M. D. Ungrin, R. Neuschafer-Rube, G. P. Puschel, K. M. Metters, and M. Abramovitz. "Molecular cloning and characterization of the four rat prostaglandin E_2 prostanoid receptor sites." *Eur J Pharmacol* 340:227–241 (1997).

Bordoni, A., P. I. Biagi, E. Turghette, and S. Hrelia. "Aging influence on delta 6-desaturase activity and fatty acid composition of rat liver microsomes." *Biochem Int* 17:1001–1009 (1988).

Bourre, J. M., M. Piciotti, and O. Dumont. "Delta 6 desaturase in brain and liver during development and aging." *Lipids* 25:354–356 (1990).

Brenner, R. R. "Nutrition and hormonal factors influencing desaturation of essential fatty acids." *Prog Lipid Res* 20:41–48 (1982).

Burr, G. O., and M. R. Burr. "A new deficiency disease produced by rigid exclusion of fat from the diet." *J. Biol Chem* 82:345–367 (1929).

———. "On the nature and role of the fatty acids essential in nutrition." *J Biol Chem* 86:587–621 (1930).

Carattoli, A., D. Fortini, C. Rozera, and C. Giorgi. "Inhibition of HIV-1 transcription by cyclopentenone prostaglandin A_1 in Jurkat T lymphocytes." *J Biol Regul Homeost Agents* 14:209–216 (2000).

Chakrin, L. W., and D. M. Bailey, eds. *The Leukotrienes*. New York: Academic Press, 1984.

Chapkin, R. S., S. D. Somer, and K. L. Erickson. "Dietary manipulation of macrophage phospholipid classes: Selective increase of dihomogamma linoleic acid." *Lipids* 23:776–770 (1988).

Cho, H. P., M. Nakamura, and S. D. Clarke. "Cloning, expression, and fatty acid regulation of human delta-5 desaturase." *J Biol Chem* 274:37335–37339 (1999).

Clarke, S. D. "Polyunsaturated fatty acid regulation of gene transcription: A mechanism to improve energy balance and insulin resistance." *Br J Nutr* 83:S59–S66 (2000).

Cleland, L. G., M. J. Jones, M. A. Neuman, M. D'Angel, and R. A. Gibson. "Linoleate inhibits EPA incorporation from dietary fish oil supplements in human subjects." *Am J Clin Nutr* 55:395–399 (1992).

Coleman, R. A., and P. P. A. Humphrey. "Prostanoid receptors." In *Therapeutic Applications of Prostaglandins,* ed. J. R. Vane and J. O'Grady, pp. 15–25. London: Edward Arnold, 1993.

Conquer, J. A., and B. J. Holub. "Dietary docosahexaenoic acid as a source of eicosapentaenoic acid in vegetarians and omnivores." *Lipids* 32:341–345 (1997).

El Boustani, S., J. E. Gausse, B. Descomps, L. Monnier, F. Mendy, and A. Crastes de Paulet. "Direct *In Vivo* characterization of delta-5 desaturase activity in humans by deuterium labeling: Effect of insulin." *Metab* 38:315–321 (1989).

Euler, U. S. von "On the specific vasodilating and plain muscle stimulating substances from accessory genital glands in men and certain animals (prostaglandins and vesiglandin)." *J Physiol* (London) 88:213–234 (1936).

Fan, Y-Y., K. S. Ramos, and R. S. Chapkin. "Dietary gamma linolenic acid enhances mouse macrophage-derived prostaglandin E_1 which inhibits vascular smooth muscle cell proliferation." *J Nutr* 127:1765–1771 (1997).

Ferreria, S. H., S. Moncada, and J. R. Vane. "Indomethacin and aspirin abolish prostaglandin release from the spleen." *Nature New Biol* England 231:237–239 (1971).

Garg, M. L., A. B. R. Thomson, and M. T. Clandinin. "Effect of dietary cholesterol and/or omega-3 fatty acids on lipid composition and delta 5-desaturase activity of rat liver microsomes." *J Nutr* 118:661–668 (1998).

Gilmour, R. S., and M. D. Mitchell. "Nuclear lipid signaling: Novel role of eicosanoids." *Exp Bio Med* 226:1–4 (2001).

Giron, D. J. "Inhibition of viral replication in cell cultures treated with prostaglandin E_1." *Proc Soc Exp Bio Med* 170:25–28 (1982).

Gordon, D., M. A. Bray, and J. Morley. "Control of lymphokine secretion by prostaglandins." *Nature* 262:401–402 (1976).

Hamberg, M., and B. Samuelsson. "Detection and isolation of an endoperoxide intermediate in prostaglandin biosyntheses." *Proc Nat Acad Sci USA* 70:899–903 (1973).

Hamberg, M., J. Svensson, T. Wakabayashi, and B. Samuelsson. "Isolation and structure of two prostaglandin endoperoxides that cause platelet aggregation." *Proc Nat Acad Sci USA* 71:345–349 (1974).

Hamberg, M., J. Svensson, and B. Samuelsson. "Thromboxanes: A new group of biologically active compounds derived from prostaglandin endoperoxides." *Proc Nat Acad Sci USA* 72:2994–2998 (1975).

Herman, A. G., P. M. Vanhoutle, H. Denolin, and A. Goossons, eds. *Cardiovascular Pharmacology of Prostaglandins*. New York: Raven Press, 1982.

Hill, E. G., S. B. Johnson, L. D. Lawson, M. M. Mahfouz, and R. T. Holman. "Perturbation of the metabolism of essential fatty acids by dietary partially hydrogenated vegetable oil." *Proc Nat Acad Sci USA* 79:953–957 (1982).

Horrobin, D. F. "Loss of delta 6 desaturase activity as a key factor in aging." *Med Hypotheses* 7:1211–1220 (1981).

———. ed. *Omega 6 Essential Fatty Acids*. New York: Wiley-Liss, 1990.

Hwang, D. "Fatty acids and immune responses." *Ann Rev Nutr* 20:431–456 (2000).

Johnson, M. M., D. D. Swan, M. E. Surette, J. Stegner, T. Chilton, A. N. Fonteh, and F. H. Chilton. "Dietary supplementation with gamma linolenic acid alters fatty acid content and eicosanoid production in healthy humans." *J Nutr* 127:1435–1444 (1997).

Johnson, R. A., D. R. Morton, J. A. Kinver, R. R. Gorman, J. C. McGuire, F. F. Sun, N. Whither, S. Bunting, J. Salmon, S. Moncada, and J. R. Vane. "The chemical structure of prostaglandin X (prostacyclin)." *Prostaglandins* 12:915–928 (1976).

Jump, D. B., A. Thelen, and M. Mater. "Dietary polyunsaturated fatty acids and hepatic gene expression." *Lipids* 34:S209–S212 (1999).

Kurihara, Y., H. Endo, and H. Kondo. "Induction of IL-6 via the EP2 subtype of prostaglandin E receptor in rat adjuvant-arthritic synovial cells." *Inflamm Res* 50:1–5 (2001).

Lam, B. K., and F. Austen. "Leukotriene C_4 synthase: A pivotal enzyme in the biosynthesis of the cysteinyl leukotrienes." *Am J Respir Critical Care Med* 161:S16–S19 (1999).

Lands, W. E. M. "Stories about acyl chains." *Biochim Biophys Acta* 1483:1–15 (2000).

Luthria, D. L., B. S. Mohammed, and H. Sprecher. "Regulation of the biosynthesis of 4,7,10,13, 16, 19 docosahexaenoic acid." *J Biol Chem* 271:16020–16025 (1996).

Lynch, K. R., G. P. O'Neioll, Q. Liu, D. S. Im, N. Sawyer, K. M. Metters, N. Colombe, M. Abramovitz, D. J. Figueroa, Z. Zeng, B. M. Conolly, C. Bai, C. P. Austin, A. Chateauneuf, R. Stocco, G. M. Greig, S. Kargman, S. B. Hooks, E. Hosfield, D. L. Williams, A. W. Ford-Hutchinson, C. T. Caskey, and J. F. Evan. "Characterization of the human cysteinyl leukotriene CysLTI receptor." *Nature* 399:789–793 (1999).

Mancini, J. A., H. Waterman, and D. Riendeau. "Cellular oxygenation of 12-hydroxyeicosatetraenoic acid and 15-hydroxyeicosatetraenoic acid by 5-lipoxygenase is stimulated by 5-lipoxygenase-activating protein." *J Biol Chem* 273:32842–32847 (1998).

Metz, S., W. Fujimoto, and R. O. Robertson. "Modulation of insulin secretion by cyclic AMP and prostaglandin E." *Metab* 31:1014–1033 (1982).

Metz, S., M. van Rollins, R. Strife, W. Fujimoto, and R. P. Robertson. "Lipoxygenase pathway in islet endrocrine cells: Oxidative metabolism of arachidonic acid promotes insulin release." *J Clin Invest* 71:1191–1205 (1983).

Moncada, S., R. Gryglewski, S. Bunting, and J. R. Vane. "An enzyme isolated from arteries transforms prostaglandin endoperoxides to an unstable substance that inhibits platelet aggregation." *Nature* 263:663–665 (1976).

Murota, S., T. Kanayasu, J. Nakano-Hayashi, and I. Morita. "Involvement of eicosanoids in angiogenesis." *Adv Pros Throm Leuko Res* 21:623–625 (1990).

Nakamura, M. T., H. P. Cho, and S. D. Clarke. "Regulation of hepatic delta-6 desaturase expression and its role in the polyunsaturated fatty acid inhibition of fatty acid synthase gene expression in mice." *J Nutr* 130:1561–1565 (2000).

Narumiya, S., Y. Sugimoto, and F. Ushikubi. "Prostanoid receptors: Structures, properties, and functions." *Physiol Rev* 7:1193–1226 (1999).

Nassar, B. A., Y. S. Huang, M. S. Manku, U. M. Das, N. Morse, and D. F. Horrobin. "The influence of dietary manipulation with n-3 and n-6 fatty acids on liver and plasma phospholipids fatty acids in rats." *Lipids* 21:652–656 (1986).

Nicosia, S., V. Capra, S. Ravasi, and G. E. Rovati. "Binding to cysteinyl-leukotriene receptors." *Am J Respir Crit Care Med* 161:S46–S50 (2000).

Ninnemam, J. L. *Prostaglandins, Leukotrienes, and the Immune Response.* New York: Cambridge University Press, 1988.

Oates, J. A., G. A. FitzGerald, R. A. Branch, E. K. Jackson, H. P. Knapp, and L. J. Roberts. "Clinical implications of prostaglandin and thromboxane A_2 formation." *N Engl J Med* 319:689–698 (1988).

Parker-Barnes, J. M., T. Das, A. Leonard, J. M. Thurmond, L-T. Chaung, Y-S. Huang, and P. Mukerji. "Identification and characterization of an enzyme involved in the elongation of n-6 and n-3 polyunsaturated fatty acids." *Proc Nat Acad Sci USA* 97:8284–8289 (2000).

Pek, S. B., and M. F. Walsh. "Leukotrienes stimulate insulin released from rat pancreas." *Proc Nat Acad Sci USA* 82:2199–2202 (1984).

Pelikonova, T., M. Kohout, J. Base, Z. Stefka, J. Kovar, L. Kerdova, and J. Valek. "Effect of acute hyperinsulinemia on fatty acid composition of serum lipids in non-insulin dependent diabetics and healthy men." *Clin Chim Acta* 203:329–337 (1991).

Peluffo, R. O., and R. Brenner. "Influence of dietary protein on delta 6- and delta 9-desaturation of fatty acids in rats of different ages and in different seasons." *J Nutr* 104:894–900 (1974).

Phinney, S. "Potential risk of prolonged gamma-linolenic acid use." *Ann Intern Med* 120:692 (1994).

Portanova, J. P., Y. Zhang, G. D. Anderson, D. Scott, J. L. Masferrer, and K. Seiber. "Selective neutralization of prostaglandin E_2 blocks inflammation, hyperalgesia, and interleukin-6 production." *J Exp Med* 184:883–891 (1996).

Quilley, J., and J. C. McGiff. "Is EDHF an epoxyeicosatrienoic acid?" *TIPS* 21:121–124 (2000).

Raz, A., N. Kamin-Belsky, F. Przedecki, and M. Obukowicz. "Dietary fish oil inhibits delta-6 desaturase activity In Vivo." *J Am Oil Chem Soc* 75:241–245 (1998).

Rossi, A., G. Elia, and M. G. Santoro. "Inhibition of nuclear factor kappa B by prostaglandin A_1: An effect associated with heat shock transcription factor activation." *Proc Nat Acad Sci USA* 94:746–750 (1997).

Rossi, A., P. Kapahi, G. Natoll, T. Takahashi, Y. Chen, M. Karin, and M. G. Santoro. "Anti-inflammatory cyclopentenone prostaglandins are direct inhibitors of kappa B kinase." *Nature* 403:103–108 (2000).

Roth, G. J., and P. W. Majerus. "The mechanism of the effect of aspirin on human platelets." *J Clin Invest* 50:624–632 (1975).

Roth, G. J., and C. J. Siok. "Acetylation of the NH2-terminal series of prostaglandin synthetase by aspirin." *J Biol Chem* 253:3782–3784 (1975).

Rozera, C., A. Carattoli, A. De Marco, C. Amici, C. Giorgi, and M. G. Santoro. "Inhibition of HIV-1 replication by cyclopentenone prostaglandins in acutely infected human cells." *J Clin Invest* 97:1795–1803 (1996).

Sacca, L., G. Perez, F. Pengo, I. Pascucci, and M. Conorelli. "Reduction of circulating insulin levels during the infusion of different prostaglandins in the rat." *Acta Endocrinol* 79:266–274 (1975).

Sack, S. "Prostaglandin: A pluralistic hormone embracing divergent signal properties." *Cardiovasc Res* 40:438–439 (1998).

Samuelsson, B. "On incorporation of oxygen in the conversion of 8, 11, 14 cicosatrienoic acid into prostaglandin E." *J Am Chem Soc* 89:3011–3015 (1965).

Santoro, M. G., B. M. Jaffe, and M. Esteban. "Prostaglandin A inhibits the replication of vesicular stromatitis virus: Effect on virus glycoprotein." *J Gen Virol* 64:2797–2801 (1983).

Sato, M., Y. Adan, K. Shibata, Y. Shoji, H. Sato, and K. Imaizumi. "Cloning of rat delta-6 desaturase and its regulation by dietary eicosapentaenoic or docosahexaenoic acid." *World Rev Nutr Diet* 88:196–199 (2001)

Schofield, J. G. "Prostaglandin E_1 and the release of growth hormone in vitro." *Nature* 228:179 (1970).

Schror, K., and H. Sinziner, eds. *Prostaglandins in Clinical Research.* New York: Liss, 1989.

Sears, B. *The Zone.* New York: Regan Books, 1995.

———. *The Anti-Aging Zone.* New York: Regan Books, 1999.

Singer, P., I. Berger, M. Wirth, W. Godicke, W. Jaeger, and S. Voigt. "Slow desaturation and elongation of linolenic and alpha-linolenic acids as a rationale of eicosapentaenoic acid–rich diet to lower blood pressure and serum lipids in normal, hypertensive, and hyperlipidemic subjects." *Prostaglandins Leukot Med* 24:175–193 (1986).

Sinzinger, H., and W. Rogatti, eds. *Prostaglandin E_1 in Atherosclerosis.* New York: Springer-Verlag, 1986.

Smith, D. L., A. L. Willis, N. Nguyen, D. Conner, S. Zahedi, and

J. Fulks. "Eskimo plasma constituents, dihomo gamma linolenic acid, eicosapentaenoic acid, and docosahexaenoic acid inhibit the release of atherogenic mitogens." *Lipids* 24:70–75 (1989).

Sprecher, H. "Metabolism of highly unsaturated n-3 and n-6 fatty acids." *Biochim Biophys Acta* 1486:219–231 (2000).

Sprecher, H., Q. Chen, and F-Q. Yin. "Regulation of the biosynthesis of 22:5 n-6 and 22:6 n-3: A complex intracellular process." *Lipids* 34:S1453–S156 (1999).

Stone, K. J., A. L. Willis, M. Hurt, S. J. Kirtland, P. B. A. Kernoff, and G. F. McNichol. "The metabolism of dihomo gamma linolenic acid in man." *Lipids* 14:174–180 (1979).

Sugimoto, Y., S. Narumiya, and A. Ichikawa. "Distribution and function of prostanoid receptors: Studies from knockout mice." *Prog Lipid Res* 39:389–314 (2000).

Tang, L., K. Loutzenhiser, and R. Loutzenhiser. "Biphasic actions of prostaglandin E_2 on the renal afferent arteriole: Role of EP3 and EP4 receptors." *Circ Res* 86:663–670 (2000).

Ulmann, L., J. P. Blond, C. Maniongur, J. P. Poisson, G. Durand, J. Bezard, and G. Pascal. "Effects of age and dietary essential fatty acids on desaturase activities and on fatty acid composition of liver microsomal phospholipids of adult rats." *Lipids* 26:127–133 (1991).

Vane, J. R. "Inhibition of prostaglandin synthesis as a mechanism of action of aspirin-like drugs." *Nature New Biol* England 231:232–235 (1971).

Vane, J. R., and J. O'Grady, eds. *Therapeutic Applications of Prostaglandins.* London: Edward Arnold, 1993.

Wallace, J. L. "The arachidonic acid pathway." In *Drug Development: Molecular Targets for GI Diseases,* ed. T. S. Gaginella and A. Gugliett. Totowa, N.J.: Humana Press, 1998.

Watkins, W. D., M. B. Petersen, and J. R. Fletcher, eds. *Prostaglandins in Clinical Practice.* New York: Raven Press, 1989.

Willett, W. C., M. J. Stampfer, G. A. Colditz, F. E. Speizer, B. A. Rosner, L. A. Sampson, and C. H. Hennekens. "Intake of trans fatty acids and risk of coronary heart disease among women." *Lancet* 341:581–585 (1993).

Williams, L. L., D. M. Doody, and L. A. Horrocks. "Serum fatty acid proportions are altered during the year following acute Epstein-Barr virus infection." *Lipids* 23:981–988 (1988).

Willis, A. L. *Handbook of Eicosanoids, Prostaglandins, and Related Lipids.* Boca Raton, Fla.: CRC Press, 1987.

Yam, D., A. Eliraz, B. Eliraz, and M. Elliot. "Diet and disease: The Israeli paradox: Possible dangers of a high omega-6 polyunsaturated fatty acid diet." *Isr J Med Sci* 32:1134–1143 (1996).

Yamamoto, N., M. Fukushima, T. Tsurumi, K. Maeno, and Y. Nishiyama. "Mechanism of inhibition of herpes simplex virus replication by prostaglandin A_1 and prostaglandin J_2." *Biochem Biophys Res Comm* 146:1425–1431 (1987).

Yokomizo, T., T. Izumi, and T. Shimizu. "Leukotriene B_4: Metabolism and signal transduction." *Arch Biochem Biophys* 385:231–241 (2001).

Index

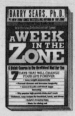

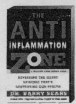

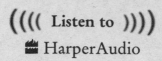
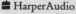
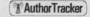
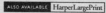